# Optimizing Health: Improving the Value of Healthcare Delivery

# Optimizing Health:
# Improving the Value
# of Healthcare Delivery

Franz Porzsolt, MD, PhD
University Hospital Ulm, Clinical Economics
Ulm, Germany

Robert M. Kaplan, PhD
University of California, Los Angeles, Schools of Public Health and Medicine
Los Angeles, California

With technical assistance from Barbara Herzberger, MD

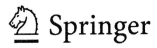 Springer

Franz Porzsolt
Clinical Economics
University Hospital Ulm
Frauensteige 6
89075 Ulm
Germany
franz.porzsolt@uniklinik-ulm.de

Robert M. Kaplan
UCLA School of Public Health
Los Angeles, CA, 90095-1772
USA
mkaplan@ucsd.edu

Library of Congress Control Number: 2006925255

ISBN-10: 0-387-33920-5          e-ISBN-10: 0-387-33921-3
ISBN-13: 978-0387-33920-7          e-ISBN-13: 978-0387-33921-4

Printed on acid-free paper.

© 2006 Springer Science+Business Media, LLC

9 8 7 6 5 4 3 2 1

springer.com

# Foreword

Health care expenditures have risen about 150% in Germany during the past decade. Laws designed to limit these costs have not been able to reverse this trend. During the same time period, the average hospital stay and the number of hospital beds have decreased, and the number of employed physicians has considerably increased. These changes indicate a dramatic restructuring of the health care system. Medical progress in prevention, diagnosis, therapy, and follow-up is closely related to all these developments. Without confirmed benefit, the financing of medical progress will not be included in the catalogue of services provided by obligatory health insurance. The challenge to clinical research is to provide the unprejudiced evidence necessary to include new knowledge in medical treatment and to remove procedures from the catalogue of services provided that offer no value for patients in an evidence-based process.

Clinical economics is the interdisciplinary branch of medical science that provides the concepts and problem-solving approaches required to address these problems. Interest is centered on benefit to patients and not the effectiveness of a treatment. This patient-benefit orientation is exceptional and sometimes appears to conflict with benefit to the hospital or service provider (profit-oriented point of view) and the economic assessment. Generally speaking, patient benefit and benefit to the hospital and the economy are not mutually exclusive. Contradictions, however, cannot be avoided and permanently provide points of conflict. This is the inherent challenge in the development of health care systems based on social consensus and medical ethics.

The data, concepts, and ideas presented in this book, which has been written by an international panel of experts, should help make the medical progress aimed at patient well-being affordable.

Reinhard Marre
Medical Director
Ulm University Clinic
Ulm, Germany

# Preface

This is an important and timely book. As health care costs soar, there is increasing interest in examining what society and particularly patients receive in return for these expenditures. *Optimizing Health* brings together the best thinking from both sides of the Atlantic to explore these issues. It employs disciplinary perspectives from economics, ethics, philosophy, psychology, clinical practice, and epidemiology to explore various ways by which the value for patients have and can be determined. It concludes with a discussion of changes required in practice, research, and health care systems to maximize the outcomes received from the provision of medical care services from the patient's perspective.

The first section of the book provides theoretical perspectives from economics and systems thinking that help us to focus on how one might determine the value of medical care for patients. The next section considers the ethical and philosophical dilemmas that face developed countries in distributing medical care. How is justice served and evidence-based medicine employed to increase the value of medical care for patients?

The section on psychology deals with measuring outcomes from the patient's perspective and involving patients in medical decision making. Measuring quality of life and gaining valid quality of life information when patients cannot respond for themselves are important topics covered by these chapters. Other chapters consider ways that patients can become more involved in medical decision making with the expectation that it will increase the value of medical care for patients.

A major section of the book about clinical practice discusses problems that can reduce the value to patients of medical care. The problems discussed include overdiagnosis, aggressive treatments that do not result in better patient outcomes, findings that an early diagnosis does not always result in a better outcome, and the extent of medical error in treatment.

The final sections deal with cost-effectiveness analyses and applications of clinical epidemiology. The chapters include a number of original investigations and applications of new methodologies. All-in-all, the volume is must reading for practitioners, policy makers, and researchers who want to find in one place the state-of-the-art thinking and future directions of valuing medical care from the patient's perspective.

Ronald Andersen
Wasserman Professor Emeritus
Departments of Health Services and Sociology
University of California School of Public Health Los Angeles
Los Angeles, Calfornia, USA

# Table of Contents

# Contributors

Franz Porzsolt
Clinical Economics, Ulm University
  Hospital, Germany

Robert M. Kaplan
Department of Health Services and
  Medicine
University of California, Los Angeles

Lawrence J. Schneiderman
Department of Family and
  Preventive Medicine,
University of California, San Diego

Heike Leonhardt-Huober
Clinical Economics, Ulm University
  Hospital, Germany

Peter Strasser
Institute for Legal Philosophy,
  Sociology, and Informatics,
Karl-Franzens University,
Graz, Austria

Hans Ruß
Clinical Economics, Ulm University
  Hospital, Germany

Johannes Clouth
Clinical Economics, Ulm university
  Hospital, Germany
Lilly Germany GmbH, Corporate
  Affairs and Health Economics

Marina Kojer
Department of Palliative Geriatrics,
  Wienerwald Geriatric Center,
  Vienna, Austria

Martina Schmidl
Department of Palliative Geriatrics,
  Wienerwald Geriatric Center,
  Vienna, Austria

Elfriede R. Greimel
Department of Obstetrics and
  Gynecology, University of Graz,
  Austria

Jörg Sigle
Clinical Economics, Ulm University
  Hospital, Germany

Jörg Richter
Clinic of Psychiatry and
  Psychotherapy, Rostock
  University, Germany

Martin Eisemann
Department of Psychology,
  University of Tromsø, Norway

Susan B. Rifkin
Tropical Institute of Community
  Health and Development in
  Africa,
London School of Economics

Hana Kajnar
Clinical Economics, Ulm University
  Hospital, Germany

E. Jane Maher
Mount Vernon Centre for Cancer
  Treatment, Mount Vernon
  Hospital, Northwood, Middlesex,
  England
University College London, and
  Centre for Complexity &
  Management, Herts University,
  Hertfordshire, England

Gemma Gatta
Epidemiology Unit,
Istituto Nazionale per lo Studio e la
  Cura dei Tumori,
(National Institute for the Study and
  Cure of Tumors)
  Milan, Italy

Joseph E. Scherger
Department of Family and
  Preventive Medicine,
  University of California, San Diego

Manfred Müller
Flight Safety, Lufthansa,
  Frankfurt/Main Airport, Germany

Horst Kunhardt
Mainkofen District Hospital,
  Deggendorf, Germany
University of Applied Sciences,
  Deggendorf, Germany

Scott D. Ramsey
Fred Hutchinson Cancer Center
  Seattle, Washington

Reinhold Kilian
University of Ulm, Department of
  Psychiatry II, Army Hospital,
  Günzburg, Germany

Amit K. Ghosh
Department of General Internal
  Medicine, Mayo Clinic College of
  Medicine,
  Rochester, Minnesota

Dirk Stengel
Clinical Epidemiology Division,
  Department of Trauma and
  Orthopedic Surgery,
  Unfallkrankenhaus Berlin,
  Germany

Nancy Spector
National Council of State Boards of
  Nursing, Chicago, Illinois

Narayana S. Murali
Mayo Clinic College of Medicine,
  Rochester, Minnesota

Sidney L. Saltzstein,
Departments of Family & Preventive
  Medicine and Pathology,
  University of California, San
  Diego

Bernhard T. Gehr
Evidence-Based Health Care,
  Human Studies Center,
  Ludwig-Maximilian University,
  Munich, Germany

Christel Weiss
Department for Medical Statistics,
  University of Heidelberg,
  Heidelberg University Hospital in
  Mannheim, Germany

Jalid Sehouli
Department of Gynecology and
  Obstetrics, Charité Medical
  Center, Berlin, Germany

# Authors' Biographies

**Ronald Anderson** is Wasserman Professor Emeritus of the Departments of Health Services and Sociology at the University of California School of Public Health in Los Angeles.

**Johannes Clouth** studied business administration, romance languages, and English before working in advertising and industry. He has worked in market research and health outcomes research for pharmaceutical companies and is head and founder of the health outcomes group of the Gesellschaft für Recht und Politik im Gesundheitswesen [Society for Jurisprudence and Politics in the Health-Care System]. Jophannes Clouth is also co-founder of the Wilsede Quality of Life Group and guest lecturer for health economics at the Rheinischen Fachhochschule [Rhein Technical University].

**Gemma Gatta** trained as a medical doctor and received a postdoctoral degree in hygiene and preventive medicine. She has performed research in the Epidemiology Unit of the National Cancer Institute in Milan, Italy, in the following fields: Lombardy Cancer Registry in Varese Province, methodology of case-control studies for screening evaluation, evaluation of an educational program on tobacco, diet, and breast feeding; EUROCARE: European cancer registries based study of cancer patients survival and care (in the coordinating and analysis group and steering committee) and EUROPREVAL: European cancer registries study of cancer patients prevalence (in the analysis group and steering committee), cancer survival comparison between North America and Europe; CONCORD project (analysis group and steering committee, descriptive epidemiology of rare tumors; European task force for rare diseases, childhood cancer survival, and evaluation of late outcomes in cancer patients.

**Bernhard Gehr** studied medicine at the Ludwig-Maximilian University in Munich and continued his studies in Edinburgh and New York City (where he received a US-EU-MEE scholarship). His interest in medical journalism grew with his years of activity in the news section of the health information pages for medical laypersons (www.netdoktor.de). He received the media prize from the German Diabetes Foundation in 2000. His book (together with Ulrike Thurm) *Diabetes-und Sportfibel* [Diabetes and Sport Primer] was published in 2001.

The topic of his medical dissertation is the FORE-Bias, which is also the topic of his contribution in this book. Bernhard Gehr is presently performing part of his training to become a general physician at the district hospital in Mühldorf am Inn in the Department of Surgery.

**Amit K. Ghosh** is Associate Professor of Medicine in the Division of General Internal Medicine at the Mayo Clinic in Rochester, Minnesota. He received his postgraduate training at the Post Graduate Institute of Medical Education and Research in Chandigarh, India and at the University of Minnesota Medical School in Minneapolis. Amit Ghosh is the Associate Program Director of the General Internal Medicine Research Fellowship at the Mayo Clinic College of Medicine. He is board certified in internal medicine and nephrology and a fellow of the American College of Physicians. His research interests include evidence-based medicine (EBM), risk communication, and understanding medical uncertainty. He has also taught and delivered numerous lectures on evidence-based medicine and complex medical decision making in the United States and Europe. He has been a tutor at the University of London Medical School, the Centre for Evidence-Based Medicine in Oxford, England, and the Oxford Workshop; and he teaches EBM at the Mayo Clinic College of Medicine.

**Hana Kajnar** was born in the Czech Republic and studied medicine at the Ludwig-Maximilian University in Munich. She wrote her doctoral thesis on qualitative meta-analysis dealing with "Shared Decision Making in Medicine" while she was a member of the Franz Porzsolt's working group in Ulm. She is presently performing an internship at the City Hospital in Sindelfingen.

**Robert M. Kaplan** is Professor and Chair of the UCLA Department of Health Services and Professor of Medicine at the UCLA David Geffen School of Medicine. He is a past President of several organizations, including the American Psychological Association Division of Health Psychology, the International Society for Quality of Life Research, the Society for Behavioral Medicine, and the Academy of Behavioral Medicine Research. Kaplan is Editor-in-Chief of *Health Psychology* and former Editor-in-Chief of the *Annals of Behavioral Medicine*. In 2005 he was elected to the US Institute of Medicine of the National Academies of Sciences.

**Reinhold Kilian** is a sociologist and previously worked as research assistant and lecturer of medical sociology and public health at Bielefeld University in Germany, research assistant at the Central Institute of Mental Health, Mannheim, Germany, and senior researcher and lecturer of public health at the Department of Psychiatry at the University of Leipzig, Germany. Since 2003 he has held the position of senior researcher and lecturer of health economics at the Department of Psychiatry II at the University of Ulm, Germany. His main research interests are medical sociology, mental health service research, quality of life research, health economic evaluation, epidemiology, and qualitative and quantitative research methods. Since 1998 he has been vice president of

Research Committee 49, Sociology of Mental Health and Illness of the International Sociological Association.

**Horst Kunhardt** is a member of the staff at the Department of Informatics at the University of Passau in Germany and CIO at the district hospital in Mainkofen. He is cofounder of the Society for Solutions in Informatics and completed his doctoral degree in the area of public health at the University of Ulm under Franz Porzsolt. He is head of the Institute for Health Management and MBA studies in health management. Since 2004 he has been professor for operational systems at the University of Applied Sciences in Deggendorf. His main professional interests include the conception of networks and server systems and the implementation of hospital information systems, evidence-based medicine, and evidence-based information technology. He has served a consultancy in the area of information technology (IT) security and organization.

**Heike Leonhardt-Huober** completed her medical studies in Ulm, Germany in 1996. She then studied teaching methods in medicine using new media. Since her graduation, she has taught various medical subjects in schools of physiotherapy. She recognized early that many conventional medical practices lack evidence, resulting in severe, undesired side effects of medical interventions. As a result, she began attending courses in evidence-based medicine in 1999 and has been involved in retrieving appropriate medical information and passing it on to her students ever since.

**Reinhard Marre** studied medicine at the Kiel, Graz, and Lübeck universities. He specialized in medical microbiology and moved to the University of Ulm in 1992, where he chaired the Department of Medical Microbiology and Hygiene. In 2000 he became Dean of the Medical Faculty of the Ulm University and Chief Executive Officer of the Ulm University Hospital in 2004.

**E. Jane Maher** completed medical studies at Kings College London, Westminster Medical School and her oncology training at Mount Vernon Cancer Centre, Middlesex Hospital, Harvard Medical School and The Royal Marsden Hospital. She is now Consultant Oncologist at the Mount Vernon Cancer Centre, Senior Lecturer at the University College, London and Visiting Professor of Cancer & Supportive Care at the Complexity and Management Centre, Hertfordshire University in England. She co-founded the Lynda Jackson Macmillan Centre for Support and Information, which is recognized internationally as a model for integrating complementary approaches and therapies into mainstream research and service activities and leads the Supportive Oncology Research Programme at Mount Vernon Cancer Centre, England. She is Chief Medical Officer at Macmillan Cancer Support (a large UK development charity) responsible for supporting 300 physicians in primary and secondary care with an interest in cancer.

**Manfred Müller** has been Manager of Flight Safety for Lufthansa since 2002 and lectures on risk management at the University of Bremen in Germany. After studying physics and mathematics for five semesters at the Ludwig-Maximilian University of Munich, he completed airline pilot training at the Lufthansa Pilot School in Bremen, Germany, and Phoenix, Arizona. He has served as first officer on Boeing 737, Boeing 747/400, and Airbus A340. In 1991 he completed Aircraft Accident Investigator Training at the University of Southern California in Los Angeles. He has been a flight captain since 1994 and has served as Flight Management System Instructor for HITEC-Aircraft (A320, B737/300) and a Simulator Instructor. He has worked in the development of Crew Resource Management programs since 1998. Since 1995 he has cooperated with Professor Hans Troidl in the Department of Experimental Surgery at the Surgical University Clinic of Köln-Merheim on risk reduction in medicine and developed risk management seminars for medical personnel. His working goal is evidence-based risk management.

**Narayana S. Murali** is a fellow in the Division of Nephrology and instructor at the Mayo Clinic College of Medicine in Rochester, Minnesota. He is pursuing an academic career as a physician-investigator bringing research from the bench to the bedside. After completing his postgraduate training under the auspices of the National Board of Examinations in India, he worked as a registrar at the Royal Canberra Hospital, University of Sydney, Australia. His research interests include evidence-based medicine, rhabdomyolysis, and the role of endothelial progenitor cells in alleviating renal diseases. He was involved in starting the Evidence-Based Physical Diagnosis Club for the internal medicine residents at the Mayo Clinic, where he is also course facilitator for evidence-based medicine (EBM) and tutors students in the art and science of EBM. He has given talks and presentations on EBM-based research at various state, national, and international scientific meetings.

**Franz Porzsolt** completed his medical studies at the University of Marburg and was research fellow of the Deutsche Forschungsgemeinschaft [German Research Association] at the Princess Margaret Hospital in Toronto, Ontario, in Canada. He completed his training as hematologist and medical oncologist at the medical school of Ulm University in Germany, completed several projects on natural killer cells and biological response modifiers such as interferons, and conducted clinical trials in advanced breast and renal cell cancer in Germany and Austria. Over the years his interest in defining the goals and value of treatment in incurable disease has continually increased. He also developed a growing interest in the general description of the value of health care from the patient's point of view, which led to the publication of *Klinische Ökonomik* [Clinical Economics] in Germany in 2003. The present book focuses on the value of health care with the aim of contributing to the development of a new research and teaching area (CLINECS) at the interface of clinical medicine and economics.

**Scott D. Ramsey** is a general internist who holds an MD degree from the University of Iowa and a PhD from the University of Pennsylvania. He is an

Associate Member of the Fred Hutchinson Cancer Center and Professor of Medicine at the University of Washington. Scott Ramsey's research focuses on cost-effectiveness analysis and cancer screening. He headed the evaluation of cost-effectiveness for the National Emphysema Treatment Trial.

**Susan B. Rifkin** is a social scientist specializing in lay persons' involvement in health care and has vast experience developing, carrying out, and assessing projects in developing countries as well as in Europe. She teaches health policy at the London School of Economics and the London School of Hygiene and Tropical Medicine. She has helped establish two Masters' degree courses in health policy and management—one at the University of Heidelberg in Germany and the other in Kisumu, Kenya. Her research interests at the moment focus on empowerment and equity, on which she has published a framework for assessing these factors on improving health outcomes.

**Hans Günther Russ** studied sciences and sociology in Mannheim and wrote his doctoral thesis in philosophy on scientific theory. He then took a position at the cultural-philosophical department at the European University Viadrina in Frankfurt am Oder, where he wrote a postdoctoral thesis on the problems of what is and what should be. His main field of interest is ethics in scientific theory. He presently is a professor at the University of Mannheim and a member of the Institute of Clinical Economics.

**Sidney Saltzstein** is professor emeritus in the departments of pathology and family and preventive medicine at the University of California in San Diego. He trained as a pathologist and as an epidemiologist. Prior to his retirement, he headed the tumor registry for San Diego and Imperial Counties in California.

**Joseph E. Scherger** is clinical professor in the Department of Family and Preventive Medicine at the University of California School of Medicine in San Diego (UCSD), director of the San Diego Center for Patient Safety, and director of Quality Improvement in Correctional Medicine at UCSD. From 2001 to 2003 he served as founding dean of the Florida State University College of Medicine and is a member of the Harvard Kennedy School of Government Health Care Delivery Policy Project. His main focus is on the redesign of office practice using the tools of information technology and quality improvement. His has been repeatedly awarded Outstanding Clinical Instructor in the School of Medicine at the University of California, Davis, and was chosen Family Physician of the Year by the American Academy of Family Physicians and the California Academy of Family Physicians in 1989. In 2000 he was nominated by the University of California Irvine medical students for the AAMC Humanism in Medicine Award. He served on the Institute of Medicine Committee on the Quality of Health Care in America from 1998 to 2001. Joseph Scherger has served on the board of directors of the American Academy of Family Physicians and the American Board of Family Practice and was editor-in-chief of *Hippocrates*, published by the Massachusetts Medical Society, from 1999 to 2001. He was the first medical editor of *Family Practice*

*Management.* He has authored more than 300 medical publications, has given more than 600 invited presentations, and is a marathon runner.

**Lawrence J. Schneiderman** is professor in the Departments of Family and Preventive Medicine and Medicine at the University of California School of Medicine in San Diego. He received his MD degree from Harvard and has been a visiting scholar and professor at many institutions around the world. He was the founding co-chair of the Bioethics Committee of the University of California Medical Center in San Diego and has served as an ethics consultant there and at the San Diego Children's Hospital. Lawrence J. Schneiderman's teaching and research activities focus on the areas of medical ethics, literature, and medicine. He is a fellow of the American College of Physicians and a member of the Physicians for Social Responsibility, American Society for Bioethics and Humanities, and American Society of Law and Medicine. Lawrence J. Schneiderman has written more than 150 medical and scientific publications, including the textbook *The Practice of Preventive Health Care* and, with Nancy S. Jecker, *Wrong Medicine: Doctor's Patients and Futile Treatment.*

**Jalid Sehouli** attended medical school at the University of Berlin and completed his training in gynecology and obstetrics at the Charité Hospital in Berlin. His specialty is the clinical management of advanced gynecological malignancies. In this context he completed several projects on aspects of surgical and systemic therapies and conducted several multicentric Phase I, II, and III clinical trials in primary and relapsed ovarian cancer. He is also interested in the principles of evidence-based medicine and health care. Jalid Sehouli is an active member of several societies, secretary of the North Eastern German Society of Gynecologic Oncology (NOGGO), vice-president of the International Institute of Clinical Economics (ICE), and treasurer of the self-help cancer organization Onkologisches Patientenseminar [Oncologic Patient Seminar].

**Nancy Spector** is Director of Education at the National Council of State Boards of Nursing (NCSBN). She received her BSN from the University of Wisconsin in Madison, her MSN from the University of California in San Francisco, and her doctorate from Rush University in Chicago. She joined NCSBN after teaching undergraduate and graduate nursing for 20 years. During her years of teaching, Nancy Spector researched quality of life in cancer patients and managed the nursing care of respiratory diseases She also taught courses related to improving evidence-based nursing practice. At NCSBN Nancy Spector has developed an interest in evidence-based regulation. She is now working with a group to identify evidence-based indicators of quality nursing education programs for the boards of nursing to use when approving schools of nursing.

**Dirk Stengel** trained in surgery in Berlin, Germany. After board certification, he worked as a senior trauma surgeon at the Department of Trauma and Orthopedic Surgery of the Unfallkrankenhaus Berlin (UKB) Trauma Center, a 600-bed metropolitan level I trauma center and academic teaching facility. He attended courses in molecular biology and biostatistics until he finished his postgraduate master of science studies in epidemiology. Together with Professor Franz Porzsolt, he founded the Institute of Clinical Economics (ICE) and was recently appointed head of the Center for Clinical Research at the UKB. He is a member of the scientific panel of the German Association of Trauma and Orthopedic Surgeons, the Cochrane Injuries Group, and various other national and international societies. He is also a peer reviewer for several international biomedical journals and assistant professor for theoretical surgery, clinical chemistry, biostatistics, and epidemiology at the Charité University Medical Center. His major research interests are efficacy, effectiveness, and efficiency of diagnostic tests, meta-analyses, and the development of methodologically sound, pragmatic study designs in surgery.

**Peter Strasser** teaches philosophy and legal philosophy at the Karl-Franzens University in Graz, Austria. He was visiting professor at the University of Arizona in 1999 and regularly teaches at the Institute for Philosophy of the Klagenfurt University in Austria as guest professor. Since 2002, together with Adolf Holl and Thomas Macho, he has published the *Bibliothek der Unruhe und des Bewahrens* [Library of Unrest and Preservation] (Styria Publishing Company). His present interests focus on questions concerning the theory of the person, bioethics, and philosophy of religion. Recent publications: *Gut in allen möglichen Welten. Der ethische Horizon"* [Good in All Possible Worlds. The Ethical Horizon], *Gibt es ein Leben nach dem Tod? Gehirne, Computer und das wahre Selbst* [Is There Life After Death? Brains, Computers, and the True Self], and *Verbrechermenschen. Zur kriminalwissenschaftlichen Erzeugung des Bösen* [Criminals. The Criminologic Creation of Evil].

**Christel Weiss** studied mathematics and physics at the University of Mainz in Germany before becoming assistant at the Institute for Experimental Surgery at the University of Heidelberg. She holds degrees in both mathematics and medical informatics. Christel Weiss is presently head of the Institute for Medical Statistics at the University Hospital in Mannheim (faculty of the University of Heidelberg) and lecturer on biomathematics and epidemiology. She provides support to medical doctors performing clinical studies.

# 1
# "CLINECS": Strategy and Tactics to Provide Evidence of the Usefulness of Health Care Services from the Patient's Perspective (Value for Patients)

Franz Porzsolt and Robert M. Kaplan

## Point of Departure

Most attempts to describe the value of health care were market oriented and left the aspects of effectiveness with the care providers (Roberts, 1989; van de Ven, 1996). A recent approach entitled "Evidence-Based to Value-Based Medicine" (Brown et al., 2005) provides an elegant link between health economics and evidence-based medicine but does not include the final step from evidence-based to everyday medicine. In this chapter, we define the term "CLINECS." The term was created by fusing the names of the disciplines that contribute to the assessment of useful health care services, that is, clinical practice, clinical epidemiology, health economics, psychology, ethics, and philosophy (Table 1.1).

We characterize a health care service as *useful* if the patient or service recipient and other members of society recognize it as valuable. When applying the term *value*, we refer to various characteristics: a perceived and quantifiable change in the state of health; an objectively determined change in the state of health; and a change in the state of health as assessed in longitudinal studies.

Accordingly, the value of a health care service from the patient's perspective is a perceived value. This value has no absolute dimension. It depends on the context in which it occurs and may change over time.

Of course, health care services are valued by persons other than patients. Because they are publicly financed, their value must also be defined from the viewpoint of other stakeholders in the system. The opinion of the responsible patient must, however, be given priority. Otherwise, we do not fulfill the goal of a health care system and pay too little attention to the ethical principle of patient autonomy.

When evaluating health care services, we must recognize that there may be discrepancies in the perspectives of observers. This means that an observer's

TABLE 1.1. "CLINECS": strategy for applying clinical epidemiology, economics, psychology, and ethics to create and evaluate value for patients in clinical practice

| Parameter | Perspectives of clinical practice (patients' perspectives) | |
| --- | --- | --- |
| | Outputs | Outcomes |
| **Clinical Epidemiology** | | |
| Validity and efficacy | Effects detected by laboratory tests or imaging procedures in clinical trials | Effects on quantity and/or quality of life demonstrated in clinical trials—referred to as "utility" if described in quality-adjusted life years (QALYs) |
| Validity and effectiveness | Effects detected by laboratory tests or imaging procedures in daily clinical practice. | Effects on quantity and/or quality of life demonstrated in daily clinical practice. |
| **Health Economics** | | |
| Efficiency | Ratio of monetary cost and consequences. Results of laboratory tests or imaging procedures, mostly assessed in clinical trials (cost-effectiveness analysis). | Ratio of monetary cost and consequences. Effects on quantity and/or quality of life mostly assessed in clinical trials (cost-utility analysis). |
| Insurance, reimbursement, and payment | Insurance and reimbursements mostly cover only outputs. Patients have little or no interest in payment for only outputs. "Bridge principles" support the decisions when outputs can replace outcomes. | Insurance and reimbursement almost never cover outcomes. Patients have an interest in payment for outcomes but are rarely willing to pay for health care services out of pocket. |
| **Psychology and Ethics** | | |
| Value for patients and society, justice and equality | Ratio of intangible and tangible costs and consequences associated with surrogate parameters for quantity and/or quality of life | Ratio of intangible and tangible costs and consequences associated with patients' preferences/expectations about the quantity and/or quality of life (perceived assurance & health) |

"Bridge principles" address the importance of a clear definition of the goal of health care services and provide necessary rules when output can replace missing outcomes data for evaluation of health care services.

description of the value of a health care service does not have to coincide with the evaluation by the patient. When evaluating health care services, the expected health condition is compared with the observed one. There is often (but not always) agreement on the patient's state of health, which is observed by two persons at the same time after treatment. In other words, the observed health condition is identically perceived by these two persons. If we compare the health conditions these two people expected as results before the treatment began, we can predict with some certainty that in most cases these expectations diverge. If one of the two people is the patient and the other a relative, a physician, or a member of the public,[1] the patient assesses the value of the health care service differently from his or her relatives, the physician, or the member of the public.

Perceived gains or losses of health assessed in longitudinal before/after comparisons are also valuable for the assessment of health care services. We call the value perceived by the patient as *value for patients* (VFP).

A discussion of VFP is long overdue. Health and health care services have become the most important economic sectors in all industrialized countries. Globalization of the economy makes it necessary to reach decisions concerning health and health care services together with neighboring countries and international partners. To enlighten the discussion, we must use terms that have been mutually agreed upon, name common goals, and have transparent strategies and tactics for achieving these goals.

## Semantic Hygiene

International discussions are often hindered because different cultures attach different meanings to identical terms. A classic example is the term *evidence*. In English, evidence means the data that support a statement. In German and all Mediterranean languages, the term evidence is used to indicate that a statement does not need the support of data, that is, it is obvious. Even within one culture different disciplines use identical terms with different meanings, such as the term *effectiveness* as used in epidemiology (Last, 1988) and in health economics. Terminologic confusion is complete when, in addition, individual scientists in a culture and in one discipline associate terms with their individual scientific concepts. We encountered this unfortunate situation during the early 1990s when we began comparing existing data for describing the usefulness of health care services. We need not explain that misunderstandings can be avoided only if we accept the necessity of semantic hygiene and agree on common standards.

The necessary differentiations are listed in Figure 1.1. For an economic assessment, both components of a possible action, the *input* and the *output*, must first

---

[1]We mention the public and publicly financed health care services because our statements should also apply to health care systems which, in contrast to the German system, are not financed by a health insurance program.

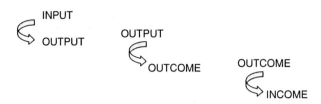

FIGURE 1.1. "Doctor's dictionary." Important differences among economic terms.

be considered. Both components can be measured in any number of dimensions. Input need not always be measured in monetary terms, and output can be expressed as an improved laboratory value or lengthening of life expectancy. When comparing input and output, each of these terms is used as a higher category, which contains every kind of input or output.

At the second level, in which different kinds of results are considered, we differentiate between *output* and *outcome*. Here the term output has a different meaning at the first and second levels. At the first level, we used the term output to differentiate between input and output. At the second level, at which we consider the output more carefully, it can be represented in dimensions that are relevant to patients, that is, (re)gained years of life or improved quality of life. In this case, we refer to the result as an *outcome*. If the result has dimensions other than years of life or quality of life, we refer to it as an *output*. Applying common definitions can advance discussions about health care services and allow us to distinguish between effective and useful health care services. Three examples are presented to further explain this difference.

- Lowering elevated blood pressure describes an output. If, as a result of lowered blood pressure the rate of strokes, heart attacks, and kidney damage are reduced, they can be described as different outcomes of lowered blood pressure.
- Improved diagnostic possibilities (including screening) increase our knowledge by providing a diagnosis. This kind of result we call output because it does not necessarily lead to the desired effects on the quantity and quality of life for the patient. If, however, as a result of the output (lowered blood pressure) strokes, heart disease, and kidney disease are avoided and quality of life improves or length of survival increases, we call these additional results outcomes. This problem must be taken into consideration regarding the results of early disease diagnosis, which almost always fulfills the criteria of an output but not necessarily those of an outcome.
- The third example concerns prevention. Most prevention programs produce outputs but not outcomes. Whether the goal of prevention—avoiding an undesired event—is achieved, such a when taking aspirin to prevent another heart attack, is not easy to confirm. Not everyone who takes aspirin after an infarct can avoid another infarct. We are well advised, not only for financial reasons, to choose those programs in which achievable benefit for the patients can be confirmed with clearly measured outcomes.

The last of the important differentiations applies to outcome and income. Even if the discussion of this pair of terms generally causes amusement, it can quickly become reality. The terms conceal the problem that the public financing of health care services should be limited to effective services, as was demanded in the 1930s by the British epidemiologist Archie Cochrane and later confirmed by Warren & Mosteller (1993). This means that not all health care services can be publicly financed. The health care systems of industrialized nations are no longer in a position to support all effective health care services. Because the resources are limited, we must apply principles of equality and justice to allocate the resources in a way that offers the most health for the most people.

## Treading on Thin Ice

Psychological effects are probably much more powerful than ever expected. This means that many effects we attributed to chemical (internal medicine) or physical (surgery, radiotherapy) interventions are only related to, but not necessarily caused by, pharmacological or surgical treatment. It is more likely that the observed effects are mediated by psychological effects, such as "knowledge framing"[2] (Porzsolt et al., 2004). As a consequence, the value of many medical services appear in a different light; their specific values decrease while their nonspecific values increase. We foresee that a considerable portion of our health care services, including medications, are not really as valuable as they are claimed to be.

Our German book *Klinische Ökonomik* [Clinical Economics] (Porzsolt et al., 2003) offered concrete examples of inappropriately evaluated health care services in many fields of medicine. We need not avoid a controversial topic—in the coming years there will be considerable reshuffling of health care services. Without going into details, classic medical services will increase in importance. These services comprise not only biomolecular knowledge and technical abilities but also communicative capacities and empathy—in short, the attitudes patients expect when they seek medical help and do not just want to be "serviced" by a hired physician with excellent credentials.

How far we are willing to go is our own decision. Even if the concept seems clear, its practical application must be prepared with utmost care. We are talking about remodeling the most powerful market segment in our economic system on which innumerable jobs and even our prosperity depends. If we agree that the health care system needs a fundamental reform of its outcomes and outputs, it would be foolish to hinder these reforms only because we fear adverse economic results for individual stakeholders.

---

[2]Knowledge framing effects are observed in daily clinical practice and are desirable in this setting. They are conceptually identical to placebo effects, which are observed in clinical trials, where they are considered bias and are therefore undesirable.

The most effective and important parameter is time. Rash decisions and actions do not help anyone. Carefully prepared concepts that provide all stakeholders with the possibility of adjusting to the changed conditions and preparing the required solutions can induce the necessary corporate identity that is lacking in nearly all industrial nations but is necessary to overcome the present economic stagnation. If we realize that we can decide how pressing the need for change is, we will no longer need to tread so gingerly.

## Bridge Principles

The differentiation between outputs and outcomes was offered as a criterion in the evaluation of publicly financed services. Measures that improve outcomes should be candidates for public funding, whereas others should not. This inviting rule, which sometimes bears the decorative adjective *evidence-based* is, unfortunately, not feasible because only a pathetic pile of publicly financed health care services would be left. For most of the provided health care services, the desired outcomes have not been systematically documented, or the validity of the data is so weak that only slogan sadists[3] are able to deal with such complex concepts without difficulty.

This leads to the equally critical, as well as ethically, medically, economically, and legally important, question. Under which conditions should we accept outputs in the place of outcomes to avoid withholding potentially useful health care services from patients while simultaneously minimizing the heath and economic risks of a treatment for individuals and society as a whole as much as possible? To help answer this question, we have worked up Hans Albert's bridge principles (1985) and present them in the second part of our discussion (see Chapter 6).

## *Goal*

The bridge principles have shed light on the importance of defining goals. The field of medicine can profit tremendously from this because goal definitions are more criminally neglected in medicine than in other fields. For outsiders it is difficult to believe (insiders are too close to notice) that concrete treatment goals are far too rarely determined prospectively during the daily clinical routine. Most of our health care systems envisage no explicit remuneration for common agreement on treatment goals reached in advance. It is justifiably feared that general financing of communicative medicine could be abused as a license to print money. If, however, the agreement on a common treatment goal could legally be remunerated, important components in the provision of health care could be suggested. A structured conversation between patient and physician would also be stimu-

---

[3]Slogan sadists are contemporaries who use the contents of frightening slogans (such as evidence-based medicine) without digesting the meaning, thereby creating problems for others.

lated, such as the prospective determination of an individual's goal of health care provision, which could later be examined. It is almost predictable that improved initial communication between doctor and patient could achieve various desired effects. We offer two examples: A considerable portion of low-value diagnostic procedures, which often ineffectively but lucratively make up for a lack of communication, would be omitted by a clear definition of goals. Moreover, determining a concrete goal of health care provision would guarantee the prerequisites that are necessary to decide under which conditions outcomes can be replaced by outputs.

## Solutions

Once common goals and a common language have been identified, possible solutions for optimizing health care services can be discussed. Our proposed solution is shown in Figure 1.2 and is based on a simple principle. The value of health care services from the patient perspective and, thereby, from the viewpoint of clinical practice, presents a necessary but not sufficient condition. The points of view represented in other disciplines must also be taken into consideration.

The assessment of usefulness or value is divided into two parts by the differentiation between outputs and outcomes from the patient/clinical-practice perspective (vertical division in Figure 1.2). This division emphasizes the importance we place on this difference. The horizontal division is influenced by the viewpoints of the various scientific disciplines.

The first horizontal level describes the viewpoint of clinical epidemiology, which offers a methodological tool with which to confirm the validity of scientific statements. As it is likely that only 20% of all medical statements are based on hard scientific facts, we believe that testing the validity by clinical epidemiology is of great importance for subsequent decisions concerning public funding of health care services.

The second contribution of clinical epidemiology concerns the differentiation between efficacy and efficiency. The efficacy of a measure is proven if the data derive from the special conditions in a clinical study (such as defined inclusion and exclusion criteria and standardized procedures according to the study protocol). If the data were gained under everyday conditions, we speak of proof of efficiency. This important difference has been overlooked because we gather data in clinical studies and apply them under everyday conditions without first having tested whether the recorded effects collected under "ideal" conditions (such as the effects of lowering blood fat levels) can also be found under everyday conditions. If we want to regain control over the financing of our health care systems, we must create transparency at these unclear interfaces.

The second horizontal level, health economics, introduces efficiency and reminds us that, in addition to outputs and outcomes, we must consider what investment or input that is required to achieve the desired results must be taken into consideration. This input can be measured in monetary or nonmonetary units. Because the patients' perspective has the highest priority in this approach, we believe that the burdens and undesired effects of diagnosis and therapy the patient has to accept and the limitations in health-related quality of life are of great importance.

This second level contributes two aspects to the concept of "CLINECS." The second aspect of health economics concerns questions of health insurance, remuneration, and additional patient fees. These aspects make up a considerable portion of traditional health economy but are of only secondary importance for our discussion.

The third horizontal level consists of the fields of psychology, ethics, and philosophy. We hope to demonstrate that psychological guidance of health and illness should be given considerably more attention. The quality of the doctor–patient relationship has a central position and must be recognized as an important economic factor. Discussions about the (unfortunately still controversial) concept of subjective health (felt assurance, perceived health), which are fundamental, have just begun. Medical care controlled by economic restraints is required to achieve health benefits for the entire population under the constraints of available resources. An intrinsic part of this requirement is the need for evaluation. No matter what one thinks of the "economization" of medicine, it has become unavoidable because the service providers require remuneration, and resources are limited.

The core of our project is the concept of *value for patients*. To improve the health of entire populations, we must attend to the values created by our health care services. Only when the concepts of the value of a health care service have become concrete can reasonable negotiations about the monetary value of this service be possible.

A second, special aspect of this level concerns the bridge principles. Hardly anyone would have expected that these considerations, which originally were developed from moral philosophy, would gain importance for economic decisions in the health care system. These bridge principles are discussed by Hans Russ in Chapter 6. They provide a structured introduction to the choice of appropriate criteria to apply so one can identify the value of health care services.

In the following chapters, authors describe these three levels and present concrete examples. We cannot offer a perfect prototype for solving problems, but we do offer a matrix that allows multiple possibilities for improvement.

## References

Albert, H. (1985). *Treatise on critical reason*. Princeton: Princeton University Press.

Brown, M.M., Brown, G.C., Sharma, S. (Eds.) (2005), *Evidence-based to value-based medicine*. Chicago: American Medical Association Press.

Last, J.M. (1988). *Dictionary of epidemiology* (2nd ed.). New York: Oxford University Press.

Porzsolt, F., Williams, A.R., Kaplan, R.M. (2003). *Klinische Ökonomik: Effektivität und Effizienz von Gesundheitsleistungen*. [Clinical economics: effectivity and effeciency of health care services.] Landsberg am Lech, Germany: Ecomed.

Porzsolt, F., Schlotz-Gorton, N., Biller-Andorno, N., Thim, A., Meissner, K., Roeckl-Wiedmann, I., et al. (2004). Applying evidence to support ethical decisions: is the placebo really powerless? *Science and Engineering Ethics*, 10, 119–132.

Roberts, C.S. (1989). Conflicting professional values in social work and medicine. *Health and Social Work*, 14, 211–218.

Van de Ven, W.P. (1996). Market-oriented health care reforms: trends and future options. *Social Science and Medicine*, 43, 655–666.

Warren, K.S., Mosteller, F. (1993). In K.S. Warren, F. Mosteller (Eds.). Doing more good than harm: the evaluation of health care interventions [Preface]. *Annals of the New York Academy of Science*, 703, 1–4.

# 2
# Systems View of Health Care

ROBERT M. KAPLAN

The art of medicine concentrates on diagnosis (finding problems) and treatment (fixing problems). The task of physicians might be described as "find it and fix it." The find-it/fix-it model exemplifies what engineers call linear thinking. The linear model has been the predominant view of the world since the time of Sir Isaac Newton, who focused his attention on discrete components of the world and assumed that these components operated independently from one another. Many things work in a linear fashion. For a complex machine or organism, linear function means that each component operates independently of the others. The environment receives relatively little attention. Ackoff (1994) explained that the industrial revolution, which began in England during the 18th century, ushered in new ways of thinking that dominated nearly all fields for several centuries. This thinking was dominated by three concepts: reductionism, analysis, and mechanism.

*Reductionism* is the belief that everything we experience is made up of component parts. Just as an automobile represents contributions from many factories, we assume that humans are also a conglomeration of component parts. Science has involved the study of taking things apart. The parts become smaller and smaller until the scientist arrives at the ultimate parts, which are no longer divisible. These are the basic elements. Reductionists believe that to understand something it must be disassembled into its component parts. It is usually assumed that these parts function independently of one another.

*Analysis* is the process by which things are divided into their components. These things may be tangible, such as the human body or a machine. However, ideas can also be disassembled.

*Mechanism,* the third basic component of linear thinking, is the belief that cause and effect can be described by one relationship. If $x$ causes $y$, we may understand the mechanism of $y$ by manipulating $x$. For example, if sun exposure causes red skin, we can recreate the red skin by placing a person in the sunlight. The sunlight is the mechanism that causes sunburn. Investigators rarely accept explanations at this global level. Instead, they search for finer mechanisms that explain relationships at a more basic level. In contrast to this linear thinking, a recent and more popular trend is toward "systems" thinking.

Understanding complexity is a fundamental goal of science. During the 19th century, Descartes proposed reductionism as a remedy to being overwhelmed by information. According to Descartes, complicated phenomena could be understood by dividing them into their component parts. It was assumed that this division would not distort the phenomenon that was being studied. This approach has led to many productive sciences. It is also apparent, however, that there are dense interconnections among the component parts of most phenomena. Virtually all sciences have come to this same conclusion (Checkland, 1994).

In contrast to mechanistic understanding, systems thinking considers the whole rather than the individual parts. A *system* is defined as a whole that cannot be divided into independent parts. The functioning of each part cannot be understood independently of the functioning of other parts. The value of individual parts is lost when the whole is disassembled. For example, an automobile broken down into component parts cannot be used to transport people. A human eye cannot see if it is removed from the body, just as a steering wheel does not direct an automobile when it is removed from the machine (Gharajedaghi & Ackoff, 1984).

Traditional scientific analysis represents an attempt to understand organisms by taking them apart and examining each part separately. This can be useful in determining the structure but may not inform about function. The traditional "find it and fix it" medical model builds upon traditional linear thinking. If a prostate gland is too large, it must be surgically reduced, high blood pressure must be lowered, and hyperactive children must be made less active. Mechanistic thinking has certainly produced some sensational successes. Many patients benefit from hernia repairs, total joint replacement, and pharmaceutical control of blood pressure. However, finding and fixing one problem often creates a new one. Easy solutions, even those derived from understanding basic mechanisms of disease, might invite new problems.

Systems thinking has now found its way into virtually all sciences. It has had a profound effect in manufacturing industries and was used to create the astounding rebound in the Japanese economy following World War II. Systems analysts studied variation using formal statistical methods. Many of these ideas were influenced by Shewhart, a physicist and self-trained statistician who worked for the Western Electric Company. Shewhart realized that many resources were used to inspect products. During the 1920s, one in four employees in the Western Electric laboratories were inspectors. Identification of a faulty product might lead to a reprimand of the responsible employee. Shewhart recognized that, even under relatively primitive conditions of manufacturing, there was predictable variation in defects. The distribution of defects remained constant over time. Shewhart recognized that there are random sources of variation that cause some defects. Inspectors and managers were often reacting to random variation. The way to improve the product was to separate the sources of variation that were random from the sources that could be controlled. Inspection alone was not enough to improve the products.

One of the key components in Shewart's thinking was that quality was associated with reproducibility. Reproducibility meant reducing variation through the standardization of procedures. He emphasized that a certain amount of variability is expected and that managers or inspectors should understand random variation and not attend to variations within an expected range. Many of the problems, he argued, were caused by overattention to random variation. Shewhart was the intellectual father of many important leaders in the business and manufacturing communities. Most notably, Demming (1994) and Juran (1993) have promoted Shewhart's ideas and have had a profound effect on industries throughout the world. American companies, such as Xerox, Ford, Motorola, McDonnell Douglas, Hartford Insurance, and others, have implemented these ideas. Demming promoted the ideas in Japan, and many believe that the remarkable success of the Japanese economy has benefited from systems thinking.

What does this have to do with health care? Many doctors and patients are offended by the suggestion that concepts from manufacturing science could have anything to do with medical care. Doctors save lives, they do not manufacture bicycles. The difficulty is that many of the problems that characterize poor manufacturing also exist in medicine. For example, consumers want products on which they can depend. If you buy an automobile, you expect it to function for a certain period of time, and you assume it was manufactured under a clearly defined protocol. The manufacturers might be confident enough in their production process to offer a warranty guaranteeing that it will operate for a certain number of miles or a fixed duration of time. We expect that a certain model of automobile manufactured in different plants would have the same level of reliability.

In health care, we expect that a patient with a defined medical problem who appears in the offices of different doctors should get the same diagnosis and treatment. We also assume that the treatment is administered in a standardized way that leads to the best result. However, diagnoses differ among places, and there is high variability in the use of medical procedures and the way they are applied. Consumers cannot expect that the services they purchase will be delivered in a reliable way.

Consider clinical decision making and clinical variation in treatment for the same disease. Berwick (1991) offered the case of Brian, a 16-year-old patient suspected of suffering from osteomyelitis.[1] Although the clinical picture and a bone scan were consistent with the diagnosis, no organism could be recovered from Brian's bloodstream. Antibiotic therapy was started on an empirical basis, but Brian continued to spike fevers for a week. He was transferred for further evaluation. The clinical question of greatest importance was this: Did Brian really have osteomyelitis caused by an organism sensitive to the current antibiotic, or was another entity involved, such as osteomyelitis with a resistant organism or even a different disease, such as lymphoma? The diagnostic strategy included careful observation. Over the next 14 days, Brian was closely monitored, and his temperature was repeatedly measured. During this period, his antibiotic regimen was changed three times, he underwent numerous radiological examinations, and had a biopsy of both the bone and the bone marrow. During those 2 weeks,

---

[1]Osteomyelitis: inflammation of the bone marrow and the adjacent bone.

100 temperature measurements were recorded in Brian's chart on 22 pages of nursing notes (Berwick, 1991). On what evidence was Brian's treatment based?

While working at the Bell laboratories, Shewhart observed how machine operators overreacted to variations over which they had little control. When operating machines, different personnel reacted differently to changes on machine gauges. Furthermore, Shewhart noticed that the same technician would react differently to the same changes on a gauge when studied at different points in time. When they overreacted to changes in gauges, they often produced more variability by tampering with the system.

Berwick's patient may be similar. Six house officers and five consultants adjusted antibiotic doses based on a stream of 101 temperament measurements. Is this reminiscent of manufacturing technicians overreacting to changes on gauges? Medical management involves a stream of decisions about starting antibiotics, changing antibiotics, obtaining laboratory tests, repeating tests, and so on. How much of this effort is wasted because it responds to random variation? Berwick challenged his colleagues to think about some of the ramifications of their practice (Berwick, 1991, pp. 1219–1220).

What do clinicians measure and respond to clinically based on what measurements? The list is endless. Measure prothombin[2] and change anticoagulants. Measure oxygen tensions and change respirator settings. Measure fever and change antibiotics. Measure blood pressure and change antihypertensive agents. Measure leukocytes and change chemotherapies. Measure pain and change analgesia. Measure electrolytes and change intravenous fluids. Measure and change, measure and change.

The art of medicine requires each physician to use his or her intuition when ordering measurements and deciding on changes. As a result, different physicians might react to the same case in different ways. Furthermore, because some of the variation is random, the same patient might receive different treatments for the same condition on repeated visits to the same doctor. Physicians are overwhelmed with data and are required to take decisive action, even when they are uncertain about the exact nature of the problem. Random variation may lead to decisions that, in turn, produce more variation. In some cases, this places patients at risk.

## Conclusions

This chapter introduces systems thinking. These ideas are clearly not new in health care and, in fact, are now common in discussions of quality improvement and health care reform. However, it may be valuable to reframe some of the discussion in the "CLINECS" terminology. Much of clinical medicine still uses linear thinking and considers simple inputs and outputs. We manipulate single variables (inputs) and look for responses on output variables. However, some of the

---

[2]Prothrombin (factor II) is produced in the liver and is part of the process resulting in blood coagulation.

responses or outputs may not clearly be related to patient outcomes. Inputs may be related to outputs. In the example of Berwick's patient, more tests were related to changes in treatment regimens. Yet, variations in inputs may not lead to better patient outcomes. In the following chapters these issues are explored in greater detail.

## *References*

Ackoff, R.L. (1994). *The democratic corporation*. New York: Oxford University Press.

Berwick, D.M. (1991). Controlling variation in health care: a consultation from Walter Shewhart. *Medical Care, 29*, 1212–1225.

Checkland, P. (1994). Systems theory and management thinking. *American Behavioral Scientist*, 38(1), 75–91.

Deming, W.E. (1994). *The new economics* (2nd ed.). Cambridge: Massachusetts Institute of Technology.

Gharajedaghi, J., Ackoff, R.L. (1984). Mechanisms, organisms, and social systems. *Strategic Management Journal*, 5, 289–300.

Juran, J.M. (1993). *A tale of the 20th century: the quality scrapbook*. New York: Jurand Institute.

# 3
# Seeking Justice in Health Care

LAWRENCE J. SCHNEIDERMAN

The simplest definition of justice is the fair distribution of burdens and benefits. A just society seeks to implement this principle for all its citizens. Within *spheres* of justice is an array of *resources*, such as money, honors, food, shelter, health care, welfare, and education, that a just society attempts to distribute justly (Walzer, 1983). Within *fields* of justice is an array of *criteria*, such as urgency of need, capacity to benefit, value to society, future potential, and past services rendered, that a just society would consider when distributing a scarce resource (Schneiderman & Jecker, 1996). How can we proceed from these generalities to the specifics of health care justice?

In his book *A Theory of Justice*, the philosopher John Rawls (1998) proposed a thought experiment that provides a good place to start. He asks us to imagine behind a "veil of ignorance" (that is, before we are born) the kind of society we would want to enter. We would not know anything about the strengths and weaknesses we would bring into the world. We would not know, for example, whether we would be rich or poor, highly intelligent and strong, endowed with a sturdy constitution or predisposed to life-long illness, or severely disabled, mentally or physically.

What kind of society would we want to enter? Would we not want a society that enabled us to live as best as reasonably possible no matter what our capacities or limitations? If we were lucky enough to be healthy and strong and gifted physically or mentally, we would want to have the opportunity to exercise these capacities and prosper and be successful. If we were not so lucky and were dependent on others to make use of our limited capacities, we would want those who were more fortunate to help us.

Thus, we would want society to distinguish between what is *unfortunate* and what is *unfair* (Englehart, 1996). When illness strikes, it is *unfortunate*. (Just look around; despite our worthy efforts to make people feel responsible for their own states of health, cancer and drunken drivers strike the slim and fit, as well as the overweight and slothful.) We would regard a society that fails to take responsibility for assisting a citizen in recovering from this misfortune as *unfair*. In other words, we would consider health care an obligation of a just society—a fundamental matter of fairness. As Daniels stated, "[h]ealth care is of special moral importance because it helps to preserve our status as fully functioning citizens" (Daniels, 2002). Or, as noted by Zollner (2002), "Equity should be everybody's concern, because inequities in health are everybody's loss. They harm many people, operate on a socioeconomic gradient, and put a strain on economic development and social cohesion."

Unlike most European countries, the United States does not seem to recognize health care as a matter of both ethics and economics. How does one account for this difference? Despite contrasts drawn by social critics who emphasize elements of North American capitalism versus European socialism, there is, in fact, great similarity in the values shared by all liberal democracies: politically— respect for individual rights and the rule of law; economically—belief in a free market and free enterprise to maximize society's material benefits. At the same time, all these societies, including the United States, recognize that restraints must be imposed on economic freedom to "eliminate or compensate for natural variations or for the contingencies of social life" (Rhodes, 2005). At the present time, no European country attempts to support its citizens with a totally regulated, centralized economy; nor has the United States ever had a totally unregulated, free market economy. All these countries recognize that to safeguard a liberal democracy, to maintain what in Europe is called "solidarity," it is necessary to redistribute material goods actively from the more fortunate to the less fortunate.

Why has the United States failed to apply this notion to universal health care? Exploring this question and examining the problems encountered by the United States in addressing what most European nations consider an essential obligation of a just society gives us an opportunity to examine the notion of justice itself.

We have to look to history and culture, as well as the economic and political systems, for answers. Quite obviously, the North American and European continents have had vastly different historical experiences. Among the features that characterize North American culture and history is a self-image of rugged individualism best symbolized by a solitary, heroic figure who in reality rode the plains only briefly, yet has continued to ride the plains for over a century in mythology—the American cowboy. Along with this self-image is the distrust of a centralized bureaucracy (especially because it usually demands the cowboy's tax support), a preference for private enterprise as opposed to government entitlements, even to the point of believing in the free market approach to addressing all sorts of social needs, including health care. Thus, many Americans have come to conceive of justice in a way that is peculiarly American. To them, justice exists in the lavish, widespread wealth and high standard of living that have been achieved by calling forth each person's best efforts and allowing the benefits of these efforts to be distributed in an unfettered way. The material successes of capitalism have confirmed the beliefs of the true believers. Small wonder that these true believers—and there are many—view with suspicion if not alarm any hand other than the "unseen hand" that "unjustly" tries to alter this state of affairs.

The American economist Henry Aaron dourly summarized the above perspective (Aaron, 2003).

The U.S. health care administration, weird though it may be, exists for fundamental reasons, including a pervasive popular distrust of centralized authority, a federalist governmental structure, insistence on individual choice (even when, as it appears to me, choice sometimes yields no demonstrable benefit), the continuing and unabated power of large economic interest, and the virtual impossibility (during normal times in a democracy whose Constitution potentiates the power of dissenting minorities) of radically restructuring the nation's largest industry—an industry as big as the entire economy of France.

Two other features of the U.S. society have interfered with achieving universal health care. Far more than European countries, the United States is inhabited by people who have emigrated from many parts of the world. They constitute many religions, ethnic groups, and races. Unlike the more homogeneous societies of Europe, such as Scandinavian countries, whose citizens tend to share similar physical and cultural traits, they could almost be (and, more than Americans, are) blood relatives, many Americans have difficulty seeing (and having empathy for) other, very different Americans, as members of the same family. They do not easily embrace what is a standard concept in Europe, "solidarity." Although this indifference is distressing, it may prove not to be a failing unique to the United States. The European concept of solidarity is being severely tested as more and more countries experience their own waves of immigrants and rising health care costs. In fact, it will be interesting to see which comes first: achievement of an all-inclusive universal health care by the United States or abandonment of the principle of all-inclusive solidarity in Europe.

Another feature of U.S. society that has interfered with achieving universal health care is a toxic side-effect of the belief in the superiority of the free market as a solution for social problems—powerful, self-interested, profit-oriented health care institutions. This is a risk for European countries that are beginning to look at this approach as a way to deal with their own mounting health care costs. How effective is the market- and profit-oriented approach to providing a just health care system? In the United States, this idea was given its most expansive test during the 1970s and 1980s under the rubric "managed competition." The idea was to encourage large health care institutions to compete with each other for the health care dollar of consumers under limited guidelines intended only to keep the process on track. Consumers (or their representatives) were expected to choose what they considered the best health care plans based on quality and price. Competition was expected to favor the most desirable health care plans and weed out the less desirable ones and, most importantly, reduce health care costs. The underlying premise was that choosing a health care plan was no different than choosing a car. Products of varying value and price would be presented to the informed consumer, who would choose at a preferred intersection of these two variables—just like choosing between a Volkswagen and a Porsche.

Many problems soon became apparent, some of which were readily predictable. Patients rarely are as capable of making informed choices about their future health care needs as they are about a car. This is so whether they are healthy and unable to imagine what they will require when they become sick or if they are forced to choose under the stress of an active illness. Many patients discovered too late that the cheap health care plan they had chosen did not cover treatments they later needed.

- In some instances, patients, unwilling to accept any cost tradeoff, sued to receive the more expensive treatments, and the courts agreed, thus undermining an important element of cost control. For example, patients went to court to obtain costly bone marrow transplantation for metastatic breast cancer, whose value had not been established and, in fact, was later disproved. The courts, moved more by the pleas of desperately ill patients than by the cold calculations of medical evidence, forced health care plans to ignore contract limitations and cover the costs.
- Health care did not fit into the standard notion of production and consumption. In the usual business transaction, the producer offers and the consumer chooses. In medicine, however, the physician makes the diagnosis and determines the treatment—hence in every important respect controlling both production and consumption.
- As health care plans struggled to control costs, they engaged in various strategies of risk selection ("cherry picking"), seeking the healthy and avoiding the sick, especially the really sick.
- For-profit health care plans had a conflict of fiduciary obligation, often focusing on raising the value of their stock to please their shareholders at the expense of serving their patients.
- A paradox emerged that distinguishes health care from the usual market model. Whereas a successful business increases productivity and efficiency as it gathers more experience over time, in medicine it is just the opposite. As medicine improves, it produces more survivors of once-fatal illnesses, thereby creating a negative feedback by "plugging the system" with more elderly, disabled, and chronically ill persons.

As can be seen from the above, the struggle over health care in the United States has led to experiences that may soon plague countries that already have universal health care, but are undergoing similar strains on the system owing to social, technological, and economic changes. From these experiences arise certain inescapable questions.

- Can policy makers reconcile the obligations of society to all its citizens (universality) by allowing freedom of choice (individualism)?
- Can policy makers reconcile the inevitable necessity of health care rationing with the rising expectations of citizens in a liberal democracy?

An experiment in the state of Oregon attempted to do what no country has done: It openly sought citizen input for determining health care treatment priorities. The experiment was directed at improving the range of options for patients who were dependent on state-funded welfare and had the most difficulty affording health care. Through a series of community meetings, an "Oregon Health Plan" was devised that aggregated individual preferences and placed conditions and treatments in a hierarchy, depending on the expressed preferences of those who took (and had) the time to participate in these community meetings. It was agreed that all treatments above a certain level of the state's budgetary limit would be insured, and all those below it would not. Although the process met with considerable criticism and controversy (including its limitation to poor patients on welfare), one certain benefit was that, by granting priority to the most cost beneficial treatments and eliminating marginally or rarely beneficial treatments that were very expensive, the roster of qualified patients could be enlarged and the range of useful treatments expanded. One conceptual flaw, however, was that the cost-benefit analyses were aimed only at the cost to society and the benefit to the individual. Benefit to society was not considered. As a result, one important consideration was neglected: the interdependence between the individual and society. Justice, you recall, is the fair distribution of *both* benefits and burdens. In this case, the fact that individualism cannot survive without the support of the community was overlooked—an unfortunate characterization of many American choices and perhaps of future European choices.

One of the most serious problems in the pursuit of a just health care system is that politicians and policy makers in all countries tend to be preoccupied with how to *pay* for health care—for example, how much should remain a public obligation and how much should be privatized, how much should be guaranteed by the state, and how much should be an individual's responsibility. Little to no thought is given to *what* should be paid for—as though health care is a commodity that needs no examination with regard to what health outcomes should be achieved.

In the end, all societies have to acknowledge that the soaring costs of health care are inevitable. Better health will always be an infinite demand, becoming more and more pronounced as more and more treatments for ailments and conditions once accepted as normal are deemed to be serious—albeit curable—*medical* problems. As the social critic Ivan Illich (1976) predicted, people who are preoccupied with the ordinary fatigues, aches, and pains of living rarely want to acknowledge that they are unhappy with their jobs or their relationships or that they are despondent because they are trapped in stressful, unfulfilling life pursuits or experiencing existential despair. Rather, they want to hear that they are physically ill, for which medicine must assume responsibility. "Diagnosed ill-health," says Illich, "is infinitely preferable to any other form of negative label or to no label at all." It relieves people of social and political responsibilities and enables them to cash in on their insurance policies.

What, then, is the ethical solution that could provide for individual desires, as well as societal responsibilities? First, we must accept that everyone is *not* entitled to everything. Everyone *is* entitled to a so-called fair opportunity, namely a decent minimum level of health care. What is a decent minimum? In my opinion, it is a level of health care that enables a person to acquire an education, hold a job, and raise a family. Alternatively, if the person, because of ill health, is unable to meet these goals, the goal is to attain a reasonable level of function within the person's limits, as well as a reasonable level of comfort, whether it be from pain or other forms of suffering.

This ensures that society's needs for productive citizenry are recognized. How about the individual's freedom of choice? Would there be different levels of health care if we allow this? Yes. Is this not unethical? In my view, no—for the simple reason that if all citizens have at least sufficient health care, that is, a decent minimum that enables them to participate in society, inequalities can be ethically justified for those who wish to obtain more expensive and elaborate health care on their own because their privilege does not deny others their rights.

## References

Aaron, H. (2003). The costs of health care administration in the United States and Canada: questionable answers to a questionable question. *New England Journal of Medicine,* 349, 801–803.

Daniels N. (2002). Justice, health, and health care. In: R. Rhodes, M.P. Battin, A. Silvers (Eds.), *Medicine and social justice: essays on the distribution of health care*. New York: Oxford University Press. p. 8.

Englehart, H.T. (1996). *The foundations of bioethics*. New York: Oxford University Press.

Illich, I. (1976). *Medical nemesis: the expropriation of health*. New York: Pantheon Books.

Rawls, J. (1998). *A theory of justice*. Cambridge, MA: Belknap Press of Harvard University Press.

Rhodes, R. (2005). Justice in medicine and public health. *Cambridge Quarterly of Healthcare Ethics*, 14, 13–26.

Schneiderman, L.J., Jecker, N.S. (1996). Should a criminal receive a heart transplant? Medical justice versus societal justice. *Theoretical Medicine*, 17, 33–44.

Walzer, M. (1983). *Spheres of justice: a defense of pluralism and equality*. New York: Basic Books.

Zollner, H. (2002). National policies for reducing social inequalities in health in Europe. *Scandinavian Journal of Public Health*, 59 (Suppl), 6–11.

# 4
# Evidence-Based Medicine and Ethics: Desired and Undesired Effects of Screening

Franz Porzsolt and Heike Leonhardt-Huober

## Ethical Dilemma

When 1000 women undergo mammography, breast cancer is diagnosed in 33 of them. Without mammography, breast cancer would be found in only 20 women. With mammography 4 of 1000 women die of breast cancer; without mammography 5 of 1000 women die of breast cancer. These facts present the difficult question of whether is it justified to save the life of 1 woman and burden 13 with the diagnosis of breast cancer and the consequent therapy and follow-up. We scientists have the duty to present facts lucidly. The interpretation of these facts and the conclusions drawn from them are not the task of science but of the society concerned.

## Mammography Saves Lives

Nyström and colleagues (2002) demonstrated that mammographic screening can reduce the risk of dying of breast cancer by 21%; that is, every fifth woman could be saved by screening. In a Cochrane review, Olsen and Gotzsche (2001) found the data insufficiently convincing to support a general recommendation for mammographic screening. Nevertheless, it is now available throughout Germany beginning in 2006. The biologic advantages seem to have convinced other experts (http://www.krebsgesellschaft.de/re_mammographie 2005). If one in five women can be saved, it is indeed an impressive number that coincides with the expectations of an effective measure, as shown in Figure 4.1.

From this point of view, one must assume that all women die of breast cancer, and of course this is not true. General mortality statistics show that about 4% of all women die of breast cancer. In Germany this adds up to about 18,000 women annually and about 40,000 in the United States (Todesursachenstatistik, 2004 and American Cancer Society, 2004). This means that about every 20th woman dies of breast cancer. Because mammographic screening does not protect women from dying of a heart attack or a severe infection, it cannot save one of five women; at most, it saves one of five of every 20th women because only every 20th woman

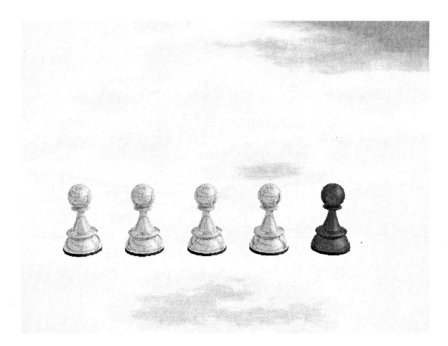

FIGURE 4.1. Mammography screening reduces the risk of dying of breast cancer by 21%. Does this mean that every fifth woman is saved or only every fifth woman at risk—or that every fifth woman without mammography would die of breast cancer? It is not easy to interpret epidemiologic statements without exact data.

dies of breast cancer. Actually, 1 of 100 women can be saved from dying of breast cancer by mammography, as shown in Figure 4.2.

To better understand this mathematical example, remember that mammographic screening is not only performed on diseased women but on all women in a certain age group. If we wish to assess the efficiency of mammography, its success must be measured on all women who are examined. We are not talking about making special measures available to a certain population or withholding them. The question is the efficiency of mammography. Because we offer far more services in the health care system than we can pay for, we have no other choice but to evaluate the various public services, compare them, and then choose those that provide the best relation between effort and outcome for the patients.

It is obvious that not all women profit from mammography—only those with breast cancer and, among them, only every fifth woman. If these two limitations are added up, 1 of 100 women profit from mammographic screening for breast cancer.

The risk of dying of breast cancer in the study by Nyström et al. (2002) was only 0.5%, not 4% to 5%, as stated in the general mortality statistics on which we based our initial assumption. Now we see that not every 20th woman risks getting breast cancer, only every 200th.

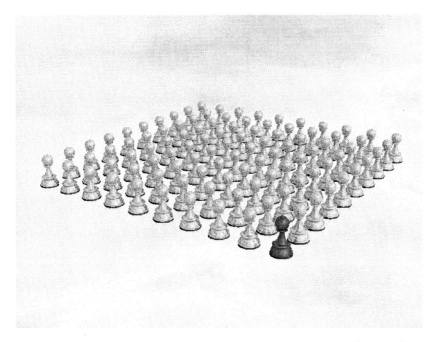

FIGURE 4.2. If all women who took part in a screening program were included in the calculation, only 1 of 100 women could be saved.

We wonder how this considerable difference arose. All persons die have the cause of death recorded in mortality statistics. The average age of women when they die is 80 years. In the study by Nyström et al. (2002), however, only women between the ages of 50 and 69 were screened, which is a considerably younger population. Breast cancer is more common in older women than in younger ones. This explains the discrepancy in the prevalence.

If only every 200th woman risks dying of breast cancer and every fifth of these can be saved, only 1 per 1000 women can be saved, as demonstrated in Figure 4.3. Further variables, such as whether mammography is performed annually or every 2 years and which subgroups are included, are not considered in this discussion of the general problem.

Nyström et al. (2002) reported a relative risk reduction of 21%, which is impressive; but because he used the relative, not the absolute, risk reduction, the prevalence must be taken into consideration. Nyström et al. (2002) also followed this rule. Without considering the prevalence, the absolute risk reduction was 0.1%, or a reduction in mortality from 0.5% to 0.4%. When applied to individuals, this means that 1 of 1000 women profit from breast screening.

The calculation of relative risk often leads to overestimation of the effects. Gerd Gigerenzer (2002) impressively described this problem in numerous statements and books with concrete examples (Gigerenzer et al., 1989, 1999). Of course, only a portion of the involved individuals are affected, and importance is

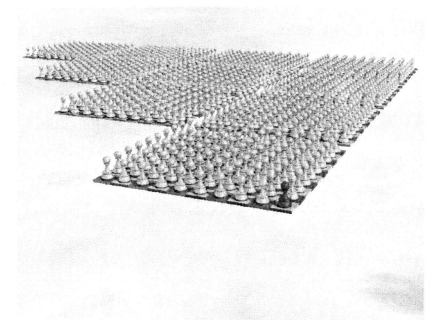

FIGURE 4.3. If, in addition, the risk in every age group for which data exist is considered, only 1 of 1000 women can be saved.

placed on demonstrating medical progress. If 1 of 1000 women has a survival advantage through mammographic screening, 999 women undergo mammography to no advantage or even with disadvantages.

## Disadvantages

Even if the benefit of a medical measure is minimal, considering the individual concerned one could say that every, even small, success must be supported. What about side effects? A fundamental principle in medicine is *nihil nocere*, or "do no harm." Every medical intervention has undesired effects, which can be severe and affect many patients. Mammography is no exception.

One undesired effect is frequent misdiagnosis. After mammography, 242 of 1000 women screened are initially suspected of having breast cancer. In most of these 242 "patients" this is a false-positive result, which is indisputably upsetting, even if the initial diagnosis is often corrected by a second opinion. During a careful evaluation one must consider that 999 women undergo mammography to no advantage, and 242 of these suffer considerable anxiety for a short time (Barratt et al., 2005). We have only touched on a technical problem that should soon be solvable. Nonetheless, only 64 of these 242 women with suspected breast cancer have biopsies. In such cases, biopsy is the correct measure to clarify the situation.

Many women experience suspicion of having breast cancer. Other women who really do have breast cancer, however, are missed by the procedure. The breast cancers of 10 of the 1000 women who undergo mammography is not discovered. Most of these 10 women discover their breast cancer themselves by self-examination during the screening intervals. Mammography does not benefit these 10 women at all.

Table 4.1 shows only the successful diagnoses in women who have undergone mammography. Of the 33 breast cancers in this group, only 23 were discovered by mammography; 10 additional breast cancers were discovered during the screening interval. Anxiety due to false-positive diagnoses was temporarily suffered by 219 women.

Calculation of the likelihood radio (LR) for the diagnosis of breast cancer by mammography from Table 4.1 results in a positive LR(+) of 10 [LR+ = (23:10) ÷ (219:967) = 10] and a negative LR(−) of 0.4 [LR− = (10:33) ÷ (748:967)]. A positive LR of 10 means the chance of diagnosing breast cancer by mammography in a patient with breast cancer is 10 times greater than the chance of diagnosing breast cancer by mammography in a healthy woman. A negative LR of 0.40 means the chance of missing a breast cancer during mammography in a woman with breast cancer is 0.40 times greater than the chance of not diagnosing a breast cancer in mammography in a healthy woman.

A positive or negative LR expresses the gain in information if the test result is positive. The closer the LR is to 1, the less information is gained from the test. A positive test result (for example, to prove the existence of a disease) is valuable if the LR of this test exceeds 3.0 and is extremely valuable if the LR exceeds 10.0. During mammography screening we can calculate a LR of 10, which means that the procedure is valuable from a statistical point of view. Analogously, a negative test result to exclude the existence of a disease is valuable if the LR of this test is below 0.3 and is extremely valuable if the LR is below 0.1. The negative LR of mammography screening is 0.4, which means that an unsuspicious finding does not exclude breast cancer with sufficient certainty.

Table 4.1 does not show that there are 33 diagnosed breast cancers in the group with mammography and 20 cases diagnosed in the group without mammography. These numbers describe the successes of the diagnostic procedure. If therapeutic

TABLE 4.1. Results for 1000 women who underwent screening mammography.

| Condition | Breast cancer discovered | Breast cancer not discovered | Total |
|---|---|---|---|
| Breast cancer discovered by mammography | 23 | 219 | 242 |
| Breast cancer not discovered by mammography | 10 | 748 | 758 |
| Total | 33 | 967 | 1000 |

successes are considered, which are also not shown in Table 4.1, one finds that death resulting from breast cancer in the mammography group could be prevented in 4 of 1000 women and in 5 of 1000 women without mammography if all women at risk of death from breast cancer could be saved.

## Ethical Problem

The unnecessary biopsies and the false-negative results are recognized problems that, however, can be reduced with increasing experience, better techniques, and general medical progress. The ethical dilemma, then, arises because more women are stigmatized as having breast cancer "diagnosed" by mammography screening than can be saved through the consequences of this stigma.

Expressed in numbers, this means that among 1000 women who undergo mammography 33 breast cancers are discovered, whereas only 20 are discovered without mammography. If one considers this diagnostic success, the difference adds up to 13 women. However, if treatment success is considered, the difference is only 1 of 1000 women because four of the women diagnosed by mammography die of breast cancer. Without mammography five of the affected women die of their breast cancer. The ethical dilemma is usually not perceived because diagnostic successes are discussed separately from therapeutic successes. The consequences resulting from the difference between diagnostic and therapeutic success receive too little attention. If our assumption that there are just as many breast cancers in the groups with and without mammography is correct, we must conclude from the data that without mammography not every breast cancer is discovered and not every undiscovered breast cancer causes death.

If breast cancer is confirmed by mammography, these women receive treatment and lead the rest of their lives as diseased, even if they would never have been aware of their cancer without the mammography. Every overdiagnosis is, unfortunately, accompanied by overtreatment. Zahl et al. (2004) have shown that the rate of overdiagnosis is about 50% in Sweden and Norway. These women are treated only because they have breast cancer. They are treated according to the same principles as are applied to every other women with breast cancer: operation, radiotherapy, and hormone or chemotherapy. These women in the overdiagnosed group would never have been disadvantaged by their cancer if it had not been discovered.

In all medical fields we have to live with the problem that it is almost impossible to predict with certainty whether an individual patient will profit from a certain treatment. We can, however, quote the probability of successful treatment in many diseases. When screening, an additional problem is that a biologically irrelevant disease (pseudodisease) is often discovered (see Chapters 11 and 23). When breast cancer is diagnosed, 12 of 1000 women become cancer patients through mammography but without gaining any recognizable advantage from the diagnosis or the subsequent therapy. In 1 of 1000 women, the diagnosis and following therapy prevent death as a result of breast cancer.

The ethical problem that must be accepted in this case—to save one life with many cases of overdiagnosis—cannot be solved scientifically. The decision must be made by those involved. Physicians and scientists can and must provide information and give advice to the best of their knowledge. The involved population cannot, however, answer the question alone whether the diagnostic measure and therapy is to be paid for through public funding or privately. Because the question must be answered by the general public, it becomes obvious that these decisions can be reached only with great care, circumspection, and self-critical reflection.

## Prostate Cancer

A similar situation exists with prostate cancer, the only difference being that up to now there are fewer data available. About 11,000 men die of prostate cancer every year in Germany (Todesursachenstatistik, 2004) and approximately 30,000 in the United States (American Cancer Society, 2004). The average age at diagnosis is 71 years, and 80% of these men survive 5 years after diagnosis; the general life expectancy for men is 75.59 years at birth in Germany (Lebenserwartung, 2004). This indicates that most men with prostate cancer survive just as long as those without it.

Screening with prostate-specific antigen (PSA) has been generally available for the past decade and a half. The recommended screening age is 50 to 69 years. Compared with breast cancer studies, there are relatively few studies on prostate cancer. In a study involving 10,000 men, Hugosson et al. (2004) demonstrated that 640 of these men in the screened group were found to have prostate cancer. In the unscreened group, only 224 cases of prostate cancer were discovered. Nevertheless, in the two groups only 227 and 224 men, respectively, received treatment for their prostate cancer. The diagnosis had no therapeutic consequence. However, more men were caused anxiety in the screened group than in the unscreened group.

Coldman et al. (2003) showed that the number of men with prostate cancer has doubled in some regions in Canada during the previous 15 years. The survival times in men with prostate cancer discovered through PSA screening have generally increased. However, in regions in which more prostate cancers have been discovered through more intensive PSA screening, survival gains are slightly shorter than in regions in which less intensive screening is carried out. This result also indicates that, as with breast cancer, many of these patients do not die of prostate cancer.

If screening does not provide survival benefits, it remains for us to examine if there are improvements in quality of life. According to Penson et al. (2005), aggressive operative therapy of prostate cancer leads to urinary incontinence in 10% to 14% of the men and to impotence in 72% to 78%.

## Possible Consequences

The consequences that can be deduced for the solution of this ethical problem affect various stakeholders in the health care system. It could be deduced that the pool of reliable data must be greatly increased. This can be achieved by more public funding of health care services that offer not only health benefits but data on the effectiveness of these health services. This demand is less a cost-cutting measure than an obligatory caution. Because the additional work must be taken into consideration, costs would initially rise. In the midterm, data would become available that enable decisions to be reached that presently cannot be made owing to a lack of appropriate information.

Improved data provide better information to involved patients, decision makers, and service providers. Improved data also enable us to identify the subgroups among involved patients who would profit from medical progress. As an important side effect we increase the chance of being able to continue financing the health care system with appropriate financial means.

## Summary

The value of screening procedures has hitherto been measured by their effectiveness. The sensitivity and specificity of the measure are evaluated. False-positive and false-negative results are regularly included in the discussion. Further potential disadvantages of screening are direct injuries caused by the investigation (such as radiation exposure during radiographic examinations or possible injuries during endoscopy or biopsy). These are included in the considerations.

Improvements in our diagnostic technologies should also remind us that diseases are discovered and treated that, even without diagnosis and treatment, would influence neither the patient's survival nor his or her quality of life, even if only positive cases were correctly identified and the examinations could be carried out without risk.

Current data on the examples of breast and prostate cancer show that these considerations are not only theoretically correct but also have practical consequences. The aim of this chapter was to collect the figures necessary to reflect reality. This analysis has nothing to do with discrediting or praising an established screening method. It is simply the task of science to produce transparency. Interpretations of the findings and the conclusions drawn from them exceed scientific competence. These decisions must be reached by the general public.

## References

American Cancer Society (2004). *Cancer facts and figures*. Washington, DC: American Cancer Society (http://www.cancer.org/docroot/PRO/content/PRO_1_1_Cancer_Statistics_2004_presentation.asp).

Barratt, A., Howard, K., Irwing, L., Alkeld, G., Houssami, N. (2005). Model of outcomes of screening mammography: information to support informed choices. *British Medical Journal*, 330, 936.

Coldman, A.J., Phillips, N., Pickles, T.A. (2003). Trends in prostate cancer incidence and mortality: an analysis of mortality change by screening intensity. *Canadian Medical Association Journal*, 168 (1), 31–35.

Gigerenzer, G. (2002). *Calculated risks: how to know when numbers deceive you.* New York: Simon & Schuster.

Gigerenzer, G., Swijtink, Z., Porter, T., Daston, L.J., Beatty, J., Krueger, L. (1989). *The empire of chance: how probability changed science and everyday life.* Cambridge, UK: Cambridge University Press.

Gigerenzer, G., Todd, P.M., ABC Group (1999). *Simple heuristics that make us smart.* New York: Oxford University Press.

Hugosson, J., Aus, G., Lilja, H., Lodding, P., Pihl, C.G. (2004). Results of a randomized, population-based study of biennial screening using serum prostate-specific antigen measurement to detect prostate carcinoma. *Cancer,* 100(7), 1397–1405.

http://www.krebsgesellschaft.de/re_mammographie Deutsche Krebsgesellschaft e.V., Steinlestr. 6, 60596 Frankfurt am Main: Qualität muss durch Krebsregister gesichert werden. Mammographie: Aufnahme in Früherkennungsprogramm gefordert by Prof. Dr. Rolf Kreienberg, Pastpräsident der Deutschen Krebsgesellschaft, aktualisiert 16.2.2005

Lebenserwartung und Sterblichkeit, Stand 9.11.2004 (http://rki.de). Berlin: Robert Koch Institute.

Nystrom, L., Andersson, I., Bjurstam, N., Frisell, J., Nordenskjold, B., Rutqvist, L.E. (2002). Long-term effects of mammography screening: updated overview of the Swedish randomised trials. *Lancet,* 359, 909–919.

Olsen, O., Gotzsche, P.C. (2001). *Screening for breast cancer with mammography.* The Cochrane Library. The Cochrane Database of Systematic Reviews 2005, Issue 4. New York: Wiley.

Penson, D.F., McLerran, D., Feng, Z., Li, L., Albertsen, P.C., Gilliland, F.D., Hamilton, A, et al. (2005). 5-Year urinary and sexual outcomes after radical prostatectomy: results from the prostate cancer outcomes study. *Journal of Urology,* 173(5), 1701–1705.

Todesursachenstatistik [Statistics on causes of deathProzentualer Anteil der Krebsformen in Deutschland [percentage of different forms of cancer in Germany] *(http://www.rki.de).* Acquired November 30, 2004. Berlin: Robert Koch Institute.

Zahl, P.H., Strand, B.H., Maehlen, J. (2004). Incidence of breast cancer in Norway and Sweden during introduction of nationwide screening: prospective cohort study. *British Medical Journal,* 328, 921–924.

# 5
# Paradoxes of Medical Progress: Abandoned Patients, Physicians, and Nurses

PETER STRASSER

Johann Nepomuk Nestroy, Austrian author and actor (1801–1862), said of progress that it appears to be much greater that it really is. This is not only because no one wants to contradict the promise that the term itself implies— advancing toward improvement. Above all, it concerns the fact that every advance of a certain dimension is accompanied by undesired collateral results, which in extreme cases can invalidate the benefit of the progress.

In relation to medical progress, which cannot be denied, I am going to discuss a series of typical collateral results that certainly must be viewed as undesired. I conceive the dynamics of progress/collateral results as a kind of practical paradox. If you increase the progress, you also increase the undesired collateral results. Four such paradoxes are discussed in relation to medical "progress": (1) the person as a virtual patient; (2) the disappearance of the "good" doctor; (3) the apparently autonomous patient; and (4) the overburdening of the "good helper."

## The Person as a Virtual Patient

*The more medicine is available, the more people feel sick or threatened by disease.* This is not only because humans are constantly becoming older on average. Even if you ignore the illnesses and misery of the aged, the paradox "more medicine, more disease" remains. The reasons are manifold.

- Improved diagnostic methods and lowering the thresholds for initiating treatment cause an increasing number of persons at increasingly younger ages to join the company of those who already consider themselves patients, so-called future patients. This is especially true in societies such as ours, which widely promote, offer, and expand examinations for screening and disease prevention.
- Increasing health consciousness in all segments of society has resulted in a large portion of leisure activities being devoted to disease prevention, whether one eats healthy food, avoids legal drugs, or practices sports to increase fitness or compensate for deficits. Although essential illnesses do exist, regardless of

what one thinks or how one talks about them, there are also many marginal, intermediate, and preliminary areas that can be semantically manipulated. We live in a culture in which entire industries profit from people who define themselves not as healthy but as not yet sick and, accordingly, learn to lead their entire healthy lives as disease-prevention existences. This is the origin of the virtual patient, who lives to avoid becoming ill.

- In addition, with the increase in treatment possibilities in modern medicine the probability also increases of embarking on a "treatment career" according to the motto, "Something can always be done." The term treatment career means that one learns to feel like a sick person in the long term even when an illness has already been overcome. An individual lives not as someone who is healthy again but as a formerly ill person, in the shadow of a temporary disease remission, so to speak.
- Risk research increases the number of disease-causing situations. On the patient side, on which we all virtually stand, the feeling intensifies of living in a situation that could cause disease until something that would conventionally be enjoyed even seems suspicious (for example, one must consult a nutrition advisor before enjoying food). The fact that the French drink more red wine than other Europeans is no longer considered part of a specific French hedonistic culture but as a national health factor—people who drink red wine live longer.
- Owing to the diverse offers for psychotherapy, ever more normal human conflicts are considered abnormal, whether they concern child-raising problems, marital conflicts, sex, or fear of dying. There are now quasi-medical professionals for all these problems.

In general, we can say that the well-being of the virtual patients always remains equivocal, as exemplified by the popularity of continually new healthy types of sports, diets, spiritual activities, and so on. The mood of the consumers generally worsens with the constant fear of not having done enough to stay healthy and, if one reaches old age, to have to live the life of a useless, permanently multimorbid individual.

## Disappearance of the Good Doctor

*The more importance attributed to ethics in medicine, the less place there is for the traditional role of the "good doctor." The Good Doctor* is the title of a book by Klaus Dörner (2001), the long-term superintendent of the Psychiatric Clinic in Gütersloh, Germany, who demands that more attention be paid to physicians' virtues instead of abstract ethical principles. The good doctor is defined as one who approaches his or her patients with good will, which exceeds the purely professional physician's role of practicing the art of medicine. The "family physician" is the role model for a good doctor and is often mentioned. This physician reacts in the broadest sense of the term as a family member and not as a handworker who enters the home to repair a technical defect.

- Medical progress brings with it a series of changes in the doctor–patient relationship, whereby the transformation of many previously trusting relationships into those of a contractual nature, involving the eventuality of law suits, is decisive. The more thoroughly and detailed these treatment contracts legalize the relation between doctor and patient, the more difficult it becomes for the physician to behave holistically toward the patient, that is, according to the traditional model. This model is continually being fobbed off onto the lower levels of hospital hierarchy, especially the nursing staff.
- When relationships are legalized, good will, which is characteristic of the good doctor, becomes increasingly rare. Good will, or benevolence, becomes an abstract ethical and legal norm. Moreover, good will is imitated in service industry slogans to guarantee patient satisfaction. Accordingly, the duty of the hospital is to be like a hotel in that physicians (but especially other health professionals) react in a customer-oriented, friendly manner. This excludes a holistic relationship similar to that in a restaurant, where the staff learns to give the customer the feeling of being at the center of gastronomic good will but without inner conviction.
- In an advertisement in Austrian Television, the actor Tobias Moretti could be seen sitting on a bench on the lawn in front of an inn. He asked the audience "Do you know what the best inns in the world are?" After taking a sip of red wine, he answered, "Hospices." This example shows how the lack of a good doctor and the repression of death are connected in our society. A good doctor is necessary for a good death and, for many, a priest or pastor as well. If these companions are lacking in hospital rooms, the fantasy of the living demands something be made of death that resembles spending a pleasant summer afternoon on a sunny bench. It is unnecessary to mention that Moretti's view has nothing in common with the reality of the multitude of elderly who live in increasing misery until they finally die owing to the demographic change in our society.
- These developments also explain the boom in medical ethics, which has hardly anything to do with the actual results of ethics in medicine. Whereas power lies in the technical apparatus, the dexterity of the physicians, and the economic resources, ethicists and ethics commissions are required to compensate for the increasing lack of good doctors and their intrinsic authority with the authority of ethical principles. Moreover, technical advances and the legalization of the doctor–patient relationship leads to a multitude of morally sensitive questions that have hitherto not arisen. (An extreme example is the "wrongful-life" trials, in which individuals with severe handicaps go to court to sue doctors for not having diagnosed their handicaps before birth and aborted them but allowed them to be born and burdened with life. Lawyers still have enough common sense to agree unanimously that no one has the right not to be born.)
- The crux of the matter is that the ethics boom in hospitals is not only the result of increased moral sensitivity but also an expression of a structural crisis in the doctor–patient situation. The causes of this crisis cannot, however, be effectively compensated by ethics experts and certainly cannot be eliminated by them.

## The Apparently Autonomous Patient

*The more insistence is placed on patient autonomy, the less rational and psychological freedom patients have in some circumstances.* In addition to the principle of benevolence, the principle of patient autonomy is a fundamental principle of modern medical ethics. In reality, however, one must assume that the greater the value placed on autonomy, the more difficult it is for the patient to practice his or her autonomy and to apply it in his or her own interest.

- Individuals who are seriously ill seek medical assistance also by demanding authoritative advice on what is best for them. They want to be released from the burden of making a decision which they are not competent to make as laypersons. The advice of the good doctor, who is both competent in his or her medical field *and* humanely caring instead of just orienting himself or herself to the ethical and legal norms helps the patient initially develop something like autonomy in the face of the existential depths of his or her own suffering.
- The fewer good doctors there are, the greater is the importance placed on informed consent of the patients. The model is the completion of the contract that occurs between the well informed parties to their mutual advantage. However, informed consent, which burdens the patient with the load of weighing risk, does not make an autonomous decision possible because abstract risks and chances cannot be weighed. There exists no "scale" laypersons could use for such purposes. Even if the patient, for example, makes a decision after reading pages of information on the ways to remove a brain aneurysm operatively, such a decision, regardless of the objective advice of a physician, is primarily the expression of the individual patient's personality, support from friends or family, or private loneliness. (One could call such a decision "autonomous" based on the information provided, but this is more of a linguistic label to justify the physician's actions than a warranted decision per se.)
- This also affects so-called shared decision making. Undoubtedly, there are diagnostic situations in which the responsible physician cannot provide a definite treatment recommendation as long as she or he merely adheres to the available empirical evidence because of a lack of prognostic clarity or the presence of a poor prognosis (for example, prostate screening in elderly men or chemotherapy for advanced-stage cancer with metastases). Many factors support the following argument: In such situations, patient preference should be accorded greater importance than the professional opinion of the physician. It is certainly a characteristic of the good doctor that she or he considers this when dealing with patients. It is also true, however, that patient preference, whenever she or he must make a vital decision as a medical layperson, is more often influenced by such factors as personality, family, and momentary mood than by objective information.
- The lack of autonomy of the patient who is obligated to be autonomous is also reflected in the fact that his or her will to live forces him or her to grab at every pharmacological and surgical straw of hope, regardless of the reasonableness of

such interventions. The patient unavoidably becomes a slave of medicotechnical possibilities that are dutifully offered by specialists, beyond the help of the good doctor. (An inherent difficulty of informed consent is that even the most zealously informing physician represents postoperative suffering or, for example, life after heart transplantation, summarily and merely as a possibility. Otherwise, the doctor could be accused of wanting to influence the patient negatively.)

- This makes the widespread desire for actively assisted death understandable. It expresses a justified desire in light of the fear of being dragged through further medical interventions as a terminally ill patient. Faced with death, patients demand autonomy over their lives, which was demanded of them the entire time. Whether one *should* advocate the authorization of actively assisted death is an altogether different question. The answer to this question depends on the possibility of abuse of a liberal regulation, the social side effects (such as brutalization), and of course religious attitudes.

## Overburdening the Good Helper

*Lacking good doctors, more holistic care is expected to be practiced by other health professionals, with the inherent danger that their professionalism can be practiced only by distancing themselves from the patients.* In 1989 Waltraud Wagner and three other nursing aides admitted to having murdered a number of patients in Pavilion V for the Elderly in the Medical Department of the Lainz Hospital in Austria. Initially Wagner was an exceptionally committed, competent nurse. She was highly trusted by the physicians, who apparently hardly concerned themselves with her psychological situation.

- The first of these murders was actually committed out of pity, which indicates that good help could no longer be compensated by professional distance. Owing to constant overstress, a reactive mixture of destructive feelings mixed with fantasies of power over the patients' fates developed from holistic care. As later investigation revealed, good doctors, whose caring relationships with the elderly patients could have provided a stabilizing setting for the nurses in their nursing duties, were lacking. All supportive auxiliary measures to help the nurses learn to deal with their destructive impulses, their loneliness, and their exhaustion were also missing.
- Holistic care is one of the most complex human activities that occurs in hospitals, sometimes under conditions of extreme pressure. There are reports in the literature that show how the nursing staff turn to measures of ritual self-protection before entering and after leaving a ward for the elderly (Schützenhof, 1999).

The staff of a ward I know practice an equilibrium ritual every day after the early shift. Before they leave the realm of nursing . . . a bottle of wine is opened, and every nurse drinks a glass. In this way they symbolically rinse away the filth, the noise, and the smells and prepare for normality.

Although elderly wards are a special case, the general fundamental problems of good help can be studied there especially well. Whoever show themselves to be particularly caring to the patients without support from the entire hospital surroundings, including the doctors, are in danger of damaging their own mental health, which can have disastrous results for the patients.

• In her book *Entweihung und Scham, Grenzsituationen in der Pflege alter Menschen* (Defilement and Shame: Precarious Situations in Nursing of the Elderly), Katherina Gröning (2000) dramatically illustrates the above-mentioned situation.

The ward was mostly occupied by elderly, long-term patients. Some patients had been operated, and the anesthesia caused states of severe confusion with the corresponding additional conditions of disorientation and phenomena which we refer to as regression of libido. . . . An elderly patient smeared himself with his own feces, whereby the nursing staff punished him in the following manner. They cleaned his body, but not his face, so that he lay in bed for a long time with feces on his face.

Gröning commented:

Obviously the nurses experienced the patient's smearing himself with feces as an attack on their honor and as a defilement of the clean hospital. The patient had . . . polluted the institution and dishonored the nurses by his behavior. The behavior of the nurses also constituted a counterdefilement. The patient was paid back in kind.

If Gröning's interpretation is correct, the incident described is even consoling when considered a second time. One recognizes to what a high degree the patient is perceived as a person, even by those for whom it probably would be easier to view him in a sort of neutral working situation that must be brought back into order. But would not the ability to distance oneself here be a sign of greater professionality? This question is double-edged. Although distancing oneself belongs to the role of professionality in nursing, it can just as well turn a person into an object as a result of an inability or unwillingness to approach patients in a holistic manner (that is, with the required respect as well as humane care).

• The described precarious situations provide no conclusions concerning the beneficent mixture of professionality and devotion, which allows so many of the hospital personnel to both endure *and* master difficult interpersonal situations. One could even argue that with the increasing importance accorded the nursing staff the typical phenomena of overcontrol and overburden can be observed among highly motivated but relatively inexperienced rotating ward physicians.

## References

Gröning, K. (2000). Entweihung und Scham, Grenzsituationen in der Pflege alter Menschen. [Defilement and shame: precarious situations in nursing of the elderly.] Frankfurt am Main: Mabuse.

Schützenhof, E. (1999). *Das Recht der Alten auf Eigensinn.* [The right of the elderly to obstinacy.] Munich: Reinhardts Gerontologische Reihe. p. 142.

# 6
# Theory Behind the Bridge Principles

HANS RUSS, JOHANNES CLOUTH, AND FRANZ PORZSOLT

Decisions must be made constantly in all areas of life. This is also true for medical research and health care, when, for example, one must decide which parameters to apply to measure effectiveness (output) or value for patients (outcome) of medical interventions. In patients with diabetes mellitus, lowering elevated blood glucose is an output. We accordingly call *outputs* the results of all health care services. If the result of a health care service can be described as (re)gained years of life or (re)gained improvement in quality of life, we refer to it as an *outcome*.

One could ask whether new drugs to treat malignant diseases should be judged by the lengthening of survival (outcome), the remission rate (output), or both. It becomes clear that the evaluation of health care services is hardly possible without an underlying theoretical concept. Here we turn to philosophy, which has long dealt with such questions. If we wish to apply this knowledge from other branches of science, we must at least become familiar with some of its fundamental terms.

The so-called bridge principles are aids to answer exactly these questions, which we call normative questions. These aids make it possible to apply empirical knowledge to the assessment of norms or rules of action.

To understand the idea behind bridge principles, it helps first to take some concepts of philosophy of science and (originally) ethics into consideration. It has proved to be exceptionally problematic to develop a generally accepted and functioning procedure to find justifiable answers to these questions. An essential principle of philosophy of science states that our empirical knowledge cannot be used to *justify* norms—more factors are required for that—but to *criticize* suggested norms. Norms that withstand this criticism can be maintained in this respect. Norms that do not are to be discarded.

Whether empirical knowledge can be rendered useful in this manner depends on the character of the empirical statements and the normative propositions. Our first example, "$HbA_{1c}$ is often elevated in patients with diabetes mellitus," describes an empirical statement. The second example, "$HbA_{1c}$ should regularly be controlled in patients with diabetes mellitus," is a normative proposition.

Empirical statements and sets of statements describe or explain facts. They are *descriptive* or *explicative*. The first of the above-mentioned examples is descriptive. Our third example, "If $HbA_{1c}$ is elevated, it should be regularly controlled," is a mixed statement. "If $HbA_{1c}$ is elevated . . ." is a descriptive statement. ". . . it should be regularly controlled" is a normative statement. Descriptive or explicative statements can be fundamentally true, whereby the term "true" refers to the descriptive function of language. A statement is true if it suitably describes a fact. Empirical statements and sets of statements (for example, observational statements, hypotheses, theories, or explanations) can principally be true in the above-mentioned sense.

Normative statements, however, cannot be true. They formulate instructions for actions, for instance, characterizing actions as obligatory, forbidden, or permitted. They are not of descriptive, but *prescriptive*, character. Norms as instructions for action must be *valid* (see second example).

The difference between empirical and normative statements is clarified in our fourth example. The statement of empirical science, "Reduction of excess weight can reduce blood-glucose values of patients with type II diabetes mellitus," is fundamentally true and describes a fact. It is empirical.

The statement, "Diabetics should lose excess weight." is, from a philosophical viewpoint, a norm. It is a recommendation or an order; that is, it is prescriptive and therefore not true. It is either valid or invalid. That is one of the differences between empirical and normative statements. In brief, empirical knowledge says something about how things are, not how they should be.

This interpretation has sometimes been questioned. According to certain tenets, some descriptive terms have the same meaning as some evaluative terms, whereby correct action is to be deduced from such terms. Others believe that norms, like empirical facts, can be recognized by observation. Such opinions, however, are laden with difficulties (Moore, 1965; Harman, 1977; Czaniera, 2001; Russ, 2002).

The statement remains that empirical knowledge per se cannot answer a normative question. It is not normative in character.

If one proposes to apply empirical knowledge to the evaluation of norms, the difficulty arises that no purely normative propositions can logically be validly deduced from merely descriptive propositions. This is a formulation of Hume's law. The philosopher David Hume (1711–1776) became aware of this problem during his moral-philosophical investigations (Selby-Bigge, 1975).

Initially, descriptive or explanatory statements, which are not normative, could perhaps be used for a logically valid deduction of rules of action. Relevant norms for actions cannot, however, be deduced from empirical knowledge. "Relevant" is needed here for further explanation, as sentences with normative components can be deduced but are irrelevant in the normative sense because they do not say what should be done. For instance, scientific knowledge states that reduction of excess weight helps normalize blood glucose levels, but this does not implicitly state what should be done. Let us look at the two following examples.

One could imagine a type II diabetic who is not interested in normalizing his or her blood glucose values. The decision to lose weight does not result from the knowledge that the subject can reduce the blood glucose level when weight is lost because he or she does not aim to achieve the goal that could be attained by losing weight.

Another type II diabetic has the goal of reducing his or her blood glucose level without taking drugs. In this case, knowledge of the possible effects of weight loss *and* the goal the person has set leads to the decision to lose weight.

It is instructive here that what ought to be done is evaluated differently, although in both cases the empirical knowledge is the same. Which action is considered right depends essentially on the *goal* that has been set. This means that goal orientation itself has the character of a norm. In the first of the two diabetics, we are talking about a permission or prohibition norm; for instance, "the blood glucose level may be lowered but does not have to be" or "the blood glucose level should not be lowered." In the second case, we are talking about a command, "The blood glucose level should be lowered." Empirical knowledge itself is not normative, and it does not permit any relevant normative conclusions. Norms are prerequisite to be able to reach normative conclusions. Whoever ignores this commits a so-called is/ought fallacy.

However, empirical knowledge is not irrelevant for answering normative questions. There is a logically correct way to apply empirical knowledge to the critical examination of norm proposals. The purpose is to reject any norm that does not withstand the criticism. For this, a sort of bridge must be constructed between descriptive and normative propositions. Norms usually have a certain function. They serve to guide human action. There are various empirically determinable conditions under which norms cannot fulfill this function or cannot fulfill it in the desired manner. A sound bridge between descriptive and normative propositions exists when arguments can show that, in the face of certain empirical knowledge, a norm cannot be considered regulative for human action. Propositions that connect empirical statements with norms in this manner are called bridge principles (Albert, 1985; Russ, 2002).

Bridge principles must be founded; otherwise they would be unfounded and thereby arbitrary. The justifications can be connected to the just-mentioned regulative function of norms. To avoid is/ought fallacies, founded bridge principles are necessary. Let us assume that a norm has been suggested that requires something humanly impossible. One can argue that such a demand cannot guide human action because the required action cannot be performed. Therefore, this norm is to be rejected; it is invalid. What is humanly possible and what is not, however, is an empirical question. Therefore, certain empirical knowledge about human nature would be used to criticize norms. Critical rejection of a norm cannot, however, be immediately deduced from empirical knowledge. It is descriptive and states only that a certain action cannot be carried out. A specific premise is required to criticize a norm, a bridge principle, which is founded on the understanding of the nonfunctionality of the norm and establishes a relationship between empirical knowledge and the norm in question. An action required by a certain norm, which, according to our empirical knowledge, cannot be performed, does not have to be performed. The norm is invalid.

This kind of criticism of norms can be applied to different empirically assessable requirements of norms, which results in different bridge principles. It is useful to state them in a detailed, conditional way to state clearly the kind of criticism that is being applied. In short, we are talking about judging a certain norm using our empirical knowledge. Norms that do not withstand such criticism are no longer considered. It is justified to reject them.

A bridge principle was just named: the *ought-implies-can principle*, which is also referred to as the *practicability principle* or *realizability postulate*. A variation can be formulated as follows: If, according to empirical knowledge, the action required by the norm is not possible, the norm does not come into consideration from an empirical point of view.

The formulation stating that the norm "cannot be considered from an empirical viewpoint" indicates that norms must fulfill further criteria to be acceptable, such as the criterion of logical consistency. A justification of this bridge principle has already been implied. Norms have the function of guiding human action. If an action is required that is not realizable (the reduction of serious results caused by diabetes mellitus is not always measured), the norm cannot be practically effective; that is, its function cannot be fulfilled. In view of this fact, it makes no sense to maintain this norm. It is rejected. A practical example is a diabetic who is urgently advised to perform more physical activity but who is not able to follow this recommendation.

Three kinds of a lack of realizability can be differentiated. First, a nonrealizable action is required. Second, it is required to reach a nonreachable goal. Third, an action is required that is not suitable to achieve the required goal. In the second case, the norm in question cannot become practically effective because it demands that something be realized that cannot be realized. The norm cannot lead to the effect it is intended to produce. It is rejected. The third case, in which the norm's intended effect cannot be produced in the manner required, is similar. This norm no longer comes into consideration.

In all three cases, the actual critical instances are of empirical nature. Assertions that an action is not realizable, a goal is not attainable, or a goal cannot be reached in a certain way, are descriptive and per se do not say anything about what should be done. Normative conclusions can only be reached with the relevant bridge principles, that is, instructions for action can be accepted or rejected.

Sometimes allegations that are false according to our empirical knowledge are included in justifications for rules of action. Because the justifications are incorrect, the norms are unfounded. This creates problems in their function for the regulation of human action. Unfounded norms are confronted with a general compliance problem. This is especially obvious when norms are doubted or conflicts between norms arise. If no reasonable answer can be given to the question of why a certain rule should be followed or why one rule of action is preferred over another, no one would understand why it should be followed. Experienced clinicians immediately think of the problems inherent in the application of guidelines. Either such norms are not followed, which would make them ineffective, or their observance is forced. This requires sanctions, which, however, lead to compliance with rules of action only to a certain degree. In this case, their practical application is continually endangered. Insufficient justifications undermine the willingness to follow norms; they thwart or endanger at least their practical effectiveness.

Justifications for norms can be erroneous, among other things, in view of empirical facts. For the above-named reasons, they undermine the action-regulating function of a certain norm. The norm is not longer valid. The relevant bridge principle is called the *congruence principle* and can be formulated as follows: If the justification for a certain norm is not valid according to our empirical knowledge, this norm does not come into consideration from an empirical point of view.

Moreover, some norms of action, if they are practically effective, can have results that are unacceptable. They can be associated with implications that make it appear prudent to reject them. Approval of a certain drug demands that it has been proved to reduce certain complaints. However, side effects generally occur with this drug that are believed to be considerably more serious than the original complaints. In view of these unacceptable negative consequences, approval is to be rejected.

Such considerations are, of course, possible only for such implications that are recognized. In such cases the norms in question cannot become practically effective in the desired manner, that is, without causing unacceptable negative results. This is the reason for the so-called *connecting principle*. This bridge principle can thus be briefly described as: Norms should only be applied if their expected consequences are accepted. Because estimating the consequences also presents an empirical problem, and the known results belong in the domain of empirical knowledge, the following bridge principle is needed to apply the known implications to norm criticism: If, according to empirical knowledge, unacceptable consequences are to be expected from following a certain norm, this norm does not come into consideration from an empirical viewpoint.

Norms are not only expected to guide our actions but also to be more appropriate than possible alternative norms. What do we mean by "more appropriate"? This refers to different aspects of a discussion about norms. For example, diverse norms permit a certain goal to be realized equally whereby the use of resources differs. The application of one norm requires, for example, fewer financial resources than another. It is generally expected to use resources wisely. This is part of the desired way of doing things, which can hardly be contested. Some norms can be superior to others in this aspect.

Norms can also be tested for whether they are more conductive to that which is recognized to be right than the competing norms (for instance, if they create a lesser degree of psychological resistance). There certainly are further facets of "more appropriate." Norms that prove to be weaker in such cases are omitted because they cannot provide practical guidance in the desired manner. They are not efficient enough. It is an empirical problem to discern whether and to what degree instructions for action use resources appropriately and whether the norms are more conducive. Statements such as, "This rule of action is more efficient than that one" are descriptive. A bridge principle is required to be able to apply norm criticism to them (that is, the *principle of comparative assessment*). We summarize the various kinds of norm evaluation under the term "effectiveness":

When a certain norm does not represent the most effective alternative from the empirical point of view, this norm does not come into consideration from an empirical standpoint. We want to assess norms according to their effectiveness. Difficult questions can result when some norms are better in certain aspects of effectiveness but worse in others when compared to alternative suggestions. What is considered effective in these circumstances must be decided according to the individual situation.

To provide the reader with instructions for practical application of the described principles, Table 6.1 demonstrates with the aid of bridge principles which endpoints for the evaluation of health care services (in this case, therapeutic success

TABLE 6.1. Applicability of various endpoints for evaluating therapeutic success in patients with diabetes mellitus.

| Parameter | Endpoint: death | Endpoint: $HbA_{1c}$ | Endpoint: HRQoL |
|---|---|---|---|
| **Bridge Principle:** Should implies can (realizability postulate). If something is required, it must be achievable. | A study investigating the endpoint "death" would require observation for longer than 10 years and would be very expensive. *Inappropriate* | $HbA_{1c}$ is easy to measure *Appropriate* | HRQoL is easy to measure and the costs are acceptable. *Appropriate* |
| **Congruence Principle:** There is a confirmed relationship between measurement and result. | The association between early death as a result of a stroke or heart attack and poorly controlled diabetes mellitus is correct. *Appropriate* | Postprandial blood glucose peaks seem to have a higher predictive value than $HBA_{1c}$. *Uncertain* | The relationship between HRQoL and late complications is controversial. *Appropriate* |
| **Connecting Principle:** Only norms should be applied whose recognized implications are accepted; norms with unacceptable results are to be rejected. | There is no possibility to finance long-term studies, which are necessary to provide evidence. *Inappropriate* | It is known that controls should be performed regularly. The monetary costs are acceptable. *Appropriate* | Implications cannot be expected from measuring HRQoL because HRQoL data have hardly proven relevant to actions. *Uncertain* |
| **Comparative Evaluation:** Are other criteria more appropriate for the evaluation than this criterion? | Are other endpoints, such as HRQoL, blindness, amputation, or heart attack, more useful than the endpoint "death"? *Uncertain* | Measuring postprandial blood glucose peaks could be more useful than measuring $HBA_{1c}$. *Uncertain* | In comparison to other endpoints, measuring HRQoL provides fewer data that are relevant to action. *Inappropriate* |
| Sum score | Inappropriate | Appropriate (< 7 points) | Inappropriate |

Estimation of appropriateness is in italics. If an endpoint is inappropriate from the view of a single bridge principle, this endpoint is to be considered entirely "inappropriate." Otherwise, the individual points are added up for a sum score. A sum of 4–7 points means an endpoint is "uncertain"; 8–12 points indicates the endpoint is "appropriate."
HRQoL = health-related quality of life.

in diabetes mellitus) are "appropriate," "uncertain," or "inappropriate." To be able to quantify statements, we have awarded 3 points to the qualification "appropriate," 2 points to "uncertain," and 0 to "inappropriate." For the evaluation and interpretation of these results it should be taken into consideration that an endpoint is considered inappropriate when it is judged inappropriate by the application of a single bridge principle. If application of all bridge criteria results in the qualification "appropriate" or "uncertain," we recommend adding up the points into a sum score. The validity of the sum score remains to be confirmed.

In summary, the evaluation of health care services is hardly possible without a theoretical concept. We turn to philosophy and learn that the consistent formulation of the desired goal is one of the essential prerequisites for avoiding irrelevant assumptions and false conclusions. We also understand that the evaluation of health care services can receive considerable support from the application of bridge principles. The table demonstrating the application of bridge principles can be useful for the practical application of these principles. The statement attributed to Albert Einstein that "a good theory is really practical" seems to be true. We hope hereby to have placated those whom we disturbed with theoretical considerations.

## References

Albert, H. (1985). *Treatise on critical reason.* Princeton: Princeton University Press.

Czaniera, U. (2001). *Gibt es moralisches Wissen? Die Kognitivismusdebatte in der analytischen Moralphilosophie.* [Does moral knowledge exist? The cognitivism debate in analytic moral philosophy.] Paderborn: Mentis.

Harman, G. (1977). *The nature of morality: an introduction to ethics.* Oxford: Oxford University Press.

Hume, D. (1740). *A treatise of human nature: Book III (Of Morals).* In L.A. Selby-Bigge (Ed.) *A treatise of human nature: Book III (Of Morals)* (1888). Oxford: Clarendon Press.

Moore, G.E. (1903). *Principia Ethica.* [*Ethical principles.*] Republished 1965. Cambridge: Cambridge University Press.

Russ H.G. (2002). *Empirisches Wissen und Moralkonstruktion.* [Empirical knowledge and moral construction.] Frankfurt am Main, Germany: Dr. Hänsel – Hohenhausen.

# 7
# How to Measure Quality of Life

ROBERT M. KAPLAN

Throughout this book, we have considered the assessment of inputs and outputs of health care systems. Furthermore, we have suggested that measuring outputs is not enough. The goal of health care is to provide value for patients. This requires that we show the value of investments in terms of patient outcomes. But how can patient outcomes be quantified? In this chapter we consider the quantification of patient-reported outcomes.

Health is a highly valued human asset. Studies on the preference for various states of being show that virtually everyone rates good health as their most desired state. Despite the perceived importance of health, health status has remained difficult to define. There are two common themes in definitions of health. First, premature death is undesirable, so one aspect of health is the avoidance of mortality. The health status of nations is often evaluated in terms of mortality rates or infant mortality rates.

Second, quality of life is important. Disease and disability are of concern because they affect life expectancy and/or life quality (Kaplan, 2005). For example, cancer and heart disease are the two major causes of premature death in the United States. In addition, disease or disability can make life less desirable. A person with heart disease may face restrictions in activities of daily living and may be unable to work or participate in social activities. Even relatively minor diseases and disabilities affect quality of life. A cold, for example, may interfere with the ability to concentrate, work, or attend school. The cold, however, lasts only a short time. A chronic disease, such as arthritis, may affect the quality of your life for a long time (Pauwels & Rabe, 2004).

Within the last few years, medical scientists have come to realize the importance of quality of life measurement. Many major diseases, including arthritis, heart disease, and diabetes, or even digestive problems, are evaluated in terms of the degree to which they affect life quality and life expectancy (Kaplan, 2005). One can also evaluate treatments for these conditions based on the amount of improvement they produce in quality of life. Figure 7.1 summarizes the number of publications under the topic of quality of life identified in PubMed between 1972 and 2004. In 1972, PubMed did not identify any publications under the

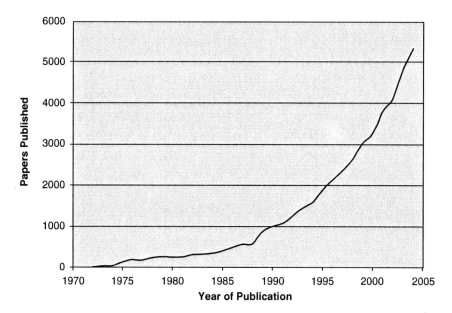

FIGURE 7.1. Quality of life publications, by year (based on PubMed).

quality of life topic heading. However, over the next 30 years, the number of articles that use the quality of life key word grew dramatically. In 2004, PubMed identified 5399 articles. Over these 30 years, the tools for quality of life measurement became more refined, allowing sophisticated analysis of patients' perceived outcomes for a variety of illnesses. Today, health-related quality of life (HRQoL) is studied in a variety of subjects throughout the stages of life and in the community. The U.S. Food and Drug Administration now considers quality of life data in their evaluations of new products, and nearly all major clinical trials in medicine use quality of life assessment measures. Several approaches to quality of life measurement are reviewed.

## What Is Health-Related Quality of Life?

There are numerous methods for assessing health-related quality of life. There is now an entire journal devoted to quality of life measurement, and several professional societies focus on the topic. Methods of assessing health-related quality of life represent at least two conceptual traditions. One grows out of the tradition of health-status measurement. Several efforts to develop measures of health status were launched during the late 1960s and early 1970s. All the projects were guided by the World Health Organization's (WHO) definition of health as a "complete state of physical, mental, and social well-being and not merely absence of disease" (WHO, 1948). The projects resulted in a variety of assessment tools, including the Sickness Impact Profile (Bergner et al., 1981), the Quality of Well-Being Scale (Kaplan et al., 1998), the SF-36 (Ware & Gandek, 1998), and the Nottingham Health Profile (Lowe et al., 1990). Many of the measures examined the effect of disease or disability on performance of social role, ability to interact in the community, and physical functioning. Some of the questionnaires have separate components for the measurement of physical, social, and mental health. The measures also differ in the extent to which they consider subjective aspects of life quality (Kaplan et al., 1993).

Perhaps the most important distinction among methods to assess quality of life is the contrast between psychometric and decision theory approaches. The psychometric approach attempts to provide separate measures for the many dimensions of quality of life. The best known example of the psychometric tradition is the Sickness Impact Profile (SIP). The SIP is a 136-item measure that yields 12 different scores displayed in a format similar to a Minnesota Multiphasic Personality Inventory (MMPI) profile (Bergner et al., 1981).

The decision theory approach attempts to weight the various dimensions of health to provide a single expression of health status. Supporters of this approach argue that psychometric methods fail to consider that different health problems are not of equal concern. A runny nose is not the same as severe chest pain. In an experimental trial using the psychometric approach, one often finds that some aspects of quality of life improve whereas others become worse. For example, a medication might reduce high blood pressure but produce headaches and impotence. Many argue that the quality of life notion is the subjective evaluation of observable or objective health states. The decision theory approach attempts to provide an overall measure of quality of life that integrates subjective functional states, preferences for these states, morbidity, and mortality.

## Common Methods for the Measurement of Quality of Life

A variety of methods have been proposed to measure quality of life, but we cannot review and critically discuss them all here. Instead, we present some of the most widely used psychometric and decision-theory-based methods. Readers interested in more detailed reviews should refer to Walker and Rosser (1993) and McDowell and Newell (1996).

### *Psychometric Methods*

SF-36

Perhaps the most commonly used outcome measure in the world today is the Medical Outcome Study Short Form-36 (SF-36). The SF-36 grew out of work by the Rand Corporation and the Medical Outcomes Study (MOS) (Kind, 1997). Originally, it was based on the measurement strategy from the Rand Health Insurance Study. The MOS attempted to develop a very short, 20-item instrument known as the Short Form-20 or SF-20. However, the SF-20 did not have appropriate reliability for some dimensions. The SF-36 includes eight health concepts: physical functioning, role–physical, bodily pain, general health perception, vitality, social functioning, role–emotional, and mental health (Kosinski et al., 1999). The SF-36 can be administered by a trained interviewer or self-administered. It has many advantages. For example, it is brief, and there is substantial evidence for its reliability and validity (Ware et al., 1981, 1992, 1995, 1999a,b; Ware & Sherbourne, 1992; Kosinski et al., 1999). The SF-36 can be machine-scored and has been evaluated in large population studies.

Despite its many advantages, the SF-36 also presents some disadvantages. For example, it does not have age-specific questions, and one cannot clearly determine whether it is equally appropriate at each level of the age continuum. The items for older, retired individuals are the same as those for children (Stewart & Ware, 1992). Nevertheless, the SF-36 has become the most commonly used behavioral measure in contemporary medicine.

### Nottingham Health Profile

The Nottingham Health Profile (NHP) is another profile approach that has been used widely in Europe. One of the important features of the NHP is that the items were originally generated on the basis of extensive discussions with patients. The NHP has two parts. The first includes 38 items divided into six categories: sleep, physical mobility, loss of energy, pain, emotional reactions, and social isolation. Items within each of these sections are rated in terms of relative importance. Items are rescaled to allow them to vary between 0 and 100 within each section.

The second part of the NHP includes seven statements related to the areas of life most affected by health: employment, household activities, social life, home life, sex life, hobbies and interests, and holidays. The respondent indicates whether a health condition has affected his or her life in these areas. Used in a substantial number of studies, the NHP has considerable evidence for its reliability and validity.

Another important strength of the NHP is that it is based on consumer definitions of health derived from individuals in the community. The language in the NHP is simple, and the scale requires only a low level of reading ability. The psychometric properties of the NHP have been evaluated in a substantial number of studies. However, the NHP, like most profile measures, does not provide weightings of relative importance across dimensions. As a result, it is difficult to compare the dimensions directly with one another (Lowe et al., 1990).

## Decision Theory Approaches

Some approaches to the measurement of health-related quality of life combine measures of morbidity and mortality to express health outcomes in units analogous to years of life. The years of life figure, however, is adjusted for diminished quality of life associated with diseases or disabilities (Kaplan & Anderson, 1996).

Modern measures of health outcome consider future as well as current health status. Lung cancer, for example, may have little impact on current functioning but a substantial impact on life expectancy and functioning in the future. Today a person with a malignant tumor in a lung may be functioning very much like a person with a chest cold. However, the cancer patient is more likely to remain dysfunctional or to die in the future. Comprehensive expressions of health status need to incorporate estimates of future outcomes as well as to measure current status (Kaplan, 1994a).

Within the last few years, interest has grown in using quality of life data to help evaluate the cost-utility or cost-effectiveness of health care programs. Cost studies have gained in popularity because health care costs have grown so rapidly in recent years. Not all health care interventions return equal benefit for the expended dollar. Objective cost studies might guide policy makers toward an optimal and equitable distribution of scarce resources. Cost-effectiveness analysis typically quantifies the benefits of a health care intervention in terms of years of life or quality-adjusted life-years (QALYs). Cost-utility is a special use of cost-effectiveness that weights observable health states by preferences or utility judgments of quality (Kaplan & Groessl, 2002). In cost-utility analysis, the benefits of medical care, surgical interventions, or preventive programs are expressed in terms of common QALYs (Gold, 1996).

If a man dies of heart disease at age 50 and we expected him to live to age 75, we might conclude that the disease precipitated 25 lost life-years. If 100 men died at age 50 (and also had a life expectancy of 75 years), we might conclude that 2500 (100 men × 25 years) life-years had been lost. Yet death is not the only relevant outcome of heart disease. Many adults suffer myocardial infarctions that leave them somewhat disabled for a long time. Though still alive, they suffer diminished quality of life. Quality-adjusted life-years take into consideration such consequences. For example, a disease that reduces quality of life by one-half takes away 0.5 QALYs over the course of each year. If the disease affects two people, it takes away 1 year (2 × 0.5) over each year. A medical treatment that improves quality of life by 0.2 for each of five individuals results in the equivalent of 1 QALY if the benefit persists for 1 year. This system has the advantage of considering both benefits and side effects of programs in terms of the common QALY units.

Of the several approaches for obtaining quality-adjusted life years, most are similar (Kaplan et al., 1998). The most commonly used methods are the EQ-5D, the Health Utilities Index (HUI), the Quality of Well-being Scale (QWB), the Health and Activities Limitations Index, and the Standard Gamble.

## EQ-5D

The approach most commonly used in the European community is the EQ-5D.[1] This method, developed by Paul Kind and associates, has been advanced by a collaborative group from western Europe known as the EuroQoL group

---

[1]General information on the EQ-5D can be located at http://www.euroqol.org/.

(Kind, 1997). The group, originally formed in 1987, comprises a network of international, multicenter, multidisciplinary researchers, originally from seven centers in England, Finland, The Netherlands, Norway, and Sweden. More recently, researchers from Spain, as well as from Germany, Greece, Canada, the United States, and Japan, have joined the group. The intention of this effort was to develop a generic currency for health that could be used commonly across Europe. The original version of the EuroQoL had 14 health states in six domains. In addition, respondents placed their health on a continuum ranging from death (0) to perfect health (1.0). The method was validated in postal surveys in England, Sweden, and The Netherlands. More recent versions of the EuroQoL, known as the EQ-5D, are now in use in a substantial number of clinical and population studies (Gudex et al., 1996; Hurst et al., 1997). Although the EQ-5D is easy to use and comprehensive, there have been some concerns about ceiling effects. Substantial numbers of people obtain the highest possible score. However, we do not anticipate this problem in the current study as all participants will be recruited because they have serious medical conditions.

Health Utilities Index

The Health Utilities Index (HUI)[2] is a family of health status and preference-based, health-related quality of life measures suitable for use in clinical and population studies (Feeny et al., 1995, 1999). Each member of the family includes a health status classification system, a preference-based multiattribute utility function, data collection questionnaires, and algorithms for deriving HUI variables from questionnaire responses. This study will use the Health Utilities Index Mark 2 (HUI-2). HUI-2 consists of six dimensions of health status: sensation (vision, hearing, speech), mobility, emotion, cognition, self-care, and pain (Feeny et al., 1995). There are five or six levels per attribute. HUI-2 focuses on capacity rather than performance. Multiplicative, multiattribute utility functions based on community preferences have been estimated for HUI-2 (Torrance et al., 1995) and HUI-3 (Feeny et al., 1999). This form of function can represent a simple type of preference interaction among the attributes.

   Evidence on test-retest reliability in the 1991 Statistics Canada General Social Survey has been reported. Agreement (kappa statistics) was high for most attributes. For the overall score, the intraclass correlation was 0.77. Evidence on agreement among assessors (self and proxy assessment) was provided by Glaser and colleagues (Glaser et al., 1997a,b, 1999). Results indicate that self and proxy assessments should not be viewed as interchangeable; agreement varies by attribute, and in general agreement was moderate to high. Evidence on responsiveness and construct validity has been published (Barr et al., 1996, 2000; Feeny et al., 1998; Furlong et al., 2001). Evidence of construct validity in the 1990 Ontario Health Survey is provided in Grootendorst et al. (2000). The HUI-3 described the

---

[2]Reference information on HUI is available at http://www.fhs.mcmaster.ca/hug/ and http://www.healthutilities.com/.

burden of morbidity for both stroke and arthritis, showing disease effects on the attributes that had been expected to be affected by these health conditions.

## Self-Administered Quality of Well-being Scale

The self-administered Quality of Well-being Scale QWB-SA[3] combines preference-weighted values for symptoms and functioning. The preference weights were obtained by ratings of 856 people from the general population. These judges rated the desirability of health conditions to place each on the continuum between death (0) and optimum health (1.00). Symptoms are assessed by questions that ask about the presence or absence of various symptom complexes. Functioning is assessed by a series of questions designed to record functional limitations over the previous 3 days within three separate domains (mobility, physical activity, social activity). The three functional domains and symptoms/problems scores are combined into a total score that provides a numerical point-in-time expression of well-being that ranges from zero (0) for death to one (1.0) for asymptomatic, optimal functioning.

The QWB has been used in numerous clinical trials and studies to evaluate medical and surgical therapies for conditions, such as chronic obstructive pulmonary disease (Kaplan et al., 1984), human immunodeficiency virus (HIV) infection (Kaplan et al., 1995, 1997a), cystic fibrosis (Orenstein et al., 1990; Orenstein & Kaplan, 1991), diabetes mellitus (Kaplan et al., 1987), atrial fibrillation (Ganiats et al., 1992), lung transplantation (Squier et al., 1995), arthritis (Kaplan et al., 1996, 2000), end-stage renal disease (Rocco et al., 1997), cancer (Kaplan, 1993b), depression (Pyne et al., 1997a,b), and several other conditions (Kaplan et al., 1998). Furthermore, the method has been used for health resource allocation modeling and has served as the basis for an innovative experiment on rationing of health care by the state of Oregon (Kaplan, 1993a,b). Studies have also demonstrated that the QWB is responsive to clinical change derived from surgery (Squier et al., 1995) or medical conditions, such as rheumatoid arthritis (Bombardier et al., 1986), acquired immunodeficiency syndrome (AIDS) (Kaplan et al., 1995), and cystic fibrosis (Orenstein et al., 1990). The self-administered form of the QWB (QWB-SA) was developed more recently. It has been shown to be highly correlated with the interviewer-administered QWB and to retain the psychometric properties (Kaplan et al., 1997b).

## Health and Activities Limitation Index

Where European investigators have invested in a standardized health-related quality of life instrument, the EQ-5D, and the Canadians have de facto adopted the HUI-3 as a national survey instrument, the United States has no one standardized instrument used broadly in national data sets. We have several national surveys of health, such as the National Longitudinal Study of Aging (LSOA), the

---

[3]General information about the QWB can be found at http://orpheus.ucsd.edu/famed/hoap/MEASURE.html/.

Health and Retirement Study (HRS), the National Health and Nutrition Evaluation Study (NHANES), the National Health Interview Survey (NHIS), and the Medical Expenditure Panel Survey (MEPS).

There has, however, been an effort to develop an ad hoc measure in association with one of our largest national data sets, the NHIS (Erickson et al., 1989). This measure is now called the Health and Activities Limitation Index, or HALex (Erickson, 1998). This index grew out of a desire to have a single summary index of health for the NHIS data to compute a health-weighted summary of life expectancy measuring achievement on the Healthy People 2000 goals. This summary was called "Years of Healthy Life" and was developed by the National Center for Health Statistics retrospectively to use the NHIS data (Erickson et al., 1995). The HALex has two dimensions, a seven-level classification of activities and function limitations ranging from "no limitations" to "limited in instrumental activities of daily living (IADLs)" and "limited in activities of daily living (ADLs)" and a self-rated overall estimation of health using the five-level, "excellent, very good, good, fair, poor" classification. The resulting classification scheme has $7 \times 5 = 35$ health states. Building on prior attempts to develop a national composite index for health states through a process using correspondence analysis, these states were weighted retrospectively to correspond to roughly what the investigators presumed they would be weighted by the HUI Mark I (Erickson, 1998).

Although its retrospective development may bring into question its validity, comparison to other indexes collected in various studies has shown favorable performance at a population level (Gold et al., 1996). This measure has two other attractive properties. First, it is computable in one of the major national data sets for health in the United States, the NHIS, so any study that collects data on activity and functional limitations and self-rated health sufficient to score the HALex can compare results to this large national survey in the United States. Second, collecting sufficient data to score the measure does not seem onerous. Accordingly, we include scoring this measure as one goal of the research proposed here.

Standard Gamble Utility

Some analysts do not measure utilities directly. Instead, they evaluate health outcomes by simply assigning a reasonable utility (Feeny et al., 2002). However, most current approaches have respondents assign weights to different health states on a scale ranging from 0 (for dead) to 1.0 (for wellness). The most common techniques include category rating scales, the standard gamble, and the time tradeoff. An important difference between methods is the incorporation of risk or preference information. Utility assessment specifically includes attitude toward risk in the judgment. These judgments under uncertainty are truly utilities (Feeny et al., 1995, 1999). The methods described above (HUI2, QWB, EQ-5D, HALex) assess health status by applying standardized weights to health states. Some investigators prefer to obtain utility ratings directly from the patient. In this study, we use the Standard Gamble to obtain a direct assessment of patient-rated utility.

The advantage of the standard gamble method is that it is clearly linked to economic theory. The standard gamble offers a choice between two alternatives: choice A—taking a gamble on a new treatment for which the outcome is uncertain. The respondent is told that a hypothetical treatment will lead to perfect health with a probability of $p$ or immediate death with a probability of $1 - p$. The alternative (choice B) is living in the current health state with certainty. In other words, the respondent can choose between remaining in a state that is intermediate between wellness and death or taking the gamble (entering a lottery) and trying the new treatment. The probability ($p$) is varied until the subject is indifferent between choices A and B.

The standard gamble has been attractive because it is based on the axioms of utility theory. The choice between a certain outcome and a gamble conforms to the exercises originally proposed by von Neumann and Morgenstern (1944).

## Disease-Specific Measures

This chapter has focused on the generic quality of life scales. However, there are significantly more disease-specific measures. Validated measures of health-related quality of life are available for illnesses, such as arthritis, diabetes, heart disease, kidney failure, and virtually every other major health condition. Two examples are the Arthritis Impact Measurement Scale (Meenan, 1982) and the University of California, San Diego (UCSD) Shortness of Breath Questionnaire (SOBQ) used in studies of patients with emphysema (Eakin et al., 1998).

The Arthritis Impact Measurement Scales (AIMS) is a health index designed at the Multipurpose Arthritis Center at Boston University. It is intended to measure physical health and social well-being for patients with rheumatoid arthritis (Meenan, 1982). The resultant scale includes 67 items with questions about functioning, health perceptions, morbidity, and demographics. The AIMS contains scales for mobility, physical activity, social activity, activities of daily living, depression, anxiety, and arthritis-related symptoms. In effect, it is an adaptation of an early version of the QWB (Kaplan & Anderson, 1996) with a series of items designed to tap more specifically the effect of arthritis on functioning and quality of life. Factor analysis of the AIMS has produced three subscales: physical function, psychological function, and pain. Most current applications of the AIMS use composite scores for these three areas.

The Shortness of Breath Questionnaire (SOBQ) includes 25 items that evaluate self-reported shortness of breath during the performance of various activities of daily living. Evaluations of the questionnaire show it to be highly correlated with other quality of life instruments, such as the Quality of Well-Being Index and the Center for Epidemiologic Studies Depression Scale. The questionnaire has high internal consistency (alpha = 0.96) and is significantly correlated with performance measures, such as the distance that can be walked in 6 minutes (Eakin et al., 1998).

# Summary

The CLINECS model requires an assessment of value for patients. To achieve this, we must go beyond the assessment of health care outputs. These outputs must be evaluated in relation to patient outcomes. A key component of patient outcomes is health-related quality of life.

Assessment of health-related quality of life has become a standard component of the evaluation of health outcomes. There are several important distinctions among commonly used approaches. Generic measures are used to evaluate health outcome for any illness or disease. Generic measures can typically be classified as derived from psychometric or decision theory. Psychometric approaches include the Sickness Impact Profile, the SF-36, and the Nottingham Health Profile. Decision theory approaches are used to estimate outcomes in terms of quality-adjusted life-years (QALYs). Methods used for this purpose include the EQ-5D, the HUI, and the QWB. Disease-specific measures are available for a wide variety of health conditions. Although disease-specific measures may be more sensitive for outcomes of a particular condition, they cannot be used for cross-illness comparisons or for cost-effectiveness analysis. Assessment of health-related quality of life is a rapidly developing field, and we anticipate major new developments over the next decade.

## *References*

Barr, R.D., Furlong, W., Feeny, D. (1996). Comments on health-related quality of life of adults surviving malignancies in childhood: Apajasalo et al. *European Journal of Cancer*, 32A, 1354–1358.

Barr, R.D., Chalmers, D., De Pauw, S., Furlong, W., Weitzman, S., Feeny, D. (2000). Health-related quality of life in survivors of Wilms' tumor and advanced neuroblastoma: a cross-sectional study. Journal of Clinical Oncology, 18, 3280–3287.

Bergner, M., Bobbitt, R.A., Carter, W.B., Gilson, B.S. (1981). The Sickness Impact Profile: development and final revision of a health status measure. *Medical Care*, 19, 787–805.

Bombardier, C., Ware, J., Russell, I.J., Larson, M., Chalmers, A., Read, J.L. (1986). Auranofin therapy and quality of life in patients with rheumatoid arthritis: results of a multicenter trial. *American Journal of Medicine*, 81, 565–578.

Eakin, E.G., Resnikoff, P.M., Prewitt, L.M., Ries, A.L., Kaplan, R.M. (1998). Validation of a new dyspnea measure: the UCSD Shortness of Breath Questionnaire; University of California, San Diego. *Chest*, 113, 619–624.

Erickson, P., Kendall, E.A., Anderson, J.P., Kaplan, R.M. (1989). Using composite health status measures to assess the nation's health. Medical Care, 27( Suppl), S66–S76.

Erickson, P., Wilson, R., Shannon, I. (1995). Years of healthy life: Healthy People 2000. *Statistics Notes*, 7, 1–15.

Erickson, P. (1998). Evaluation of a population-based measure of quality of life: the Health and Activity Limitation Index (HALex). *Quality of Life Research*, 7, 101–114.

Feeny, D., Furlong, W., Barr, R.D. (1998). Multiattribute approach to the assessment of health-related quality of life: Health Utilities Index. *Medical and Pediatriac Oncology*, Suppl 1, 54–59.

Feeny, D., Furlong, W., Boyle, M., Torrance, G.W. (1995). Multi-attribute health status classification systems: Health Utilities Index. *Pharmacoeconomics*, 7, 490–502.

Feeny, D., Furlong, W., Mulhern, R.K., Barr, R.D., Hudson, M. (1999). A framework for assessing health-related quality of life among children with cancer. *International Journal of Cancer*, 12(Suppl), 2–9.

Feeny D., Furlong, W., Torrance, G.W., Goldsmith, C.H., Zhu, Z., DePauw, S., et al. (2002). Multiattribute and single-attribute utility functions for the health utilities index mark 3 system. *Medical Care*, 40, 113–128.

Furlong, W.J., Feeny, D.H., Torrance, G.W., Barr, R.D. (2001). The Health Utilities Index (HUI) system for assessing health-related quality of life in clinical studies. *Annals of Medicine*, 33, 375–384.

Ganiats, T.G., Palinkas, L.A., Kaplan, R.M. (1992). Comparison of Quality of Well-Being scale and Functional Status Index in patients with atrial fibrillation. *Medical Care*, 30, 958–964.

Glaser, A.W., Abdul Rashid, N.F., U, C.L., Walker, D.A. (1997a). School behaviour and health status after central nervous system tumours in childhood. *British Journal of Cancer*, 76, 643–650.

Glaser, A.W., Davies, K., Walker, D., Brazier, D. (1997b). Influence of proxy respondents and mode of administration on health status assessment following central nervous system tumours in childhood. *Quality of Life Research*, 6, 43–53.

Glaser, A.W., Furlong, W., Walker, D.A., Fielding, K., Davies, K., Feeny, D.H., et al. (1999). Applicability of the Health Utilities Index to a population of childhood survivors of central nervous system tumours in the U.K. *European Journal of Cancer*, 35, 256–261.

Gold, M.R. (1996). *Cost-effectiveness in health and medicine.* New York: Oxford University Press.

Gold, M.R., Franks, P., Erickson, P. (1996). Assessing the health of the nation: the predictive validity of a preference-based measure and self-rated health. *Medical Care*, 34, 163–177.

Grootendorst, P., Feeny, D., Furlong, W. (2000). Health Utilities Index Mark 3: evidence of construct validity for stroke and arthritis in a population health survey. *Medical Care*, 38, 290–299.

Gudex, C., Dolan, P., Kind, P., Williams, A. (1996). Health state valuations from the general public using the visual analogue scale. *Quality of Life Research*, 5, 521–531.

Hurst, N.P., Kind, P., Ruta, D., Hunter, M., Stubbings, A. (1997). Measuring health-related quality of life in rheumatoid arthritis: validity, responsiveness and reliability of EuroQoL (EQ-5D). *British Journal of Rheumatology*, 36, 551–559.

Kaplan, R.M. (1993a). California Policy Seminar: allocating health resources in California: learning from the Oregon experiment. Berkeley, CA: California Policy Seminar.

Kaplan, R.M. (1993b). Quality of life assessment for cost/utility studies in cancer. *Cancer Treatment Reviews*, 19(Suppl A), 85–96.

Kaplan, R.M. (1994a). Value judgment in the Oregon Medicaid experiment. *Medical Care*, 32, 975–988.

Kaplan, R.M. (1994b). The Ziggy theorem: toward an outcomes-focused health psychology. *Health Psychology*, 13, 451–460.

Kaplan, R.M. (2005). Decision making in medicine and health care. *Annual Review of Clinical Psychology*, 1, 525–556.

Kaplan, R.M., Anderson, J. (1996). The general health policy model: an integrated approach. In B. Spilker (Ed.), *Quality of life and pharmacoeconomics in clinical trials.* New York: Raven. pp. 309–322.

Kaplan, R.M., Groessl, E.J. (2002). Cost/effectiveness analysis in behavioral medicine. *Journal of Consulting and Clinical Psychology*, 70, 482–493.

Kaplan, R.M., Atkins, C.J., Timms, R. (1984). Validity of a quality of well-being scale as an outcome measure in chronic obstructive pulmonary disease. *Journal of Chronic Diseases*, 37(2), 85–95.

Kaplan, R.M., Hartwell, S.L., Wilson, D.K., Wallace, J.P. (1987). Effects of diet and exercise interventions on control and quality of life in non-insulin-dependent diabetes mellitus. *Journal of General Internal Medicine*, 2, 220–228.

Kaplan, R.M., Feeny, D., Revicki, D.A. (1993). Methods for assessing relative importance in preference based outcome measures. *Quality of Life Research*, 2, 467–475.

Kaplan, R.M., Anderson, J.P., Patterson, T.L., McCutchan, J.A., Weinrich, J.D., Heaton, R.K., et al. (1995). Validity of the Quality of Well-Being Scale for persons with human immunodeficiency virus infection: HNRC Group; HIV Neurobehavioral Research Center. *Psychosomatic Medicine*, 57, 138–147.

Kaplan, R.M., Alcaraz, J.E., Anderson, J.P., Weisman, M. (1996). Quality-adjusted life years lost to arthritis: effects of gender, race, and social class. *Arthritis Care and Research*, 9, 473–482.

Kaplan, R.M., Patterson, T.L., Kerner, D.N., Atkinson, J.H., Heaton, R.K., Grant, I. (1997a). The Quality of Well-Being scale in asymptomatic HIV-infected patients: HNRC Group; HIV Neural Behavioral Research Center. *Quality of Life Research*, 6, 507–514.

Kaplan, R.M., Sieber, W.J., Ganiats, T.G. (1997b). The Quality of Well-Being scale: comparison of the interviewer-administered version with a self-administered questionnaire. *Psychology & Health*, 12, 783–791.

Kaplan, R.M., Ganiats, T.G., Sieber, W.J., Anderson, J.P. (1998). The Quality of Well-Being scale: critical similarities and differences with SF-36. *International Journal for Quality in Health Care*, 10, 509–520.

Kaplan, R.M., Schmidt, S.M., Cronan, T.A. (2000). Quality of well being in patients with fibromyalgia. *Journal of Rheumatology*, 27, 785–789.

Kind, P. (1997). The performance characteristics of EQ-5D, a measure of health related quality of life for use in technology assessment [abstract]. In: *Proceedings of the Annual Meeting of International Society of Technology Assessment in Health Care*, 13(5), 81.

Kosinski, M., Keller, S.D., Hatoum, H.T., Kong, S.X., Ware, J.E., Jr. (1999). The SF-36 health survey as a generic outcome measure in clinical trials of patients with osteoarthritis and rheumatoid arthritis: tests of data quality, scaling assumptions and score reliability. *Medical Care*, 37(Suppl 5), MS 10–22.

Lowe, D., O'Grady, J.G., McEwen, J., Williams, R. (1990). Quality of life following liver transplantation: a preliminary report. *Journal of the Royal College of Physicians of London*, 24(1), 43–46.

McDowell, I., Newell, C. (1996). *Measuring health: a guide to rating scales and questionnaires*. (2nd ed.). New York: Oxford University Press.

Meenan, R.F. (1982). The AIMS approach to health status measurement: conceptual background and measurement properties. *Journal of Rheumatology*, 9, 785–788.

Orenstein, D.M., Kaplan, R.M. (1991). Measuring the quality of well-being in cystic fibrosis and lung transplantation: the importance of the area under the curve. *Chest*, 100, 1016–1018.

Orenstein, D.M., Pattishall, E.N., Nixon, P.A., Ross, E.A., Kaplan, R.M. (1990). Quality of well-being before and after antibiotic treatment of pulmonary exacerbation in patients with cystic fibrosis. *Chest*, 98, 1081–1084.

Pauwels, R.A., Rabe, K.F. (2004). Burden and clinical features of chronic obstructive pulmonary disease (COPD). *Lancet*, 364, 613–620.

Pyne, J.M., Patterson, T.L., Kaplan, R.M., Gillin, J.C., Koch, W.L., Grant, I. (1997a). Assessment of the quality of life of patients with major depression. *Psychiatric Services*, 48, 224–230.

Pyne, J.M., Patterson, T.L., Kaplan, R.M., Ho, S., Gillin, J.C., Golshan, S., et al. (1997b). Preliminary longitudinal assessment of quality of life in patients with major depression. *Psychopharmacology Bulletin*, 33, 23–29.

Rocco, M.V., Gassman, J.J., Wang, S.R., Kaplan, R.M. (1997). Cross-sectional study of quality of life and symptoms in chronic renal disease patients: the Modification of Diet in Renal Disease Study. *American Journal of Kidney Diseases*, 29, 888–896.

Squier, H.C., Ries, A.L., Kaplan, R.M., Prewitt, L.M., Smith, C.M., Kriett, J.M., et al. (1995). Quality of well-being predicts survival in lung transplantation candidates. *American Journal of Respiratory and Critical Care Medicine*, 152, 2032–2036.

Stewart, A.L., Ware, J.E. (1992). *Measuring functioning and well-being: the medical outcomes study approach.* Durham, NC: Duke University Press.

Torrance, G.W., Furlong, W., Feeny, D., Boyle, M. (1995). Multi-attribute preference functions: Health Utilities Index. *Pharmacoeconomics*, 7, 503–520.

Von Neumann, J., Morgenstern, O. (1944). *Theory of games and economic behavior.* Princeton, NJ: Princeton University Press.

Walker, S.R., Rosser, R. (1993). *Quality of life assessment: key issues in the 1990s.* Dordrecht, The Netherlands: Kluwer Academic.

Ware, J.E., Jr., Gandek, B. (1998). Overview of the SF-36 Health Survey and the International Quality of Life Assessment (IQOLA) Project. *Journal of Clinical Epidemiology*, 51, 903–912.

Ware, J.E., Jr., Sherbourne, C.D. (1992). The MOS 36-item short-form health survey (SF-36). I. Conceptual framework and item selection. *Medical Care*, 30, 473–483.

Ware, J.E., Jr., Brook, R.H., Davies, A.R., Lohr, K.N. (1981). Choosing measures of health status for individuals in general populations. *American Journal of Public Health*, 71, 620–625.

Ware, J.E., Jr., Kosinski, M., Bayliss, M.S., McHorney, C.A., Rogers, W.H., Raczek, A. (1995). Comparison of methods for the scoring and statistical analysis of SF-36 health profile and summary measures: summary of results from the Medical Outcomes Study. *Medical Care*, 33(Suppl), AS 264–279.

Ware, J.E., Jr., Bayliss, M.S., Mannocchia, M., Davis, G.L. (1999a). Health-related quality of life in chronic hepatitis C: impact of disease and treatment response; the Interventional Therapy Group. *Hepatology*, 30, 550–555.

Ware, J.E., Jr., Keller, S.D., Hatoum, H.T., Kong, S.X. (1999b). The SF-36 Arthritis-Specific Health Index (ASHI). I. Development and cross-validation of scoring algorithms. *Medical Care,* 37(Suppl), MS 40–50.

World Health Organization, 1948. Preface to Charter document. Geneva: WHO.

# 8
# New Instrument to Describe Indicators of Well-Being in Old Old Patients with Severe Dementia: Vienna List

FRANZ PORZSOLT, MARINA KOJER, MARTINA SCHMIDL, ELFRIEDE R. GREIMEL, JÖRG SIGLE, JÖRG RICHTER, AND MARTIN EISEMANN

The proportions of old people and people suffering from dementia are steadily increasing in industrial societies. Consequently, the number of people depending on institutional care is growing. Such care is provided in general hospitals, geriatric hospitals, nursing homes, private homes, senior residences, and by the families. Obviously, there are large differences in costs and efficacy of these various types of care. In general, quality of life data have been increasingly appreciated as the key outcome measure for the assessment of therapeutic interventions and for the usefulness of various treatment facilities. Quality of life is defined by the World Health Organization (WHOQOL Group, 1995) as:

... an individual's perception of their position in life, in the context of the culture and value systems in which they live, and in relation to their goals, expectations, standards, and concerns. It is a broad ranging concept, effected in a complex way by the person's physical health, psychological state, level of independence, social relationships and their relationships to salient features of their environment.

Many of the instruments in use to measure quality of life represent brief global measures that cannot be applied to patients with severe dementia. The most important reason for the slow growth of empirical data in this area probably relates to the obvious methodological problems of obtaining reliable subjective accounts of individuals with severe dementia who have compromised cognitive abilities, frequently with concurrent impairment of communicative skills.

Because of these impairments in this group of patients, most of the available instruments are not applicable for assessing quality of life-related issues by means of traditional measures, such as questionnaires or interviews, which require a highly complex procedure of introspection and evaluation involving several components of cognition, including implicit and explicit memory (Barofsky, 1996).

Facing these problems, attempts have been made to develop direct observational methods (Lawton et al., 1996) that measure positive affects, such as pleasure, interest, and contentment, as well as negative affects, such as sadness, anxiety/fear, and anger according to operationalized criteria during a series of 10-minute direct observations. An alternative approach was chosen by the Bradford Research Group in the United Kingdom (Kitwood & Bredin, 1997) with Dementia Care Mapping (DCM) based on the psychosocial model of "person-centered care," which provides detailed observational ratings covering aspects of articulation, feeding, social withdrawal, passive engagement, walking, and a number of indicators of well-being.

Literature searches (up to 2003) of MEDLINE, Embase, Psyclit, and Cinahl using the keywords "dementia," "well-being," and "quality of life" were conducted. Lawton and colleagues (1998) developed the Minimum Data Set (MDS) comprising cognition, activities of daily living, time use, depression, and problem behaviors. Lawton (1994) also proposed including observations of demented patients' emotional behaviors. Most of the measurements are derived from existing instruments and are confined to a few of the following dimensions: affect, activity, enjoyment, self-esteem, and social interactions. Ready and Ott (2003) concluded from their review that the psychometric properties of most of the available instruments have to be regarded as preliminary.

As mentioned above, there existed no quality of life assessment tools for patients with severe dementia as representative of our population. Unfortunately, the instruments developed for demented patients were not found applicable to our patients, who were in advanced stages of dementia (for example, the Mini Mental State Examination could not be completed by any of our patients). For this reason, in 1998 the Department of Palliative Geriatrics at the Wienerwald Geriatric Center launched a project to develop a new instrument based on observations made by the staff (physicians, nurses, physiotherapists) completely independent on the patients' ability to cooperate.

## Methods

### Patients

In the present study, 217 consecutive patients (44 men, 173 women) were included. The average age was 84 years (range 61–105 years). Most of the patients suffered from severe dementia according to the International Classification of Diseases, 10th edition, (ICD-10) (34.5% were F00—dementia in Alzheimer's disease; 61.5% were F01—vascular dementia; 4.0% were F02—other). It appeared that more women (38%) had been diagnosed as suffering from Alzheimer's disease than men: 23% [$\chi^2$ (df 2) = 6.05; $p$ = 0.049]. As concerns age, the patients with Alzheimer's disease (87.3 ± 5.7 years) and vascular dementia (86.3 ± 7.0 years) were significantly older than those with other diagnoses (78.5 ± 15.6 years) ($t$ = 3.27, $p$ = 0.002 and $t$ = 2.74, $p$ = 0.007 respectively).

## Development of the Item Pool

Thirteen staff members comprising doctors, nurses, and therapists from the Department of Palliative Geriatrics at the Wienerwald Geriatric Center in Vienna observed severely demented patients during a 1-year period (May 1998 to April 1999). The patient's behavior was documented on one of the wards (32 beds). Based on this documentation, 65 items for the description of behavior in demented inpatients were derived and allocated to categories supposedly reflecting aspects relevant to their well-being, such as voice, language, mood, eye contact, acceptance of body contact, gait, muscular tension, hand movement, sleep, activities, communication, and independence in food intake. This approach is different from prevailing approaches, which are mainly based on the use of items from existing instruments measuring specific aspects.

Subsequently, 771 assessments of 217 inpatients in various situations, such as eating, dressing, and grooming, were obtained with this list between June 1999 and September 2000 by both physicians and nurses. Each of the original 65 items was scored on a 5-point Likert scale from 0 = never to 4 = always.

## Further Assessments

Patients were diagnosed according to the ICD-10. They were rated by means of the Brief Cognitive Rating Scale (BCRS) (Reisberg et al., 1983), the Global Deterioration Scale (GDS) (Reisberg et al., 1982), the Barthel Index (Mahoney & Barthel, 1965), and the Spitzer Index (Spitzer et al., 1981).

The BCRS describes the severity of cognitive impairment providing five main axes (concentration, short-term memory, long-term memory, orientation, self-care ability) and five coaxes (language, psychomotoric function, mood and behavior, drawing skills, calculating skills), each rated on a 7-step scale.

The GDS is a proxy rating scale to assess the severity of dementia in elderly people on a 7-point Likert-type scale (1 = no impairment; 7 = most severe impairment).

The Barthel Index was used to assess activities of daily living in 10 areas (feeding, transfers bed to chair and back, grooming, toilet use, bathing, mobility, climbing stairs, dressing, stool control, bladder control).

The Spitzer Index is a global quality of life measure covering five areas (activity, daily life, health, social relations, and future perspectives with a maximum score of 10 points.

The BCRS, GDS, and Spitzer Index were rated by physicians and the Barthel Index by nurses. All ratings, including the 65-item list, were made on the same occasion. Data collection was carried out using electronic questionnaires implemented through the Quality-of-Life Recorder technology (Sigle & Porzsolt, 1996).

## Statistical Analysis

Descriptive statistics were generated for demographic data and diagnostic categories and for the BCRS and GDS scales, the Barthel and Spitzer Indices, and the newly developed instrument. A factor analysis (principal component analysis, oblimin with

Kaiser normalization as rotation method) was performed based on these 771 assessments. The number of interpretable factors was determined by interpretation of a scree plot. The consistency of the factors was tested by Cronbach's alpha coefficients. To improve the consistency of the scales, items were deleted based on the criteria of changes in magnitude of Cronbach's alpha coefficients and on the fit of the item with the content of the core items of the factors. To test the stability of the factor structure, we conducted separate analyses for doctors and nurses. For testing construct validity, we used the two external criteria Brief Cognitive Rating Scale and the Barthel Index. Spearman rank correlation coefficients were calculated to test for interrater reliability. We included only data in which the electronic recording confirmed that it was obtained at exactly the same time.

## Results

Most patients suffered from severe dementia, as indicated by the results (all given as the mean ± SD) of the BCRS (57 ± 8.8) and GDS (5.7 ± 1.1), the low level of activities of daily living (Barthel Index 26.8 ± 29.7) in the present sample, and the distribution of diagnoses according to the ICD-10.

Of the 771 assessments, 386 were performed by nurses and 385 by physicians. Based on the electronic recordings, we identified 22 pairs of assessments made at the same time by a nurse and a physician. A planned feasibility analysis after 120 assessments resulted in the exclusion of the Spitzer Index because of a general floor effect (mean score < 3).

The factor analysis suggested five factors based on the interpretation of the scree plot. The results of the five-factor solution are provided in Table 8.1, which shows high eigenvalues and an explained variance of more than 60%. To improve the consistency of the five factors, 18 of the original 65 items were deleted based on the criteria of changes in magnitude of Cronbach's alpha coefficients and on the fit of the item with the content of the core items of the factors. In a next step, eight further items were excluded owing to different factor loadings among raters and content considerations, leaving the following five factors: communication (15 items), negative affect (10 items), body contact (5 items), aggression (4 items), and mobility (6 items). The factor structure matrix, including the single items for physicians and nurses, is shown in Table 8.2 and demonstrates a high congruency of the factor structure between the two groups of raters on the item level.

TABLE 8.1. Eigenvalues and explained amounts of variance for the five-factor solution

| Factor | Eigenvalues | | % of Variance | | Cumulative % | |
|---|---|---|---|---|---|---|
| | Nurse | Physician | Nurse | Physician | Nurse | Physician |
| 1 | 10.0 | 10.7 | 24.4 | 26.0 | 24.4 | 26.0 |
| 2 | 5.7 | 6.1 | 13.8 | 15.0 | 38.2 | 41.0 |
| 3 | 4.9 | 4.8 | 11.9 | 11.8 | 50.0 | 52.1 |
| 4 | 2.5 | 2.1 | 6.1 | 5.0 | 56.1 | 58.0 |
| 5 | 2.0 | 2.5 | 4.9 | 6.1 | 61.0 | 63.9 |

Extraction method was the principal component analysis.

TABLE 8.2. Structure matrix

| Factor | 1 Nurse | 1 Physician | 2 Nurse | 2 Physician | 3 Nurse | 3 Physician | 4 Nurse | 4 Physician | 5 Nurse | 5 Physician |
|---|---|---|---|---|---|---|---|---|---|---|
| **Communication** | | | | | | | | | | |
| ITEM 59 | 0.82 | 0.83 | −0.19 | −0.14 | 0.04 | −0.32 | 0.29 | 0.05 | 0.06 | 0.25 |
| ITEM 62 | 0.81 | 0.64 | 0.02 | 0.16 | 0.08 | −0.39 | 0.28 | 0.22 | −0.09 | 0.34 |
| ITEM 6 | 0.79 | 0.78 | −0.26 | 0.13 | −0.07 | −0.29 | 0.18 | 0.08 | 0.10 | 0.17 |
| ITEM 61 | 0.79 | 0.67 | −0.23 | −0.13 | 0.10 | −0.56 | 0.22 | 0.09 | 0.08 | 0.25 |
| ITEM 8 | 0.78 | 0.81 | −0.20 | 0.08 | −0.16 | −0.25 | 0.14 | 0.12 | 0.12 | 0.18 |
| ITEM 65 | 0.73 | 0.77 | −0.27 | −0.13 | −0.05 | −0.05 | 0.52 | 0.10 | 0.01 | 0.48 |
| ITEM 56 | 0.70 | 0.69 | −0.08 | 0.08 | −0.15 | 0.07 | 0.07 | −0.06 | 0.05 | 0.10 |
| ITEM 14 | 0.70 | 0.85 | −0.11 | −0.11 | 0.02 | −0.10 | 0.44 | −0.06 | 0.15 | 0.26 |
| ITEM 32 | 0.66 | 0.64 | −0.14 | −0.06 | 0.35 | −0.48 | 0.03 | −0.11 | 0.15 | 0.22 |
| ITEM 31 | 0.65 | 0.65 | −0.12 | 0.01 | 0.32 | −0.54 | 0.08 | 0.00 | 0.15 | 0.19 |
| ITEM 13 | 0.64 | 0.76 | −0.24 | −0.04 | 0.06 | −0.42 | 0.11 | 0.13 | 0.12 | 0.20 |
| ITEM 50 | 0.64 | 0.77 | −0.40 | −0.19 | −0.04 | −0.17 | 0.46 | −0.03 | 0.19 | 0.35 |
| ITEM 64 | 0.62 | 0.61 | 0.05 | 0.13 | 0.06 | −0.17 | 0.49 | −0.21 | 0.03 | 0.40 |
| ITEM 60 | 0.59 | 0.69 | 0.12 | 0.17 | −0.27 | 0.03 | 0.01 | 0.28 | −0.11 | 0.07 |
| ITEM 15 | 0.45 | 0.73 | 0.03 | −0.13 | −0.08 | 0.19 | 0.34 | −0.19 | 0.12 | 0.06 |
| **Negative affect** | | | | | | | | | | |
| ITEM 18 | −0.08 | 0.04 | 0.83 | 0.87 | −0.03 | −0.14 | −0.08 | 0.11 | −0.28 | −0.02 |
| ITEM 22 | −0.04 | 0.09 | 0.80 | 0.74 | 0.11 | −0.34 | −0.10 | 0.08 | −0.20 | 0.00 |
| ITEM 3 | −0.07 | 0.02 | 0.75 | 0.82 | 0.16 | −0.18 | −0.13 | 0.17 | −0.11 | −0.06 |
| ITEM 24 | −0.09 | −0.01 | 0.74 | 0.76 | −0.05 | −0.18 | −0.05 | 0.12 | −0.37 | 0.08 |
| ITEM 27 | 0.04 | 0.02 | 0.66 | 0.77 | −0.13 | −0.10 | −0.17 | 0.45 | −0.45 | −0.05 |
| ITEM 17 | −0.28 | −0.17 | 0.66 | 0.71 | −0.08 | 0.14 | −0.16 | 0.38 | −0.58 | −0.12 |
| ITEM 25 | −0.30 | 0.17 | 0.65 | 0.63 | 0.03 | −0.02 | −0.29 | −0.02 | −0.08 | −0.07 |
| ITEM 54 | −0.20 | −0.20 | 0.62 | 0.58 | −0.09 | 0.10 | 0.19 | 0.28 | −0.34 | 0.05 |
| ITEM 53 | −0.10 | −0.01 | 0.60 | 0.50 | −0.07 | 0.23 | 0.14 | 0.17 | −0.28 | 0.01 |
| ITEM 47 | −0.28 | −0.26 | 0.53 | 0.61 | 0.00 | 0.11 | −0.26 | 0.37 | −0.45 | −0.11 |
| **Bodily contact** | | | | | | | | | | |
| ITEM 35 | 0.00 | 0.17 | 0.02 | −0.03 | 0.93 | −0.76 | −0.08 | −0.13 | 0.11 | −0.11 |
| ITEM 34 | 0.01 | 0.27 | 0.00 | 0.07 | 0.93 | −0.81 | −0.09 | −0.12 | 0.12 | −0.09 |
| ITEM 33 | 0.03 | 0.37 | 0.00 | 0.14 | 0.90 | −0.77 | −0.09 | −0.06 | 0.12 | 0.00 |
| ITEM 36 | −0.06 | −0.21 | 0.01 | 0.10 | 0.89 | −0.81 | −0.13 | −0.15 | 0.16 | −0.08 |
| ITEM 37 | −0.06 | −0.27 | 0.01 | 0.15 | 0.86 | −0.76 | −0.12 | −0.16 | 0.17 | −0.06 |
| **Aggression** | | | | | | | | | | |
| ITEM 4 | −0.14 | 0.01 | 0.25 | 0.27 | −0.19 | 0.08 | 0.13 | 0.91 | −0.88 | 0.08 |
| ITEM 19 | −0.24 | −0.05 | 0.31 | 0.18 | −0.22 | 0.16 | 0.13 | 0.84 | −0.83 | 0.09 |
| ITEM 1 | 0.05 | 0.20 | 0.28 | 0.20 | −0.07 | 0.12 | 0.01 | 0.71 | −0.78 | 0.08 |
| ITEM 29 | 0.22 | 0.11 | 0.20 | 0.21 | −0.10 | 0.05 | 0.03 | 0.84 | −0.77 | 0.15 |
| **Mobility** | | | | | | | | | | |
| ITEM 40 | 0.42 | 0.56 | −0.31 | −0.23 | −0.20 | 0.08 | 0.79 | −0.14 | 0.22 | 0.80 |
| ITEM 41 | 0.49 | 0.64 | −0.28 | −0.27 | −0.23 | 0.07 | 0.71 | −0.19 | 0.23 | 0.63 |
| ITEM 57 | 0.01 | 0.01 | 0.01 | 0.08 | −0.05 | 0.00 | 0.68 | 0.14 | −0.18 | 0.70 |
| ITEM 42 | 0.04 | 0.07 | 0.07 | 0.06 | −0.02 | 0.05 | 0.68 | 0.20 | −0.18 | 0.80 |
| ITEM 43 | 0.43 | 0.63 | −0.43 | −0.15 | −0.08 | −0.09 | 0.66 | 0.00 | 0.22 | 0.64 |
| ITEM 55 | 0.41 | 0.46 | −0.14 | −0.07 | −0.10 | 0.04 | 0.42 | −0.23 | 0.03 | 0.34 |

Extraction method was the principal component analysis; rotation method was the Oblimin with Kaiser normalization.

In addition, it appeared that the factors were generally unrelated to each other except for significant correlations between the factors "communication" and "body contact" ($r = 0.25$; $p < 0.001$ each) and "mobility" and "negative affect" (physicians: $r = 0.22$; $p = 0.001$; nurses: $r = -0.33$; $p < 0.01$). Cronbach's alpha coefficients as a measure of internal consistency were high for both nurses and physicians (Table 8.3). The congruence of nurses' and physicians' ratings is further demonstrated by similar item severity (relative ratings) and selectivity of the single factors (Table 8.4).

TABLE 8.3. Cronbach's alpha coefficients

| Factor | No. of items | Nurse | Physician |
|---|---|---|---|
| 1 – Communication | 15 | 0.93 | 0.94 |
| 2 – Negative affect | 10 | 0.88 | 0.89 |
| 3 – Body contact | 5 | 0.90 | 0.90 |
| 4 – Aggression | 4 | 0.86 | 0.87 |
| 5 – Mobility | 6 | 0.81 | 0.82 |

TABLE 8.4. Item severity and selectivity

| Parameter | Item severity | | Item selectivity | |
|---|---|---|---|---|
| | Nurse | Physician | Nurse | Physician |
| Communication | | | | |
| 59 Responds to distant calls | 0.57 | 0.63 | 0.82 | 0.85 |
| 62 Seeks contact | 0.53 | 0.56 | 0.81 | 0.71 |
| 06 Speaks comprehensibly | 0.64 | 0.69 | 0.79 | 0.81 |
| 61 Contact possible | 0.83 | 0.90 | 0.79 | 0.74 |
| 08 Speaks meaningful groups of words | 0.59 | 0.68 | 0.77 | 0.82 |
| 65 Eats and drinks by him/herself | 0.66 | 0.68 | 0.79 | 0.78 |
| 56 Reads newspaper | 0.24 | 0.19 | 0.69 | 0.64 |
| 14 Carries out simple orders | 0.39 | 0.64 | 0.73 | 0.84 |
| 32 Maintains visual contact | 0.72 | 0.74 | 0.65 | 0.71 |
| 31 Visual contact possible | 0.80 | 0.85 | 0.63 | 0.72 |
| 13 Comprehends single words | 0.89 | 0.88 | 0.63 | 0.81 |
| 50 Uses both hands intentionally | 0.62 | 0.67 | 0.70 | 0.79 |
| 64 Worries about others | 0.25 | 0.23 | 0.65 | 0.63 |
| 60 Rings the bell | 0.29 | 0.31 | 0.58 | 0.67 |
| 15 Carries out complicated orders | 0.08 | 0.24 | 0.47 | 0.64 |
| Negative affect | | | | |
| 18 Full of despair | 0.40 | 0.43 | 0.82 | 0.86 |
| 22 Sad/crying | 0.32 | 0.36 | 0.77 | 0.75 |
| 03 Whining voice | 0.33 | 0.32 | 0.72 | 0.83 |
| 24 Nervous/anxious | 0.37 | 0.40 | 0.76 | 0.75 |
| 27 Wailing | 0.30 | 0.31 | 0.69 | 0.80 |
| 17 Tensed | 0.36 | 0.43 | 0.73 | 0.72 |
| 25 Resigned | 0.27 | 0.38 | 0.65 | 0.63 |
| 54 Restless/confused | 0.25 | 0.31 | 0.62 | 0.59 |
| 53 Problems falling asleep | 0.25 | 0.36 | 0.59 | 0.49 |
| 47 Muscular tension | 0.37 | 0.43 | 0.60 | 0.62 |

(*Continued*)

TABLE 8.4. (*Continued*)

| Parameter | Item severity | | Item selectivity | |
|---|---|---|---|---|
| | Nurse | Physician | Nurse | Physician |
| Body contact | | | | |
| 35 Body contact possible on shoulders | 0.77 | 0.87 | 0.92 | 0.78 |
| 34 Body contact possible on arms | 0.81 | 0.91 | 0.90 | 0.80 |
| 33 Body contact possible on hands | 0.82 | 0.94 | 0.88 | 0.73 |
| 36 Body contact possible on the head | 0.63 | 0.63 | 0.91 | 0.88 |
| 37 Body contact possible on the face | 0.56 | 0.55 | 0.88 | 0.84 |
| Aggression | | | | |
| 04 Aggressive voice | 0.27 | 0.27 | 0.89 | 0.90 |
| 19 Aggressive acts | 0.21 | 0.19 | 0.85 | 0.84 |
| 01 Loud voice | 0.32 | 0.33 | 0.80 | 0.80 |
| 29 Insults others | 0.23 | 0.22 | 0.81 | 0.88 |
| Mobility | | | | |
| 40 Walks upright | 0.37 | 0.40 | 0.92 | 0.95 |
| 41 Walks straight up to something | 0.33 | 0.36 | 0.87 | 0.87 |
| 57 Departs from ward | 0.07 | 0.05 | 0.53 | 0.46 |
| 42 Wanders around | 0.16 | 0.17 | 0.53 | 0.62 |
| 43 Sits upright | 0.57 | 0.57 | 0.80 | 0.81 |
| 55 Willing to help on ward | 0.13 | 0.09 | 0.55 | 0.54 |

For testing construct validity, we used two external criteria, the Brief Cognitive Rating Scale (BCRS) used by physicians and the Barthel Index used by nurses (Table 8.5). The correlation coefficients between the various areas of the BCRS and the two relevant scales of the new instrument (communication and mobility) indicate satisfactory validity. The second criteria, the Barthel Index (a measure of activities of daily living), was significantly correlated with the scales "communication" and "mobility" of our instrument. Furthermore, the latter correlated with the scale "negative affect" and "acceptance of body contact" in the expected direction. When testing for gender differences concerning the factors, we found significant differences for all but one factor (Table 8.6). The interrater reliability between subsamples of physicians and nurses also proved to be satisfactory (Table 8.7).

# Discussion

The special problem associated with assessing well-being in patients with severe dementia is their lack of competence, which compromises the reliability of their reports. Consequently, observer ratings are the only alternative for such self-ratings. However, observer ratings have the potential risk of overrating the well-being of patients if the provider and rater of health care services are identical. We have controlled for this risk by semiquantitatively describing the frequency of distinct behavior patterns in demented patients.

TABLE 8.5. Correlations with BCRS scores and the Barthel Index

| Parameter | Communication | Negative affect | Bodily contact | Aggression | Mobility |
|---|---|---|---|---|---|
| Physicians | | | | | |
| BCRS 1: concentration | −0.71* | 0.05 | 0.07 | −0.02 | −0.45* |
| BCRS 2: short–term memory | −0.67* | 0.02 | 0.11 | −0.01 | −0.42* |
| BCRS 3: long–term memory | −0.68* | 0.14 | 0.09 | 0.08 | −0.46* |
| BCRS 4: orientation | − 0.65* | 0.12 | 0.12 | 0.11 | −0.40* |
| BCRS 5: everyday life competence | −0.47* | −0.04 | −0.04 | −0.10 | −0.44* |
| BCRS 6: language | −0.71* | −0.02 | 0.02 | −0.09 | −0.37* |
| BCRS 7: psychomotorics | −0.41* | −0.01 | 0.06 | −0.10 | −0.59* |
| BCRS 8: mood and behavior | −0.60* | 0.10 | −0.02 | 0.03 | −0.34* |
| BCRS 9: constructive skills | −0.55* | 0.03 | 0.02 | −0.06 | −0.34* |
| BCRS 10: calculation skills | −0.59* | 0.17* | 0.09 | 0.09 | −0.35* |
| Main axis | −0.73* | 0.07 | 0.09 | 0.02 | −0.49* |
| Co-axis | −0.71* | 0.07 | 0.04 | −0.03 | −0.49* |
| BCRS total score | −0.74* | 0.07 | 0.06 | −0.01 | −0.50* |
| Nurses | | | | | |
| Barthel item 1: feeding | 0.70* | −0.21* | −0.10 | 0.02 | 0.63* |
| Barthel item 2: transfer | 0.46* | −0.27* | −0.17* | −0.08 | 0.83* |
| Barthel item 3: personal care | 0.41* | −0.17* | −0.02 | −0.12 | 0.36* |
| Barthel item 4: toilet use | 0.47* | −0.25* | −0.20* | −0.12 | 0.67* |
| Barthel item 5: bathing | 0.08 | −0.07 | 0.04 | −0.06 | 0.09 |
| Barthel item 6: moving | 0.43* | −0.28* | −0.18* | −0.09 | 0.83* |
| Barthel item 7: stairs | 0.32* | −0.23* | −0.14 | −0.03 | 0.72* |
| Barthel item 8: dressing | 0.51* | −0.23* | −0.22* | −0.09 | 0.67* |
| Barthel item 9: bowel | 0.48* | −0.20* | −0.16* | −0.15* | 0.57* |
| Barthel item 10: bladder control | 0.44* | −0.20* | −0.22* | 0.14 | 0.56* |
| Barthel Index | 0.56* | −0.28* | −0.20* | −0.10 | 0.83* |

BCRS: Brief Cognitive Rating Scale.
*$p < 0.001$.

TABLE 8.6. Factor scores of observations by gender of the patients

| Factor | Observations of males[a] (n = 123) | Observations of females[a] (n = 648) | t-score | p |
|---|---|---|---|---|
| 1 – Communication | 34.8 ± 13.2 | 33.8 ± 11.8 | 0.82 | 0.415 |
| 2 – Negative affect | 9.5± 6.7 | 14.8 ± 6.7 | −8.37 | < 0.001 |
| 3 – Body contact | 14.9 ± 4.3 | 16.7± 4.9 | −4.18 | < 0.001 |
| 4 – Aggression | 3.1± 3.0 | 4.3 ± 3.5 | −3.21 | 0.001 |
| 5 – Mobility | 8.1 ± 5.5 | 6.3 ± 5.5 | 3.38 | 0.001 |

[a]Mean ± SD.

The results of this study demonstrate that the behavior of old old patients with severe dementia can be described by the five factors of the Vienna List. By explaining more than 60% of the total variance, these five factors obviously cover a considerable part of the possible spectrum of behavior in these patients.

TABLE 8.7. Paired sample test and Spearman rank correlation coefficients between nurses and physicians concerning the same patient on the same day (22 pairs)

| Factor | Nurses[a] | Physicians[a] | t-score/p | R/p |
|---|---|---|---|---|
| 1 – Communication | 25.8 ± 10.5 | 26.4 ± 8.9 | – 0.35/0.727 | 0.71/< 0.001 |
| 2 – Negative affect | 11.9 ± 7.6 | 8.6 ± 5.0 | 2.46/0.023 | 0.57/ 0.006 |
| 3 – Body contact | 15.9 ± 5.7 | 18.4 ± 2.9 | – 2.22/0.038 | 0.53/ 0.011 |
| 4 – Aggression | 4.3 ± 3.0 | 2.2 ± 2.1 | 3.69/0.001 | 0.35/ 0.112 |
| 5 – Mobility | 6.5 ± 5.7 | 5.1 ± 5.8 | 2.03/0.056 | 0.81/< 0.001 |

[a]Mean ± SD.

R/p = rank correlation coefficient/p value.

Because nurses and physicians have contact of different intensity with patients and their corresponding different perspectives, it was surprising that their assessments correlated highly in three of the five factors. The two factors aggression and mobility yielded higher scores among nurses than among doctors.

As concerns aggression, there are mainly two explanations for this difference. First, nurses spend more time and have closer contact with the patients and consequently have a higher risk of inducing aggressive behavior. In addition, the extended period of contact increases the chance of experiencing an episode of aggressive behavior. Secondly, patients normally behave differently toward nurses and doctors owing to differences in role expectation and familiarity related to the frequency of contact. However, we consider this latter explanation as unlikely in these patients because of their cognitive impairment.

Regarding mobility, it is plausible that the doctors report lower scores for mobility of the patients because they mainly see the patients under certain circumstances, such as during rounds where the ward routines limit the mobility of the patient.

Because these five factors encompass most of the behavioral repertoire of demented old old patients, we assume that the factors can be regarded as a useful approach to describing the well-being of these patients.

*Acknowledgment.* This research was supported by the Guest Professorship Program of the University of Ulm, Germany, and a Scientific Medical Grant from the Mayor of the City of Vienna, Austria.

## References

Barofsky, I. (1996). Cognitive aspects of quality of life assessment. In: B. Spilker (Ed.), *Quality of life and pharmacoeconomics in clinical trials.* Philadelphia: Lippincott-Raven.

Kitwood, T., Bredin, K. (1997). *Evaluating dementia care: the DCM method* (7th ed.). Bradford, UK: Bradford Dementia Research Group, Bradford University.

Lawton, M.P. (1994). Quality of life in Alzheimer disease. *Alzheimer Disease Associated Disorders*, 8(Suppl 3), 138–150.

Lawton, M.P., van Haitsma, K., Klapper J. (1996). Observed affect in nursing home residents with Alzheimer's disease. *The Journals of Gerontology Series B: Psychological Sciences and Social Sciences*, 51B, 3–14.

Lawton, M. P., Carsten, R., Parmelee, P. A., van Haitsma, K., Corn, J., Kleban, M.H. (1998). Psychometric characteristics of the minimum data set II: validity. *Journal of the American Geriatric Society*, 46, 736–744.

Mahoney, F., Barthel, D.W. (1965). Functional evaluation: the Barthel Index. *Maryland State Medical Journal*, 14, 61–65.

Ready, R.E., Ott, B.R. (2003). Quality of life measures for dementia. *Health and Quality of Life Outcomes*, 1, 1–9.

Reisberg, B., Ferris, S.H., de Leon, M.J., Crook, T. (1982). The Global Deterioration Scale (GDS). *Psychopharmacological Bulletin*, 24, 629–636.

Reisberg, B., Schneck, M.K., Ferris, S.H., Schwartz, G.E., de Leon, M.J. (1983). The Brief Cognitive Rating Scale (BCRS): findings in primary degenerative dementia (PDD). *Psychopharmacological Bulletin*, 19, 47–50.

Sigle, J., Porzsolt, F. (1996). Practical aspects of quality of life measurement: design and feasibility study of the Quality-of-Life-Recorder and the standardized measurement of quality of life in an outpatient clinic. *Cancer Treatment Review*, 22, 75–90.

Spitzer, W.O., Dobson, A.J., Hall, J. (1981). Measuring the quality of life of cancer patients. *Journal of Chronic Disease*, 34, 585–597.

WHOQOL group (1995). The World Health Organization Quality of Life assessment (WHOQOL): position paper from the World Health Organization. *Social Science and Medicine*, 41, 1403–1409.

# 9
# Patient Empowerment: Increased Compliance or Total Transformation?

Susan B. Rifkin

Over the past decade, the idea of patient empowerment has been increasing in popularity. Although there is no consensus on the definition of this term, the concept contains some essential elements on which all can agree. They include involvement of the patient in decisions about personal health care and increased sharing of knowledge by health professionals to ensure that decisions are made wisely. However, it is not surprising that there is a range of views about the degree of power that patients should and do have and the context in which they should exercise this power. These views are rooted in ideological, political, and historical frameworks; and they center on ideas about professional dominance and, more broadly, on changes in structures and institutions that deliver health care.

Many reasons are given to support patient empowerment. Professionals argue that only through patient empowerment can patients comply with the advice they provide (Feste & Anderson, 1995). Advocates of equity in health care argue that only through policies that allow patients to become engaged in decisions about their own health can health needs of the poor be addressed (Anderson, 1996). Those concerned with health care costs and coverage argue patients must become involved in their own care to reduce waste and coverage (Segal, 1998). Patients themselves, especially women, are demanding information to make choices about their own health in some societies (Linden, 1994).

The literature suggests that, historically, arguments to support patient empowerment derive from two views about the role and power of patients. One view is that compliance with doctors' orders, which is critical to good health and health improvements, can best be pursued and maintained when the patient becomes actively involved in decisions about his or her own health. This view, discussed widely by medical professionals, suggests that improved compliance with medical advice is a critical element in good health. The other most widely argued interpretation of health improvements suggests that the health of individuals improves not merely by complying with doctors' orders but also by transforming patients' own ideas and attitudes about health. This transformation comes about, first, by dealing with health in the context of the social and economic situation and then by having professionals provide the knowledge and skills that build confidence for people to have power over their own lives (Anderson, 1996). The former view is one that is embedded in the biomedical interpretation of health, and the latter is embedded in the socioeconomic interpretation about how health improves. These two views are not mutually exclusive. However, the arguments and concerns that support each view do not have the same priority.

The purpose of this chapter is to explore in some detail the views that relate patient empowerment to improved health. I examine the historical development of each position and the arguments that support the importance of patient empowerment in each context. I then review the evidence that relates to improved health outcomes in the context of each view. In the discussion, I highlight practical and conceptual issues arising from the previous descriptions.

## Good Health as Compliance

Those who understand patient empowerment in the context of compliance argue that the value of patient empowerment is that it improves patients' responses to medical directives. This view is rooted in the discipline of social psychology and proposes the patient as an active participant in the management of illness and health. As Salmon and Hall (2003) discussed, this approach is historically based on the view that the body is a machine that can be supported and repaired within a scientific and Western framework. Good health is defined as the absence of disease, and the role of the medical profession is to cure or prevent disease and keep the body functioning as a well maintained organism.

Patient empowerment in the context of compliance focuses on three main issues. The first is patient acceptance of professional directives and responsibility. The second is patient education, and the third is the provision of information.

Concerning the first issue, professionals have traditionally controlled the management of disease in individuals, thus relieving patients of responsibility. However, as patients confront areas that are problematic for medicine (such as unexplained symptoms, chronic pain, and disease), the professional has difficulty accepting full responsibility, largely because the reasons for the patient's compliance and the effect of medical treatment are not clear. As a result, clinicians now encourage patients to deal with their own health problems.

Regarding the issue of patient education, Feste and Anderson (1995) examined this dialogue in the context of diseases such as diabetes, which require not only drug compliance but also a lifestyle change. They pointed to the development of an empowerment approach that is rooted in both psychology and education. This approach to disease control rejects the earlier approach of compliance, in which education is used by health professionals to persuade patients to follow specific behaviors. Instead, education is seen as a way to enable patients to increase their self-reliance and expand their freedom of choice. By focusing on the role of education and, specifically, health educators in health improvement, the new approach to compliance is broadened to take into account factors beyond the rigid biomedical view of health. These factors include the patient's lifestyle as well as the attitudes and behaviors of both health professionals and patients. However, because the approach sees health improvements as a result of individual compliance and professional dominance over patient choices, it deals with empowerment within the relatively limited context of causes and cures of disease embedded in the biomedical model of health.

Patient empowerment through education is rapidly expanding owing to access to information on the Internet (Hersh, 1999). Grol (2001) cited findings suggesting that 40% to 50% of people who access the Internet do so to find medical information. He went on to point out, however, that both the quality and accessibility for laymen is variable; and, at present, there is little research to investigate the impact of this information on patient care or doctor–patient communication. The potential of this type of information is increasingly being recognized, as reflected in the rapidly proliferating literature.

As suggested above, the area of chronic disease is highly suitable for investigating patient empowerment. The literature here is most prolific and continues to expand. The studies come mainly from research in Western industrial societies, where considerable experience and institutional support for these types of investigation exist. Investigations into behavioral changes in diabetics (Kidd et al., 2004) and people with lower-back pain (Skelton, 1997) are typical of studies of this nature. Designed as intervention studies (where patient education is the critical intervention), these investigations attempt to measure changes in behavior in individuals within the context of self-management of their illness. They focus on *outcome* rather than *process*. Those who look at education (Skelton, 1997) rather than merely the provision of information (Kidd et al., 2004) often present new theories about how patient education is conceived and implemented (Feste & Anderson, 1995).

What is the evidence that patient empowerment in the context of compliance is improving the quality of medical care and providing better health outcomes? In a study that compared different approaches, including evidence-based medicine and clinical practice guidelines, professional development, assessment and accountability, total quality management, and patient empowerment, Grol (2001) reviewed the literature to answer this question. He said that most research has been focused on doctor–patient communication, and he cited reviews that showed that patient satisfaction and compliance improve when the doctor is more involved in sharing information with the patients. However, many patients, although having positive feelings about receiving information, do not want to be involved in decision making, which could reflect a reluctance to accept responsibility for their own health. The conclusion is that the value of empowering patients by providing more information and education has yet to be demonstrated on a wide scale.

In addition, Grol pointed out two dangers. The first concerns unrealistic expectations on the part of patients, who now have access to information. These expectations include demands on professionals to provide alternative treatments and views about positive outcomes of their medical problems. The second is the expansion of consumerism through advertisement of services and medicines. Increased advertising by drug manufacturers has led to patients demanding patented medicines. Not only are these medicines more expensive than their generic counterparts, many can be bought over-the-counter (OTC) without a prescription. OTCs being taken without the indications having been discussed with the doctor have become a large public health problem. The recent example of painkillers being removed from the market by the U.S. Food and Drug Administration highlights such dangers.

## Health as Equity

Health improvements that are analyzed in the context of equity contribute another approach to the value of patient empowerment. Equity in health refers to addressing differences in health among groups of people that reflect unfairness and that are avoidable (Evans et al., 2001). Thus, any discussion about equity implies an ethical/moral judgment, which is not the case in discussions about compliance. Much of the early work concerning equity and social justice in health emerged from the developing countries in the wake of the departure of colonial governments after World War II. Evidence from The Rockefeller Foundation (Bryant, 1969) and from the experience of British medical doctors working in Africa (King, 1966) indicated that health was not only a result of the provision of health services. Poor health resulted equally from a lack of resources and limited access to the limited resources available. The socioeconomic environment also played a major role, particularly in the poor health of the impoverished.

These concerns laid the basis for the World Health Organization's conference on Primary Health Care in 1978 (WHO/UNICEF, 1978). At this time, the member nations of the WHO accepted primary health care as the policy for all nations, resulting in national policies committed to taking into account equity and participation (key to empowerment) as key elements (Rifkin, 2003). Policies supporting equity and empowerment have continued to be a concern of international United Nations agencies (WHO, 1986; World Bank, 2000). Their concern is supported by data that concludes there are wide health disparities among groups in the same geographic area and that these differences are perpetuated by socioeconomic disparities (Bravemann & Tarimo, 2002). The conclusion for some is that these gaps can be closed only by confronting the wider causes of poor health. One approach is to provide opportunities for the poor to gain knowledge, skills, experience, and confidence to change their own lives (Anderson, 1996; Rifkin & Pridmore, 2001). In this context, empowerment goes beyond mere participation in health care. It addresses the issue of transformation, focusing on patient and community changes in attitudes and behavior rooted in a shift of control from professional to lay person (Sen, 1997).

Patient empowerment in the context of equity focuses on three major issues: social justice, the distribution of health care related to resources and costs, and the role of health promotion. In the literature, the issue of social justice within the wider social context has been addressed by Rawls (1971). In the health context, the Nobel Laureate Amatya Sen, in his book *Development as Freedom* (1999), used health extensively to illustrate his arguments. Essentially, the social justice argument says that those with limited opportunities due to their economic and/or social conditions are denied their human rights to good health. To gain these rights, access to health services is a necessary, but not sufficient, condition. The circumstances that keep people in poverty must also be addressed. In the context of health, professionals have a duty to address health problems in a holistic way and to provide opportunities for the poor to transform their conditions and behaviors. To do so, professionals must examine and address the structures that contribute to inequities. Anderson (1996) provided an example of this approach in her research on immigrant women in Canada who have a chronic illness. Her investigation shows how these women were unable to make use of services provided (in this case management of diabetes) because they lacked confidence, self-esteem, and incentives. In addition, the structure of health care support did not encourage these women to seek and use the available health services.

The second issue—service provision related to resources and costs—is at the center of health system reforms in national health care systems. It has been argued that health services provided mainly by governments are inefficient and often ineffective (Kaul, 1997). Reforms that focus on decentralization have been promoted to correct these problems. A wider role for lay people who are community leaders and reflect local concerns about health services is a key element to ensure accountability and transparency at the local level. Patient empowerment in this context is discussed in terms of economic reforms of health care provision and uses the language of economists rather than of health professionals. Central to this view of empowerment is demand-driven reforms that promote a greater role for the consumers (patients) of health services. This role would be supported by access to information, including alternative assessments of problems, and mechanisms to create inputs to health budgets at the service-provider level (Segal, 1998). Segal argued that if the above conditions are met consumers (patients) will have a greater capacity to follow healthy life styles and reduce risks of poor health outcomes.

The third issue is the focus on health promotion as a means by which empowerment can develop. In his book *Health Promotion Practice: Power and Empowerment*, Laverack (2004) explored the relationship between health promotion and empowerment in detail. After a review of the literature and a discussion of the importance of WHO's Ottawa Charter (WHO, 1986) to the advocacy of empowerment of lay people, he proposed a method by which to pursue empowerment as a goal in health programs. Emphasizing both the process and outcome of transformation as the key to health improvements, Laverack provided a framework for action for health workers. The framework is useful to those concerned with structural change and demand-driven reforms in quest of improvements in health outcomes and health care provision.

Patient empowerment in the context of equity defines health in holistic terms, taking into account the socioeconomic-political environment, as well as causes of and cures for disease. The literature concerning these issues is far more encompassing than that considering empowerment with reference to compliance. Data used when presenting this view rarely come from intervention studies or from studies confined to Western industrial societies. Rather, a literature search reveals publications that cover topics from most countries in the world and look at the range of health determinants, including income, female literacy, and household expenditure, as well as health service access and utilization. A good example of the diversity of analysis can be found in Evans et al. (2001), where studies range from social inequalities and the burden of health in the United States to examining adolescent lives and livelihoods in Tanzania.

What is the evidence that patient empowerment in the context of addressing equity is improving the quality of medical care and providing better health outcomes? Although a great deal has been written about the potential improvements, the evidence to support these outcomes is weak. Authors critically reviewing the data, rather than advocating an approach, conclude that there is a major barrier in the existing health provision environment (Rifkin, 2003). Some studies have concluded that health professionals assume a dominant role in discussions with patients (Aady, 2000). They are neither trained nor prepared to surrender this role and resist changes that demand an equal partnership. Health professionals are also resistant to changes that move their understanding of health into the wider socioeconomic environment; they prefer to stay in the biomedical domain in which they have been trained and are experienced.

## Discussion

The preceding examination of patient empowerment raises a number of points for discussion. From the practical side, both health professionals and policy makers seek answers to critical questions. Professionals want to know about the interest, capacity, and ability of lay people to become involved in decisions about their own health. They also want to know whether and why the process of involvement is related to health outcomes. For the policy maker, questions focus on what changes in institutions and structures are necessary to incorporate patient involvement. They also want to know whether patient empowerment can be cost-effective and efficient or if time and money will be wasted in terms of improving health outcomes.

On the conceptual level, the issue of power and control is pivotal. The word "empowerment" has "power" at the center. Discussions about patient empowerment are, at the root, discussions about who has what power and how is it exercised. Answers to this question are ideological as well as political. The ideology revolves around the belief in the superiority of Western scientific medicine in achieving health improvements versus the value of a holistic view of health. It also revolves around the ethical issues of resource distribution to target the poor. The politics revolve around the resistance of those who have power to relinquish it. Basically, professionals and policy makers want to achieve a balance between professional and lay concerns. How this balance is to be achieved is seen differently in the context of compliance than it is in the context of equity. In addition, the differing views can be regarded as conflict rather than consensus.

Those who advocate patient empowerment in the compliance context are accused of limiting the context to biomedical concerns. It is argued that they do not wish to examine the implications of empowerment in a more holistic way because it means confronting the question of professional dominance. Such confrontation would lead to questioning the power and control of professionals and the legitimacy of the concepts on which they base their domination. The equity argument, however, raises concerns about bringing scientific decisions into an explicitly political realm. Not only can the authority of professionals be undermined, but such politicization of health care decisions could be detrimental to health care as well as unrealistic to implement.

Whereas this dichotomy has historical roots that were traced earlier in the chapter, the past decade has seen a shift from the defense of a fixed position to a search for mutual interests. During a period labeled "postmodern," the trend is to highlight the contributions of various interpretations and meanings and focus on the value of a range of views in specific situations. To be precise, we are presently experiencing exploration of an interpretation of patient empowerment in both views and the application of a mix that is most relevant to the specific problems. This approach leads to identifying commonalties rather than differences and to searching for the relevance of theory and practice. Discussions of patient empowerment for compliance and/or equity focus on both process and content, on using both "top down" (professionally led) and "bottom up" (lay-person led) solutions, on educating both professionals and patients (not merely providing information), and on recognizing change as inevitable.

## Conclusion

There is a growing interest in the role of patient empowerment in improving health care. This chapter has identified several issues that have been highlighted in the literature, including the role of the health professional, the expectations of the patient, the evidence to support the contribution of patient empowerment to health outcomes, and the questions and conflicts that focus on power and control. In a rapidly changing world where information is global, where the search is on to make health care most efficient and effective, and where transparency and accountability are both public and personal issues, the relationship between health professionals and their patients has become increasingly important. Research is still needed to help define the exact nature of this relationship and its value to personal health improvements. However, at the moment there is a window of opportunity to be creative and innovative about these changes and see a relationship in which both professional and patient become empowered through mutual learning and interaction.

## References

Aday, L. (2000). An expanded conceptual framework of equity: implications for assessing health policy. In: G. Albrecht, R. Fitzpatrick, S. Scrimshaw (Eds.), *Handbook of Social Studies in Health and Medicine*. London: Sage.

Anderson, J. (1996). Empowering patients: issues and strategies. *Social Science and Medicine*, 43, 697–705.

Braveman, P., Tarimo, E. (2002). Social inequalities in health within countries: not only an issue for affluent nations. *Social Science and Medicine*, 54, 1621–1635.

Bryant, J. (1969). *Health and the developing world*. Ithaca: Cornell University Press.

Evans, T., Whitehead, M., Diderchisen, F., Bhuiya, A., Wirth, M. (Eds.). (2001). *Challenging inequities in health: from ethics to action*. Oxford: Oxford University Press.

Feste, C., Anderson, R. (1995). Empowerment: from philosophy to practice. *Patient Education and Counseling*, 26, 139–144.

Grol, R. (2001). Improving the quality of medical care: building bridges among professional pride, payer profit and patient satisfaction. *Journal of the American Medical Association*, 286, 2578–2586.

Hersh, W. (1999). A world of knowledge at your fingertips. *Academic Medicine*, 74, 240–243.

Kaul, M. (1997). The new public administration: management innovations in government *Public Administration and Development*, 17, 13–26.

Kidd, J., Marteau, T., Robinson, S., Ukoummunne, O.C., Tydeman, C. (2004). Promoting patient participation in consultations: a randomised controlled trial to evaluate the effectiveness of three patient-focused interventions. *Patient Education and Counselling*, 52, 107–112.

King, M. (1966). *Medical care in developing countries*. Nairobi, Kenya: Oxford University Press.

Laverack, G. (2004). *Health promotion practice: power and empowerment*. London: Sage.

Linden, K. (1994). Health and empowerment. *The Journal of Applied Social Sciences*, 18, 33–40.

Rawls J. (1971). *A theory of justice*. Cambridge, MA: Harvard University Press.

Rifkin, S. (2003). A framework linking community empowerment and health equity: it is a matter of choice. *Journal of Health, Population and Nutrition*, 21, 168–180.

Rifkin, S., Pridmore, P. (2001). *Partners in planning: information, participation and empowerment*. London: Macmillian.

Salmon, P., Hall, G. (2003). Patient empowerment and control: a psychological discourse in the service of medicine. *Social Science and Medicine*, 57, 1969–1980.

Segal, L. (1998). The importance of patient empowerment in health system reform. *Health Policy*, 44, 31–44.

Sen, A. (1999). *Development as freedom* (1st ed.). New York: Knopf.

Sen, G. (1997). Empowerment as an approach to poverty. Background paper to the *Human Development Report* (revised 1997) (http://www.hsph.harvard.edu/Organizations/healthnet/Hupapers/97_or.pdf).

Skelton, A.M. (1997). Patient education from the millennium: beyond control and emancipation? *Patient Education and Counseling*, 31, 151–158.

World Bank (2000). *World development report 2000/2001: attacking poverty*. Oxford: Oxford University Press.

World Health Organization (1978). *Primary health care: report of the International Conference on Primary Health Care*. Geneva: World Health Organization.

World Health Organization (1986). *Ottawa Charter for Health Promotion*. Geneva: World Health Organization.

# 10
# Shared Decision Making in Medicine

Hana Kajnar

During the last decades, a great change has taken place in doctor–patient relationships (Shorter, 1991). Improved diagnostic and therapeutic competence among physicians has led to increasing neglect of history taking and consideration of patients' interests. The patients' biology has become more important to physicians than their psyche, and patients often do not have the opportunity to voice their concerns or express their anxieties. This often causes patient dissatisfaction with the consultation, and there is a loss of trust and mutual respect in the doctor–patient relationship. A greater consideration of patients' concerns and more information exchange between physician and patient could therefore result in a more effective health care system. Decisions have to be made based on the doctor's knowledge and the patient's preferences.

There are various ways to combine the physician's knowledge with the patient's preferences in the decision-making process, such as the "decision making models" consisting of the paternalistic model (Charles et al., 1997, 1999a,b), the informed decision-making model, the physician-as-agent model, and the shared decision-making model (Charles et al., 1997, 1999a,b, 2000; Gafni et al., 1998). These models have in common that the information flow between doctor and patient is either one-sided (informed decision-making model—information flow from doctor to patient), physician-as-agent model—information flow from patient to doctor), or nearly nonexistent (paternalistic model). The shared decision-making model contains a two-way flow of information. After having exchanged their knowledge, the two partners (patient and doctor) decide together about the next action to take. Because of its growing actuality and changing physician behavior (Vevaina et al., 1993; Gafni et al., 1998; Frosch & Kaplan, 1999), one can find a lot of information about this model in the literature. This chapter contains a systematic review of the topic. The following issues are covered.

- Components of shared decision making
- Target parameters and outcomes of fundamental components of shared decision making
- Advantages and disadvantages of shared decision making
- Prerequisites for shared decision making

- Causes for low validity of some studies
- Implementation of shared decision making and alternatives

## Methods

A systematic literature search was performed in the following databases: MEDLINE (1990–2001), Embase and Scisearch (1980–2001), Catline, Cochrane, Kluwer-Verlagsdatenbank, Medikat, Psychinfo, Psychlit, Psyndex, Russmed articles, Russmedbooks, Serline, and the Verbunddatenbank des Bibliotheksverbundes Bayern. The search was implemented by using the following terms in a standardized manner: "shared decision-making"; "evidence-based medicine"; "informed consent"; "informed patient"; "placebo effects"; "effects of informed consent"; "result of informed consent"; "impact of informed consent"; "informed consent on outcome"; "effect of shared decision-making on outcome"; "shared decision-making and outcome"; and "effects of shared decision-making."

Furthermore, a hand search for Edward Shorter (1991) and a purposive search in the *British Medical Journal* using the term "decision" were performed. The received literature was classified into "quantitative" (Giacomini & Cook, 2000a,b; Kielhorn & Schulenburg, 2000) and "qualitative" (Britten, 1995; Jones & Hunter, 1995; Keen & Packwood, 1995; Kitzinger, 1995; Mays & Pope, 1995a,b; Pope & Mays, 1995a; Giacomini & Cook, 2000a,b; Kielhorn & Schuldenburg, 2000) studies, reviews, and discussion papers. The validity of "quantitative" studies and reviews was assessed using a special question list introduced by Sackett and colleagues (1996) in their book *Evidence-based Medicine: How to Practice & Teach EBM*. Qualitative studies were evaluated analogously with the help of an appropriate question list (Keen & Packwood, 1995; Mays & Pope, 1995b; Pope & Mays, 1995; Green & Britten, 1998; Poses & Isen, 1998; Patton, 1999; Sofaer, 1999; Giacomini & Cook, 2000a,b; Kielhorn & Schulenburg, 2000). Finally, the papers were separated into valid and partly valid studies, depending on the number of obtained affirmative answers to the question lists (valid—more than half of the questions affirmed; partly valid—half or fewer of the questions affirmed).

## Results

### *Components of Shared Decision Making*

Shared decision making involves a decision being made by patient and physician together (Charles et al., 1997). The procedure of shared decision making can be divided into three main phases (Charles et al., 1999a), the first of which can be further broken down (Towle & Godolphin, 1999) into three categories.

- *Information exchange*: development of a doctor–patient relationship (Ong et al., 1995; Charles et al., 1997; Towle & Godolphin, 1999); establishment of the patient's preferences for amount and format of information (Towle &

Godolphin, 1999); establishment of the patient's preferences for his or her role in decision making (Charles et al., 1997; Towle & Godolphin, 1999); consideration of the patient's concerns and expectations, identification of choices, and evaluation of the research evidence (Towle & Godolphin, 1999); and finally presentation of the research evidence to the patient and support for his or her consideration of it in regard to treatment preferences (Entwistle et al., 1998b; Charles et al., 1999a; Towle & Godolphin, 1999)

- *Deliberation* (Charles et al., 1999a; Towle, & Godolphin, 1999)
- *Decision* (Charles et al., 1997; Towle & Godolphin, 1999)

## Target Parameters and Outcomes of Fundamental Components of Shared Decision Making

There is not much evidence in the literature with regard to the realization of all aspects of shared decision making. Only implementation of the fundamental components of this process has been widely evaluated. Those fundamental components are *information about therapy options, decision support, and deliberation*. It is often not possible to separate these three main parts, which is why they are generally summarized as "decision aids" or "patient decision support" in the literature. Articles dealing with the implementation of decision aids and the evaluation of their target parameters (often in comparison with conventional methods) are discussed in this section.

A definition of decision aids was made by O'Connor and colleagues (2002).

Decision aids are interventions designed to help people make specific and deliberative choices among options by providing information on the options and outcomes relevant to a person's health status. The specific aims of decision aids may vary slightly, but in general they seem to enable people to:

1. Understand the probable outcomes of options;
2. Consider the personal value they place on benefits versus harms;
3. Participate in deciding about their health care.

Today, making decisions about screening or therapy options is often problematic for various reasons. Therefore, decision aids should help the patient find the right solution for his or her problem. They are more detailed than the usual information leaflets and take the specific preferences and values of each patient into account. Furthermore, they consider the patient's own risk profile. In the meantime, about 80 forms of decision aids (decision boards, interactive computer programs, video and audio tapes, and so on) have been developed, but only some of them have been applied in consultations. They are usually based on the "decision analysis."

To make an evaluation of decision aids possible, so-called target parameters have been defined: the patient's knowledge about his or her problem, realistic expectations with regard to this problem, an increase or decrease in the decisional conflict, satisfaction with the decision-making process and its results, preferences and decisions for a screening or therapy option (are there differences compared to conventional methods?), effects on participation in the decision-making process, mental effects, physical effects, lasting agreement with the chosen option, agreement between personal values and the chosen option, regretting the decision, and compliance.

The target parameters—knowledge, realistic expectations, participation in the decision-making process, physical effects—were influenced in a positive way by the decision aids, whereas it was not possible to determine the effect on the other parameters, partly because of the limited amount of research done on these topics.

## Advantages and Disadvantages of Shared Decision Making

The advantages and disadvantages of shared decision making for physicians, society, and patients are explained below.

### Advantages

Physicians have to know and to implement the newest evidence, which means they are obliged to always be up to date (Bennet et al., 1997; Entwistle et al., 1998a). If patients are well informed and can participate in the decision-making process, there are fewer misunderstandings during the consultations, and the patients are more satisfied. Consequently, they do not go to see or even change their physician as often. This could lead to lower costs for the health care system (Charles et al., 1999a). An obvious advantage for patients is better outcomes, which were discussed above. With the help of shared decision-making interventions, screening options whose advantages have not yet been confirmed, such as prostate-specific antigen (PSA) screening, could be used by patients more efficiently (Bennet et al., 1997).

### Disadvantages

It is still not clear whether shared decision making takes more time than other forms of doctor–patient relationships. If this were the case, it would lead to higher costs for the health care system (Charles et al., 1999a). Furthermore, paternalistic doctor–patient relationships could be destroyed by introducing this model, and the placebo effect of "the doctor knows best" would disappear when the patients are confronted with uncertainty in medicine. Conflicts could also arise when the two participants in the shared decision-making process prefer different solutions to the patient's problem. This would be the case if the patient chose an ineffective or even dangerous option against the physician's advice (Entwistle et al., 1998a,b). The physician would be confronted with ethical and legal problems because, in the end, he or she is responsible for the implementation of the less effective, less safe therapy option (Geiselmann, 1994).

## Prerequisites for Shared Decision Making

### Demands for Research

It should be possible for patients to choose their preferences in a valid and reliable way with the help of decision aids. Unfortunately, this is often not the case.

There is a "procedural invariance in preference assessment in health care" (Sumner & Nease, 2001), which means that the *process* of choosing a health outcome preference influences the decision made.

Two decision tools for the same problem could lead a person to two different decisions (Charles et al., 1997). The content and form of information should be presented in a way that enables patients to make a valid, reliable decision (Quill & Suchman, 1993). This is difficult to realize for several reasons. Each patient interprets a verbal estimation of risk (for example, "low" risk of stroke) in a different way (Mazur & Merz, 1994b). Relative risk estimations and absolute risk estimations for the same event are interpreted differently. The sequence and particularity of information, or even the color of the presentation, can influence the patient's choice (Tymchuk & Ouslander, 1991; Mazur & Merz, 1993; Mazur & Hickam, 1997; Carrere et al., 2000; Wolf & Schorling, 2000) The scaling of information (for instance, long, detailed scale versus short, less detailed scale showing adverse events) also influences the patient's choice (Mazur & Hickam, 1994, 1996; Mazur & Merz, 1994a). It makes a difference to the patient whether the same information is presented in a positive or a negative way (O'Connor, 1989; Malloy et al., 1992). Consequently, there is still a demand for research on the preferred format and quantity of information for patients. Physicians should be taught to explain this information to patients effectively (Feldman-Stewart et al., 2000). Furthermore, it is necessary to adapt the format and content of information to special patient groups (Doyal, 2001).

Another prerequisite for shared decision making is the determination of important outcomes for the patient. Here the outcomes model plays an important role. The model considers not only measurable physiological parameters but also the quality of life and life expectation while planning therapy (Kaplan, 1999; Sieber & Kaplan, 2000). Strategies should be developed to motivate patients to participate in the decision-making process. Many patients are not able to communicate their concerns properly, which results in dissatisfaction, distrust, and more physical complaints (Barry et al., 2000; Bell et al., 2001). Not all patients profit from the model of shared decision making. For example, some patients want to be informed thoroughly but are not interested in participating in making the decision (Robinson & Thomson, 2001). Other patients are used to the paternalistic doctor–patient relationship and do not accept any change in this respect. Research on recognizing patients for whom this model is suitable and profitable is sorely needed.

Competence of Physicians and Patients

An important prerequisite for shared decision making is the ability of doctors and patients to communicate their concerns, understand each other, and take part at the decision-making level as equal partners. This process helps avoid misunderstandings (Britten et al., 2000). Towle (1999) demands "competencies for patients and physicians for informed shared decision-making." Entwistle et al. (1998a,b) reported similar competencies for physicians and patients. Finally, it is the duty of the physician to determine if the patient wants to participate (Bates, 2001). In some situations the patient is interested in sharing the decision, whereas in others she or he prefers the doctor to decide (McKinstry, 2000). In any case, the physician has to practice evidence-based medicine to be able to give the patient valid, relevant information (Rubin et al., 2000).

# Discussion

## Components of Shared Decision Making

Patient–physician communication and particularly the process of shared decision making have become increasingly important in communications research. It is assumed that the doctor–patient communication influences patient behavior, satisfaction with the consultation, compliance, understanding of medical information, quality of life, and the health outcome. However, this relationship is highly complex because it requires an interaction between individuals in different hierarchal positions, is usually involuntary, deals with essential problems, and is emotionally demanding (Ong et al., 1995).

Therefore, it is difficult to divide the process of shared decision making into consecutive components and develop a theoretical model to guide its realization. It is clear that a fixed behavior checklist is difficult to put into practice because human interactions and situations are so varied. Furthermore, the components of such a behavior checklist could not be measured easily, as they do not appear sequentially (as in a checklist) but often simultaneously or in a different sequence.

The patients' views of important components of shared decision making have not yet been investigated thoroughly. The implementation of fundamental principles of shared decision making (establishing patient preferences and their influence on the decision-making process, physicians' respect for and acceptance of patients' decisions) as orientation for the decision-making process seems to be more realistic than a fixed behavior checklist (Charles et al., 1997). Nevertheless, a precise checklist for shared decision making could provide useful guidance in physician–patient communication for inexperienced doctors.

## Target Parameters and Outcomes of Fundamental Components of Shared Decision Making

As already described, the target parameters—knowledge, realistic expectations, participation in the decision-making process, physical effects—were influenced in a positive way by the decision aids. In contrast, it was not possible to determine the effect on the other parameters partly because of the limited amount of research done on these topics.

The studies that were evaluated also had some limitations. In addition to the limited number of articles on some target parameters, the studies were extremely heterogeneous. Many different decision tools were evaluated, and the context varied. Therefore, it is not surprising that there was no clear trend toward a positive or negative effect in the outcomes of some of the target parameters. Furthermore, different decision-making models were often applied simultaneously or successively during one consultation. Among the studies included in this chapter, only one decision-making process (shared decision making or its fundamental components) was implemented and evaluated.

This probably also influenced the outcomes of some target parameters. Furthermore, the subjects who took part in the studies were not always patients who had a medical problem but healthy volunteers. Nevertheless, it is possible to say that the target parameters (knowledge, realistic expectations, participation in the decision-making process, physical effects) were influenced in a positive way because despite their inhomogeneity most of the reviewed articles did show a clear effect.

Patients' views on shared decision making were (contrary to the physicians' opinions) mostly positive. A possible explanation for this observation is the fact that they received more attention than during conventional consultations. Furthermore, they were asked to participate actively. Despite learning about risks and side effects, they were satisfied with the decision-making process. Obviously, patients can be confronted with negative information in a constructive way.

Many physicians were dissatisfied with the decision aids for several reasons. Not every decision tool is appropriate for each situation. In some situations, the decision board can be more helpful than an informational video. Therefore, it is understandable that some doctors were satisfied with a specific decision tool, whereas others thought it to be inappropriate. Whereas some physicians thought that a decision tool would take too much time, others did not. Whether a decision tool can be integrated into the consultation in a time-effective way also depends on the situation and the decision aid.

## Advantages and Disadvantages of Shared Decision Making

It is clear that shared decision making has both advantages and disadvantages. Because knowledge of the newest evidence and good cooperation among physicians constitute prerequisites for informing the patient and, thus, for shared decision making, implementation of this model could lead to a better quality of health care. Furthermore, the patients' satisfaction with their care could be increased because they have the opportunity to participate in the decision-making process and have better health outcomes. As a result, patients would not go to see or change doctors as often. Together with the well reasoned use of screening and therapy options, this could lead to a more effective health care system and lower costs.

On the other hand, it is still unknown whether the costs and the time spent on implementation of the various decision aids are acceptable. Some other established forms of the doctor–patient relationship could be destroyed by introducing this model. For each patient, the physician has to consider whether he or she would benefit from shared decision making. This model is not appropriate for every person, medical field (for example psychiatry), or situation.

## Prerequisites for Shared Decision Making

There are some prerequisites for shared decision making that should be fulfilled. Some of the methods applied for the choice of preferences do not represent real patient preferences in a valid, reliable way. Furthermore, many decision aids are demanding and require greater patient comprehension. Especially elderly patients may have problems with these complex decision tools. If the patients are not sure about how to decide, they often rely on suggestions or the subjective opinions of their physician. In such cases, the doctor should be aware of the ethical responsibility. It is still not clear what the form and amount of information for the patient should be to avoid manipulation by the way the information is presented. The information should be complete, comprehensive, and objective and should give the patient the opportunity to make a decision in accordance with his or her personal values.

Health outcomes involving quality of life are especially important to patients. Hence, they should be considered by the research more intensively. Researchers should try to find a way to motivate patients to take part in decision making. It is still not clear whether this is possible. For this purpose, patients' views on shared decision making should be particularly taken into account. Nevertheless, it is the task of the physician to decide whether the path of shared decision making should be taken.

Finally, some communication issues—such as directive, nondirective, open versus closed questions, and time spent on consultation, all of which influence the shared decision making process—and the acceptance of these issues by patients should be investigated more thoroughly. It is also important to implement follow-up studies to determine the long-term effects of shared decision making. Physicians' requirements, which are theoretical and difficult to put into practice, are also part of shared decision making. Fundamental principles, such as the ones described earlier (see Target Parameters and Outcomes of Fundamental Components of Shared Decision Making) would be easier to realize. Many patients cannot learn the required competencies. It is the task of the doctor to lead the interested patients to shared decision making.

## Causes for Low Validity of Some Studies

Quality-of-life outcomes, such as anxiety, are often used to evaluate the shared decision-making process. Unfortunately, these outcomes are difficult to measure (Coulter, 1994), and the validity and reliability of the methods applied is often questionable. Furthermore, the communication process is difficult to judge because several decision-making models may be applied during one consultation, and the patient's behavior can be interpreted differently. It is not clear whether participation in the decision-making process can be completely measured. Many instruments used for this purpose cannot distinguish between different degrees of participation (Elwyn et al., 2001). Verbal and nonverbal behavior can be interpreted in many ways. Finally, the patient's thoughts are difficult to measure, and therefore correct description of the communication process is demanding (Charles et al., 1997). Obviously, studies that deal with communication processes cannot be blinded. Consequently, systematic biases may occur (if, for example, the same physician cares for both the experimental and the control groups). Contamination among patients in different groups is also possible (if, for example, they meet in the waiting room). Many studies included healthy volunteers. Furthermore, some studies had only a small number of participants or did not have a control group. In summary, all these factors decrease the quality of the studies.

## Realization of Shared Decision Making and Alternatives

### Obstacles to Shared Decision Making

There are some obstacles to the realization of shared decision making. For various reasons, many physicians distrust the application of evidence-based medicine, which is a prerequisite for this decision-making model (Oliver et al., 1996; Elwyn et al., 1999). Furthermore, problems can also occur on the part of the organizational structures. Lack of time and continuity in the care of a patient—patients are often cared for by several doctors from different medical fields—play an important role. Another problem is the fact that for many diseases no evidence regarding appropriate screening or therapy exists, or there are fluctuations in the quality of the evidence (Entwistle et al., 1998a,b). Moreover, the research is often financed by the pharmaceutical industry, and the evidence may therefore be biased (Chatterton, 1999). It is difficult to inform the patient in these cases. Furthermore, it is also unknown what amount of information is enough. Problems can also result from the financing of the health care system (Entwistle et al., 1998a,b; Parker, 2001). Should the doctor, as the agent of the patient, support the patient's choice of an expensive but probably ineffective therapy or consider the costs to the health care system and refuse the therapy? Of course, problems can also occur regarding patients' attitudes. Some people do not want to be informed, whereas others believe in fate or are afraid of taking responsibility.

Despite of all these obstacles, the British National Health Service has developed strategies for more intensive patient participation in the decision-making process (Department of Health, 2001). Unfortunately, the German health care system still fails to promote a more patient-orientated approach to doctor–patient communication (Klemperer, 2003).

### Alternatives

As an alternative for special circumstances or a complement to shared decision making, "community informed consent" (Irwig, 2000) was suggested. Furthermore, better establishment of self-help groups (Bates, 2001) who cooperate closely with experts may create a lobby for patients. This would promote an exchange of information within the scope of shared decision making.

# Summary

It is the task of the physician to decide whether a doctor–patient relationship would profit from shared decision making or another decision-making model. This depends, of course, on the person and the situation. For example, in urgent medical situations, a different decision-making process, such as the paternalistic model, seems to be more appropriate. In summary, it can be stated that shared decision making has both positive and negative aspects. The two partners have to decide together whether this model has advantages or disadvantages for the patient in a specific situation. Nevertheless, the patient is the one who needs help, and the physician has the knowledge and power to provide it. This means that, in practice, neither can ever act as a completely equal partner. However, it is important that the physician always respect the patient.

## *References*

Barry, C.A., Bradley, C.P., Britten, N., Stevenson, F.A., Barber, N. (2000). Patients' unvoiced agendas in general practice consultations: qualitative study. *British Medical Journal*, 320, 1246–1250.

Bates, C. (2001). The good doctor. *Clinical Medicine,* 1, 128–131.

Bell, R.A., Kravitz, R.L., Thom, D. (2001). Unsaid but not forgotten: patients' unvoiced desires in office visits. *Archives of Internal Medicine,* 161, 1977–1984.

Bennet, C.L., Buchner, D.A., Ullman, M. (1997). Approaches to prostate cancer by managed care organisations. *Urology,* 50, 79–86.

Britten, N. (1995). Education and debate: qualitative research; qualitative interviews in medical research. *British Medical Journal*, 311, 251–253.

Britten, N., Stevenson, F.A., Barry, C.A. (2000). Misunderstandings in prescribing decisions in general practice: qualitative study. *British Medical Journal*, 320, 484–488.

Carrere, M-O., Moumjid-Ferrdjaoui, N., Charavel, M. (2000). Eliciting patients' preferences for adjuvant chemotherapy in breast cancer: development and validation of a bedside decision-making instrument in a French Regional Cancer Centre. *Health Expectations,* 3, 97–113.

Charles, C., Gafni, A., Whelan, T. (1997). Shared decision-making in the medical encounter: what does it mean? (or it takes at least two to tango). *Social Science and Medicine,* 44, 681–692.

Charles, C., Gafni, A., Whelan, T. (1999a). Decision-making in the physician-patient encounter: revisiting the shared treatment decision-making model. *Social Science and Medicine,* 49, 651–661.

Charles, C., Whelan, T., Gafni, A. (1999b). What do we mean by partnership in making decisions about treatment? *British Medical Journal*, 319, 780–782.

Charles, C., Gafni, A., Whelan, T. (2000). How to improve communication between doctors and patients. *British Medical Journal,* 320, 1220–1221.

Chatterton, H.T. (1999). Efficacy, risk, and the determination of value: shared medical decision-making in the age of information. *The Journal of Family Practice,* 48.

Coulter, A. (1994). Assembling the evidence: patient-focused outcomes research. *Health Libraries Review,* II, 263–268.

Department of Health. The expert patient: a new approach to chronic disease management for the 21st century (http://www.dh.gov.uk). Retrieved September 14, 2001.

Doyal, L. (2001). Informed consent: moral necessity or illusion?. *Quality in Health Care,* 10(Suppl 1), I29–I33.

Elwyn, G., Edwards, A., Gwyn, R. (1999). Towards a feasible model for shared decision-making: focus group study with general practice registrars. *British Medical Journal,* 319, 753–756.

Elwyn, G., Edwards, A., Mowle, S. (2001). Measuring the involvement of patients in shared decision making: a systematic review of instruments. *Patient Education and Counseling,* 43, 5–22.

Entwistle, V.A., Sheldon, T.A., Sowden, A., Watt, I.S. (1998a). Evidence-informed patient choice: practical issues of involving patients in decisions about health care technologies. *International Journal of Technology Assessment in Health Care,* 14, 212–225.

Entwistle, V.A., Watt, I.S., Davis, H. (1998b). Developing information materials to present the findings of technology assessments to consumers: the experience of the NHS Centre for Reviews and Dissemination. *International Journal of Technology Assessment in Health Care,* 14, 47–70.

Feldman-Stewart, D., Brundage, M.D., McConnell, B.A. (2000). Practical issues in assisting shared decision-making. *Health Expectations,* 3, 46–54.

Frosch, D.L., Kaplan, R.M. (1999). Shared decision-making in clinical medicine: past research and future directions. *American Journal of Preventive Medicine,* 17, 285–294.

Gafni, A., Charles, C., Whelan, T. (1998). The physician-patient encounter: the physician as a perfect agent for the patient versus the informed treatment decision-making model. *Social Science and Medicine,* 47, 347–354.

Geiselmann, B. (1994). Informed refusal: the patient's influence on long-term treatment. *Pharmacopsychiatry,* 27(Suppl), 58–62.

Giacomini, M.K., Cook, D.J. (2000a). Users' guides to the medical literature. XXIII. Qualitative research in health care A. Are the results of the study valid? *Journal of the American Medical Association,* 284, 357–362.

Giacomini, M.K., & Cook, D.J. (2000b, July). Users' guides to the medical literature. XXIII. Qualitative research in health care B. What are the results and how do they help me care for my patients? *Journal of the American Medical Association,* 284, 478–482.

Green, J., Britten, N. (1998). Education and debate: qualitative research and evidence based medicine. *British Medical Journal,* 316, 1230–1232.

Irwig, L. (2000). Implementing honesty about screening using community informed consent [letter]. *British Medical Journal,* 321, 450.

Jones, J., Hunter, D. (1995). Education and debate—qualitative research: consensus methods for medical and health services research. *British Medical Journal,* 311, 376–380.

Kaplan, R.M. (1999). Shared medical decision-making: a new paradigm for behavioral medicine—1997 presidential address. *Annals of Behavioral Medicine,* 21, 3–11.

Keen, J., Packwood, T. (1995). Education and debate—qualitative research: case study evaluation. *British Medical Journal,* 311, 444–446.

Kielhorn, A., von der Schulenburg, J-M. (2000). *The health economics handbook.* Amsterdam: Adis International. p. 152.

Kitzinger, J. (1995). Education and debate: qualitative research; introducing focus groups. *British Medical Journal,* 311, 299–302.

Klemperer, D. (2003). *Wie Ärzte und Patienten Entscheidungen treffen: Konzepte der Arzt-Patient-Kommunikation.* [How physicians and patients make decisions: concepts of doctor-patient communication]. Publication by the working group Public Health, research emphasis on work, social structure, and social state, Wissenschaftszentrum Berlin für Sozialforschung, Berlin.

Malloy, T.R., Wigton, R.S., Meeske, J. (1992). The influence of treatment descriptions on advanced medical directive decisions. *Journal of the American Geriatric Society*, 40, 1255–1260.

Mazur, D., Hickam, D.H. (1994). The effect of physician's explanations on patients' treatment preferences: five-year survival data. *Medical Decision-Making*, 14, 255–258.

Mazur, D., Hickam, D.H. (1996). Five-year survival curves: how much data are enough for patient-physician decision-making in general surgery? *European Journal of Surgery*, 162, 101–104.

Mazur, D., Hickam, D.H. (1997). The influence of physicians' explanations on patient preferences about future health-care states. *Medical Decision-Making*, 17, 56–60.

Mazur, D., Merz, J.F. (1993). How the manner of presentation of data influences older patients in determining their treatment preferences. *Journal of the American Geriatric Society*, 41, 223–228.

Mazur, D., Merz, J.F. (1994a). How age, outcome severity, and scale influence general medicine clinic patients' interpretations of verbal probability terms. *Journal of General Internal Medicine*, 9, 271–286.

Mazur, D., Merz, J.F. (1994b). Patients' interpretations of verbal expressions of probability: implications for securing informed consent to medical interventions. *Behavioral Sciences and the Law*, 12, 417–426.

Mays, N., Pope, C. (1995a). Education and debate: qualitative research; observational methods in health care settings. *British Medical Journal*, 311, 182–184.

Mays, N., Pope, C. (1995b). Education and debate: qualitative research; rigour and qualitative research. *British Medical Journal*, 311, 109–112.

McKinstry, B. (2000). Do patients wish to be involved in decision-making in the consultation? A cross-sectional survey with video vignettes. *British Medical Journal*, 321, 867–871.

O'Connor, A.M. (1989). Effects of framing and level of probability on patients' preferences for cancer chemotherapy. *Journal of Clinical Epidemiology*, 42, 119–126.

O'Connor, A.M., Stacey, D., Rovner, D. (2002). Decision aids for people facing health treatment or screening decisions (Cochrane Review). *The Cochrane Library*, Issue 2.

Oliver, S., Rajan, L., Turner, H. (1996). Informed choice for users of health services: views on ultrasonography leaflets of women in early pregnancy, midwives, and ultrasonographers. *British Medical Journal*, 313, 1251–1253. See also: Letters: Antenatal screening. (1999). *British Medical Journal*, 318, 805.

Ong, L.M.L., De Haes, J.C.J.M., Hoos, A.M. (1995). Doctor-patient communication: a review of the literature. *Social Science and Medicine*, 40, 903–918.

Parker, M. (2001). The ethics of evidence-based patient choice. *Health Expectations*, 4, 87–91.

Patton, M.Q. (1999). Enhancing the quality and credibility of qualitative analysis. *Journal of Health Services Research*, 34, 1189–1208.

Pope, C., Mays, N. (1995). Education and debate: qualitative research; reaching the parts other methods cannot reach: an introduction to qualitative methods in health and health services research. *British Medical Journal*, 311, 42–45.

Poses, R.M., Isen, A.M. (1998). Perspectives—qualitative research in medicine and health care: questions and controversy. *Journal of General Internal Medicine*, 13, 32–38.

Quill, T.E., Suchman, A.L. (1993). Uncertainty and control: learning to live with medicine's limitations. *Humane Medicine*, 9, 109–120.

Robinson, A., Thomson R. (2001). Variability in patients' preferences for participating in medical decision-making: implication for the use of decision support tools. *Quality in Health Care* 10(Suppl 1), I34–I38.

Rubin, G.L., Frommer, M.S., Vincent, N.C. (2000). Getting new evidence into medicine. *Medical Journal of Australia,* 172, 180–183.

Sackett, D.L., Richardson, W.S., Rosenberg, W., Haynes, R.B. (1996). *Evidence-based medicine: how to practice & teach EBM.* San Diego: Harcourt Brace (now Harcourt Trade).

Shorter, E. (1991). *Das Arzt-Patienten-Verhältnis in der Geschichte und Heute.* [The doctor-patient relationship in history and today.] Vienna: Picus.

Sieber, W.J., Kaplan, R.M. (2000). Informed adherence: the need for shared medical decision-making. *Controlled Clinical Trials,* 21(Suppl 5), 233S–240S.

Sofaer, S. (1999). Qualitative methods: what are they and why use them? *Journal of Health Services Research,* 34, 1101–1118.

Sumner, W., Nease, R.F. (2001). Choice-matching preference reversals in health outcome assessments. *Medical Decision-Making,* 21, 208–218.

Towle, A., Godolphin, W. (1999). Framework for teaching and learning informed shared decision-making. *British Medical Journal,* 319, 766–771.

Tymchuk, A.J., Ouslander, J.G. (1991). Informed consent: does position of information have an effect upon what elderly people in long-term care remember? *Educational Gerontology,* 17, 11–19.

Vevaina, J.R., Lois, M.N., Bone, R.C. (1993). Issues in biomedical ethics. *Disease-a-Month,* 39, 869–925.

Wolf, A., Schorling, J.B. (2000). Does informed consent alter elderly patients' preferences for colorectal cancer screening? Results of a randomised trial. *Journal of General Internal Medicine,* 15, 24–30.

# 11
# Overdiagnosis and Pseudodisease: Too Much of a "Good Thing?"

Robert M. Kaplan

Evidence-based medicine promotes a scientific basis for medical decisions. It often goes beyond the argument that diagnosis and treatment is always valuable. In addition to finding (diagnosing) and fixing (treating) a disease, evidence must show that a patient can benefit from diagnosis and treatment. Our CLINECS model (see Chapter 1) distinguishes outputs from outcomes. Services received do not necessarily translate into value for patients. There are occasions when diagnosis and treatment offers no benefit or when they may even produce harm. In this chapter we consider circumstances in which accurate diagnosis may not necessarily lead to better patient outcomes.

## Overdiagnosis

The "find-it-and-fix-it" medical model is concerned with the diagnosis and treatment of disease. However, the underlying objective is to extend life expectancy and improve quality of life (Kaplan, 2005). There are many cases in which a diagnosis may reduce quality of life without any clear benefit. One of the best examples is a classic paper by Bergman and Stamm (1967). These pediatric cardiologists were concerned about the overdiagnosis of heart murmurs in children. The well trained ear of a pediatric cardiologist can detect murmurs in large numbers of children. One study found that 44% of normal infants in Nashville, Tennessee, had innocent heart murmurs (Quinn & Campbell, 1961–1962). Bergman and Stamm (1967) surveyed more than 20,000 children from the Seattle schools. They identified 93 in whom either heart disease or rheumatic fever had been diagnosed at some time in their lives. Among them, 18 actually had heart disease, and the other 75 had no evidence of current problems. However, 40% of those with a previous diagnosis of heart disease were currently restricted in their activity because their parents feared potential heart attacks. The best evidence indicated that these children should not be restricted and that the reduced physical activity may actually be harmful. Confusion about heart disease and incorrect concerns about exertion played a major part in the families' decisions to restrict their children. The heart disease was not causing the restriction; instead, it was a misunderstanding of the implications of a former diagnosis.

## Mammography Controversy

In January 1997, the U.S. National Institutes of Health convened a panel to make recommendations about the use of screening mammography for women between the ages of 40 and 50 years. In contrast to the diagnostic testing used when a women belongs to a high risk group or has felt a lump in her breast, screening mammography is used to evaluate asymptomatic women. Most systematic reviews of screening mammography show little benefit of screening, particularly for women under the age of 50 (Olsen & Gotzsche, 2001). The Panel's review shocked the American Cancer Society. They called the panel's conclusion "outrageous." The headline of *USA Today* (January 24, 1997) read, "Mammogram Panel Only Adds to Furor." Commentators on morning talk shows were outraged by the committee's decision. What controversial statement could evoke these reactions? The panel concluded that each woman should decide for herself. They suggested that women consider the costs and the possibilities of being frightened by benign tumors before they decide whether they should undergo mammography. In other words, the panel said that routine mammography has some risks and some benefits, and women should take these factors into consideration. Many believe that women cannot handle these ambiguities. For example, Richard Krausner, the former Director of the National Cancer Institute, decided to disregard the report of his expert panel. He announced that he would ask another panel appointed by the President to look at the same question.

The controversy over screening mammography is similar to the controversies of screening for other types of cancer (Kaplan, 2005). Unfortunately, the issues are complex. In this chapter I spell out the rationale for taking a cautious view of screening. Admittedly, this is controversial territory. However, it is important to understand why most panels of experts, after reviewing the evidence, have suggested a cautious position on screening. I begin with the biases inherent in screening for cancer.

## Pseudodisease

Diagnostic technologies have greatly increased in number and precision. Better magnification allows pathologists to see many abnormalities that were formerly overlooked. Blood tests enable detection of abnormalities that were previously undefined. New chemical assays identify proteins and antigens that are specific to particular tumors. We have assumed that greater diagnostic acumen leads to better health because diseases can be diagnosed early. In addition to identifying more diseases, better testing might also identify more pseudodiseases.

Pseudodisease is disease that never produces clinically meaningful effects. All of us have identifiable abnormalities. However, many of these problems should not worry us because they never produce significant problems for our quality of life or life expectancy. Black and Welch (Black & Welch, 1997; Black, 2000) argued that there is a huge reservoir of pseudodisease that can be identified as diagnostic testing improves. Advances in imaging and diagnostic testing will lead to continual increases in the incidence and prevalence of cancer and other microscopic diseases.

Black and Welch (1993) used thyroid cancer to illustrate their point. Citing data from the Connecticut Tumor Registry, they noted that the prevalence of clinical thyroid cancer, defined as a tumor larger than 2 cm, was about 1 case per 1000 adults between 50 and 75 years of age. However, if microscopic inspection of the thyroid improves, more adults will have abnormalities. For example, in a study of Finnish adults, Harach and colleagues (1985) made slices at 2.5-mm intervals at autopsy. In adults of the same age, they found 36% had some evidence of thyroid cancer. More troubling was the realization that slicing the gland at 2.5-mm intervals would still leave many tumors undetected because there would be intervals of 2.5 mm between the slices. The method would detect tumors larger than 2.5 mm but would capture only one-fifth of the tumors 5 mm in size. Applying this simple logic, they realized that most, if not all, adults aged 50 or older have thyroid cancer (Black & Welch, 1993).

The thyroid cancer example is an important one. Thyroid cancer is not a major cause of death. The common assumption is that a diagnosis of cancer identifies a person on a pathway toward death. However, most of us may have cellular tumors that can be identified through improved technologies. At present, few people recommend screening for thyroid cancer. However, many physicians and organizations advocate screening for breast, prostate, and colorectal cancers. We are less concerned about the potentially identifiable thyroid cancers because they are likely to be a pseudodisease. Might there also be pseudodisease in the breast, prostate, or colon?

## Upward Spiral of Treatment Intensity

Improvements in technology and the increased detection of pseudodisease might lead to an increasing spiral of treatment intensity. Black and Welch (1997) described a cycle of increased treatment intensity.

The cycle begins when improved technology lowers the threshold for disease detection. For example, improved microscopic techniques can identify more thyroid cancer, and new developments in prostate-specific antigen (PSA) screening yield even greater numbers of prostate cancers (Kaplan, 2005). This occurs because new cases are uncovered that would have been missed with cruder technologies. As a result, the incidence and prevalence of the disease increase. However, less severe cases are also found. This increase in the number of cases detected boosts confidence in the new technology by giving clinicians the satisfaction that they are finding cases that previously would have been missed. As a result, more screening tests are conducted.

Identification of disease early in its course might improve survival. However, many of these detected cases are probably pseudodisease. In other words, they are cases that would have never caused clinical problems. These cases might be treated, and long-term follow-up might show good health outcomes. However, it is also likely that these cases of pseudodisease would never have become clinical cases had they not been detected. Autopsy studies consistently show that most young adults who died from noncardiovascular causes have fatty streaks in their coronary arteries, indicating the initiation of coronary disease (Strong et al., 1999). Cancers of the breast and prostate have been identified in as many as 30% (breast) (Kaplan & Wingard, 2000; Horton, 2001) and 40% (prostate) (Fowler et al., 2002; Vis, 2002) of older adults who died from other causes. Many people with undiagnosed disease are never harmed by the pathology; indeed, they may never know they even have the problem. As diagnostic technology improves, our ability to diagnose more of this reservoir will increase, and problems will be identified in many individuals who would not benefit from treatment. The problem has been fiercely debated in relation to cancer screening tests, such as mammography and the PSA assay (Gelmon & Olivotto, 2002; Vis, 2002). When pseudodisease is detected, there is an apparent benefit of treatment, even though treatment had no real benefit. The apparent benefit, which is an artifact, in turn leads to more screening. Refinements in testing could lead to the false impression of an epidemic. The apparent epidemic would in turn lead to even more screening.

Ironically, testing may have a greater chance of detecting pseudodisease than real disease. The chances of finding a disease through a screening program is directly proportional to the length of time the disease is in a preclinical phase. This is inversely related to the rate of disease progression (Black et al., 2002). For example, a rapidly progressing disease might be absent at the time the screening test is performed and may be beyond a point where it can be treated the next time the screening is conducted. Consider, for example, rapidly developing ovarian cancer. A women may have no evidence of the disease when screened at age 40. At age 42, she may develop a rapidly progressing tumor that is beyond intervention when screened again at age 43. Conversely, a case of pseudodisease that progresses slowly can be detected over many years. However, because the disease progresses so slowly, identification and treatment might have little or no effect because it is unlikely the disease will ever to produce clinically meaningful problems.

## Conclusions

This chapter furthers the discussion about the relationship between inputs, outputs, and outcomes. Many traditional views argue for the greater use of diagnostic tests. It has been suggested that more investment in screening (inputs) can lead to identification of more cases to be treated (outputs). However, translation of outputs to outcomes has not always been clearly established. The chapter offers examples suggesting that testing can identify cases of pseudodisease, or disease of little clinical significance. In these cases, expenditure of resources is of little value to patients. The following chapters continue to explore these issues.

## References

Bergman, A.B., Stamm, S.J. (1967). The morbidity of cardiac nondisease in school-children. *New England Journal of Medicine*, 276, 1008–1013.

Black, W.C. (2000). Overdiagnosis: an underrecognized cause of confusion and harm in cancer screening. *Journal of the National Cancer Institute*, 92, 1280–1282.

Black, W.C., Haggstrom, D.A., Welch, H.G. (2002). All-cause mortality in randomized trials of cancer screening. *Journal of the National Cancer Institute*, 94, 167–173.

Black, W.C., Welch, H.G. (1993). Advances in diagnostic imaging and overestimations of disease prevalence and the benefits of therapy. *New England Journal of Medicine*, 328, 1237–1243.

Black, W.C., Welch, H.G. (1997). Screening for disease. *AJR American Journal of Roentgenology*, 168, 3–11.

Fowler, J.E., Jr., Bigler, S.A., Farabaugh, P.B. (2002). Prospective study of cancer detection in black and white men with normal digital rectal examination but prostate specific antigen equal or greater than 4.0 ng/mL. *Cancer*, 94, 1661–1667.

Gelmon, K.A., Olivotto, I. (2002). The mammography screening debate: time to move on. *Lancet*, 359, 904–905.

Harach, H.R., Franssila, K.O., Wasenius, V.M. (1985). Occult papillary carcinoma of the thyroid; a "normal" finding in Finland: a systematic autopsy study. *Cancer*, 56, 531–538.

Horton, R. (2001). Screening mammography: an overview revisited. *Lancet*, 358, 1284–1285.

Kaplan, R.M. (2005). Screening for cancer: are resources being used wisely? *Recent Results in Cancer Research*, 166, 315–334.

Kaplan, R.M., Wingard, D.L. (2000). Trends in breast cancer incidence, survival, and mortality. *Lancet*, 356, 592–593.

Olsen, O., Gotzsche, P.C. (2001). Cochrane review on screening for breast cancer with mammography. *Lancet*, 358, 1340–1342.

Quinn, R.W., Campbell, E.S. (1961–1962). Heart disease in children: a survey of school children in Nashville, Tennessee. *Yale Journal of Biological Medicine*, 34, 370–385.

Strong, J.P., Malcom, G.T., McMahan, C.A., Tracy, R.E., Newman, W.P., 3rd, Herderick, E.E., et al. (1999). Prevalence and extent of atherosclerosis in adolescents and young adults: implications for prevention from the Pathobiological Determinants of Atherosclerosis in Youth Study. *Journal of the American Medical Association*, 281, 727–735.

Vis, A.N. (2002). Does PSA screening reduce prostate cancer mortality? *Canadian Medical Association Journal*, 166, 600–601.

# 12
# Palliative Medicine Today: Evidence and Culture

E. Jane Maher

Most people receiving chemotherapy and radiotherapy for cancer are not cured. One-third to one-half of radiation treatments delivered in Europe and North America are given with palliative, not curative, intent, with an even lower percentage for chemotherapy treatments (Coia et al., 1988; Maher et al., 1990; Lawton & Maher, 1991; Maher, 1991; Coia, 1992). Across Europe, the "cancer population" is becoming increasingly older with more co-morbidities and with changing attitudes toward cancer and its treatments.

Treatment for incurable cancer is costly. By the 1990s it was estimated that in the United States alone radiation therapy given to palliate locoregional disease from non-small-cell lung cancer (NSCLC), together with that given for bone and brain metastases from all solid tumors, cost approximately $1 billion every year (Hanks, 1992).

There are three types of palliative studies are available in the literature on which to base clinical decision making: prospective randomized trials and meta-analyses (McQuay et al., 1997; Ben-Josef et al., 1999; Ratanatharathorn et al., 1999; Roos & Fisher, 2003; Wu et al., 2003); retrospective audits; and patterns-of-care studies (Lawton & Maher, 1991; Maher et al., 1992; Lievens et al., 2000a,b; Roos, 2000; van der Linden & Leer, 2000). Interpretation of such studies is hampered by the significant variation in the type of palliative treatments offered and the aims of therapy among countries (Priestman et al., 1989; Palmer et al., 1990) and also among centers within the same country. Interpretation of all three is hampered by non-patient-, non-tumor-related factors that influence palliative practice (Chow et al., 2002).

## Variations in Palliative Therapy

Clinical trials, in particular, have had less influence on palliative treatment than in other areas. In a survey, fewer than 3% of clinical oncologists were influenced by the published literature when treating common metastatic cancers (Price et al., 1986). It is rarely acknowledged, however, that differences in culture and attitude to health care may affect the influence of a palliative trial, no matter how well designed or how significant the results. A British trial compared two fractions with ten fractions of radiotherapy for palliation of inoperable non-small-cell lung cancer (NSCLC). The results showed comparable symptom relief, side effects, and survival in the two groups; and the trial recruited more than 300 patients in less than 2 years, with the subsequent audit showing a demonstrable change in practice as a result of the trial (Bleehen et al., 1991; Goddard et al., 1991). This confirmed the willingness of the British oncologist to accept an option involving less rather than more therapy. During the same time period, however, when a series of Radiotherapy and Oncology Group (RTOG) studies in the United States suggested that low-dose radiation therapy in a few fractions was as effective for palliating bone metastases as a higher dose in more fractions, the trial was immediately reanalyzed using slightly different outcome measures, and the opposite conclusion was obtained, illustrating the American preference for more rather than less therapy (Tong et al., 1982; Blitzer, 1985).

More recent reviews have confirmed the continuing variation in the application of palliative treatments and measurement of outcomes among countries (Macbeth & Stevens, 2004). Therapy described as palliative tends to be delegated to less experienced therapists, which must inevitably lead to less rigorous audit, less carefully designed trials, and lower priority given in training programs (Crellin et al., 1989). In a survey of British clinical oncologists divided into equal groups according to seniority, 8% of those in training estimated that less than half of their workload was palliative, compared with 50% of those of more than 15 years standing. Similarly, one-third of oncologists in training estimated that two-thirds or more of their workload was palliative compared with 10% of their senior colleagues.

Different ways of organizing health care may exert different pressures. Until recently in the United Kingdom, 90% of cancer patients were treated under the state-funded National Health Service (NHS), with treatment free at the point of delivery, avoiding a "fee for service" approach. Resource limitation significantly influences choices made by British doctors. International surveys have confirmed that centers funded largely through fee for service tend to use higher doses of radiotherapy and more complex treatments for palliative patients than those reimbursed in other ways (Maher et al., 1992).

In the United States, health care has revolved around specialists, part of whose salary or departmental funds depend directly or indirectly on specific tests performed or therapy delivered, with a higher rate of procedures of all kinds. With managed care programs becoming more prevalent, the situation is changing, but in countries where the approach has historically been one of fee for service, the general population, as well as the medical profession, appears to have a more pronounced desire for intervention. For example, in the United States juries involved in litigation tended to be lenient about sins of commission, in contrast to sins of omission. This can be compared to the British approach, as Clare put it in an editorial in the *British Medical Journal*, "whereas in America it is better to do something than nothing, in Britain medicine is cautious about making matters worse" (Clare, 1988).

The precise role of specialists differs in different health care systems. Treatment policy is affected by which type of specialist sees a patient first. This is illustrated by the results of two surveys comparing North American and European practice. In one, a group of North American doctors from a variety of disciplines were asked which therapy they favored for a patient with advanced NSCLC and extensive positive regional nodes. Radiation therapy, chemotherapy, and surgery were favored by radiation therapists, medical oncologists, and surgeons, respectively. Similarly, when a variety of British health professionals were asked what benefits in terms of extension of survival and symptom relief would be required before recommending an intense regimen of palliative chemotherapy for patients with advanced solid tumors, family doctors required a 75% chance of symptom relief and/or a potential extension of survival of 24 months. Oncologists would be satisfied with a 50% chance of symptom relief and a 12-month extension of survival before recommending such therapy (Slevin et al., 1990).

## Surrogate Surveys

Surrogate surveys can be used to illustrate "invisible" differences in attitude, which may have a significant difference in the delivery of palliative treatment. During the 1990s, a number of surrogate surveys were published in which theoretical case histories were circulated to a number of specialists who were asked how they would treat these patients. Such studies have the advantage of allowing variations in attitude to be explored (Maher & Jefferis, 1990). One such questionnaire surveyed a large group of radiation oncologists, and the results illustrate a number of the problems in design and interpretation of palliative studies. Although these are now 10 years old, the points illustrated are just as relevant today.

The questionnaire was sent to all clinical members of The European Society for Therapeutic Radiology (ESTRO), the American Society for Therapeutic Radiology (ASTRO), and the Canadian College of Radiation Therapy, with 644 valuable responses (278 replies from 21 European countries, 99 from Canadians, and 268 from North Americans). It was composed of two sections. The first gave three case histories and asked respondents about the management of three theoretical patients, including radiotherapy techniques proposed, aims of treatment, whether treatment should be described as radical or palliative, estimated survival, and cure rate. The cases involved a 64-year-old man with brain metastases from small-cell lung cancer, a 59-year-old man with inoperable NSCLC and mediastinal nodes, and a 64-year-old woman with bone metastases and breast cancer (Table 12.1).

The second section concerned aspects of service organization, such as staffing equipment, patient workload, proportion of all treatments perceived to be palliative in each unit, management of terminal care, and funding. Some of the results are summarized in Tables 12.2 and 12.3.

TABLE 12.1. Case histories

| Parameter | Characteristics |
| --- | --- |
| **Case A** (brain metastases) | |
| History | Primary = small cell cancer |
| | Age 64 years, male |
| | Widower, lives alone, good general condition, |
| | Disease initially limited to mediastinum |
| | Treatment: |
| | 6 months of chemotherapy |
| | 1 month mediastinal radiotherapy |
| | Apparent complete remission |
| | Therapy complete 4 months ago |
| | Now cerebral metastases |
| Tumor | Multiple cerebral metastases on CT scan |
| Symptoms | Headache and vomiting (responded to steroids) |
| **Case B** (primary squamous cell carcinoma of the bronchus) | |
| History | Age 59 years, male |
| | Married, with adult children |
| Tumor | 4-cm hilar mass on chest radiograph |
| | Mediastinoscopy revealed positive mediastinal nodes (N2) |
| | Bronchoscopy: squamous cell cancer right main bronchus |
| Symptoms | Hemoptysis |
| **Case C** (bone metastases) | |
| History | Primary = cancer of the breast |
| | Age 64 |
| | Married housewife with adult children |
| | T2NX breast cancer treated with mastectomy |
| | 2-year symptom-free interval |
| Tumor | Multiple hot spots on bone scan |
| | Sclerotic, not lytic lesions on radiograph |
| | On tamoxifen |
| Symptoms | Pain T6-T9 |
| | Not radicular |
| | No neurological signs |

The survey confirmed the variation in therapy offered, attitude to advanced disease, differences in aims, uncertainty as to predicted survival of individual patients, and differences in the role of radiation and medical oncologists in the management of advanced cancer.

In general, Americans reported that they would give twice as much treatment in terms of total dose and number of fractions of radiation as their Canadian colleagues. The European countries came somewhere in between.

Between one-third and one-half of the total workload was considered palliative, and there was a relation between this proportion and attitude to the treatment of advanced lung cancer. Most of the departments estimating less than 50% palliative treated the NSCLC case radically and vice versa. Although there has been a closing of these gaps over the last 10 years, there are still significant differences in attitude between Canada and the United States and among the various countries in Europe

TABLE 12.2. Management of radiotherapy for non-small-cell lung cancer (case B)

| Parameter | Canada | Europe | USA |
|---|---|---|---|
| Management NSCLC | | | |
| Median dose of radiotherapy (Gy) | 40 (20–60) | 56 (8–75) | 60 (30–73) |
| Median number of sessions | 15 (5–30) | 28 (1–37) | 32 (10–60) |
| Treatment aims for NSCLC[a] | | | |
| Curative | 40% | 53% | 85% |
| Palliative | 69% | 47% | 39% |
| Relieve symptoms | 86% | 69% | 95% |
| Prevent symptoms | 58% | 50% | 94% |
| Extend life | 37% | 69% | 92% |
| Management—terminal care | | | |
| Radiotherapist | 38% | 47% | 15% |
| Medical oncologist | 2% | 53% | 60% |
| Family doctor | 60% | Not known | 26% |

From Price et al. (1986).
NSCLC = non-small-cell cancer.
[a]A small number described treatment as both curative and palliative.

TABLE 12.3. Management of radiotherapy for metastatic disease (brain metastases and bone metastases)

| Parameter | Case A (brain metastases) | | | Case C (bone metastases) | | |
|---|---|---|---|---|---|---|
| | Canada | Europe | USA | Canada | Europe | USA |
| Management | | | | | | |
| Median dose | | | | | | |
| (Gy) | 20 (10–40) | 30 (13–60) | 30 (22.5–55) | 20 (8–30) | 30 (5–50) | 30 (10–46) |
| Median no. | | | | | | |
| of sessions | 5 (1–15) | 10 (2–30) | 11 (10–30) | 5 (1–10) | 10 (1–25) | 10 (7–42) |
| Aims | | | | | | |
| Relieve | 78% | 87% | 96% | 100% | 97% | 99% |
| Prevent | 65% | 39% | 80% | 47% | 35% | 79% |
| Extend life | 22% | 23% | 48% | 1% | 5% | 11% |
| Give hope | 24% | 20% | 44% | 15% | 12% | 38% |
| Predicted survival | | | | | | |
| < 6 months | 80% | 67% | 60% | 0% | 1% | 2% |
| 7–12 months | 20% | 30% | 35% | 7% | 10% | 8% |
| 1–2 years | 0% | 2% | 3% | 36% | 40% | 38% |

From Price et al. (1986).

Differences in attitude toward the management of advanced disease were indicated by the fact that 90% of both Canadians and Americans thought the NSCLC patient would not live more than 2 years. Although 36% of Canadians considered the patient incurable, only 3% of Americans considered this to be the case. Similarly, 40% of Canadians, 53% of Europeans, and 85% of Americans described their treatment as radical, and only 10% of Canadians aimed to extend life. If treatment was described as palliative, one-fourth of Europeans and more than half of Americans aimed to extend life using palliative radiotherapy.

These differences in attitude had important effects on therapy in that those describing treatment as radical and/or aiming to extend life gave significantly higher doses and more fractions of radiation than those who did not. Another consequence of such variation is that populations participating in a palliative study would clearly vary among countries.

Although there was agreement that treatment of metastatic disease should be described as palliative, again there was significant variation in therapy. This could be related to differences in the precise aims of treatment and predicted survival. Those who aimed to prevent symptoms gave more therapy than those who aimed only to relieve them; and those who predicted a longer survival also gave more therapy. A difference in predicted survival of only a few months appears to have a significant impact on proposed therapy, but doctors are inaccurate in their predictions, as has been indicated by other studies (Sadler et al., 1992). Recent reviews have confirmed that prediction of prognosis has a significant impact on the type of treatment offered and is a very inexact science. The entry criteria for many palliative trials is a survival of more than 3 months, whereas the actual median survival is less than 3 months.

## Giving Hope

Perhaps one of the more striking differences in aims between the surveyed groups was the relative importance placed on "giving hope." For example, for the patient with brain metastases, less than one-fourth of Canadians or Europeans included this as one of their aims compared with more than one-half of Americans. Those who included it gave more radiation that those who did not. There appeared to be a preference among American therapists to use more anticancer therapy, rather than supportive care alone, in advanced disease. For example, again considering the patient with brain metastases, if palliative radiotherapy was considered inappropriate, 80% of Canadians would offer no other oncological therapy, and 2% proposed chemotherapy. Fewer than half of Americans surveyed would accept an option of no further anticancer treatment, and one-fourth would offer chemotherapy.

Giving hope persists as an important aim for palliative treatment. For example, a recent study explored the use of second-line palliative chemotherapy in the treatment of breast cancer and showed that giving hope was one of the most important aims for oncologists offering such therapy (Grunfeld et al., 2001, 2005). The involvement and training of cancer specialists in supportive care varied among countries. For management of NSCLC during the 1990s, just under half of European radiotherapists participated in the terminal care of their patients compared to 38% of Canadians and 15% of Americans. More than half of the Canadians perceived a family doctor to be involved, and 2% expected involvement a medical oncologist. In comparison, only one-fourth of American radiation therapists thought a family doctor would be involved and 60% considered a medical oncologist.

## Reimbursement to the Provider

The study provided limited support for a relation between the method of reimbursement and the type of therapy given. In Canada, 90% of departments are funded entirely through government agencies, with private or university funds making up less than 10% of the support. In the United States, most centers are primarily funded privately, with only 43% having less than 75% private funding, 59% no federal government support, and 75% no local government support. In Europe there is more varied approach: 60% receive some government funding, 23% get research-based funds, and 38% have other sources of income, including private funds. In the more mixed European situation, there was a weak but significant correlation between funding, dose, and number of fractions in that the institutions that were all partially privately funded gave higher doses and more fractions than those that were completely government funded. This relation was confirmed in later studies (van der Linden & Leer, 2000).

## Conclusions

A number of factors unrelated directly to the disease or the patients may affect palliative practice. For example, there are differences in attitude toward treating advanced disease with a small chance of cure in terms of treating disease accepted as incurable, organization of health services, medical training, litigation rate, availability of resources, and method of reimbursement. There are also differences regarding the point in the natural history of disease at which patients are referred to an oncologist and a lack of reliable prognostic factors to allow estimation of survival time.

If clinical trials are to recruit successfully and change practice, priorities might include clarification of prognoses of patients currently treated, agreement as to the most appropriate measure of outcome, and acknowledgement of the effects of cultural differences on palliative treatment.

### *References*

Ben-Josef, E., Shamsa, F., Youssef, E., Porter, A.T. (1999). External beam radiotherapy for painful osseous metastases: pooled data dose response analysis. *International Journal of Radiation Oncology, Biology, Physics*, 45, 715–719.

Bleehen, N.M., Birling, D.J., Fayers, P.M., Aber, V.R., Stephens, R.J. (1991). Inoperable non small cell lung cancer (NSCLC): A Medical Research Council randomised trial palliative radiotherapy with two fractions or ten fractions. *British Journal of Cancer*, 63, 265–270.

Blitzer, P.H. (1985). Reanalysis of the RTOG study of palliation of symptomatic osseous metastases. *Cancer,* 55, 1468–1472.

Chow, E., Wu, J.S., Hoskin, P., Coia, L.R., Bentzen, S., Blitzer, P.H. (2002). International consensus on palliative radiotherapy endpoints for future clinical trials in bone metastases. *Radiotherapy and Oncology*, 64, 275–280.

Clare, A. (1988). National variations in medical practice. *British Medical Journal,* 298, 1334.

Coia, L.R. (1992). The use of radiotherapy in the treatment of brain metastases. *International Journal of Radiation Oncology, Biology, Physics,* 23, 229–238.

Coia, L.R., Laurence, R., Hanks, G.E., Martz, K., Steinfield, A., Diamon, J.J., et al. (1988). Practice patterns of palliative care for the United States 1984–1985. *International Journal of Radiation Oncology, Biology, Physics,* 14, 1261–1269.

Crellin, A., Marks, A., Maher, E.J. (1989). Why don't British radiotherapists give single fractions of radiotherapy for bone metastases? *Clinical Oncology,* 1, 63–66.

Goddard, M., Maher, E.J., Hutton, J., Shah, D. (1991). Palliative radiotherapy: counting the cost of changing practice. *Health Policy* 17, 243–256.

Grunfeld, E.A., Ramirez, A.J., Maher, E.J., Peach, D., Young, T.E., Albery, P., et al. (2001). Chemotherapy for advanced breast cancer: what influences oncologists decision-making. *British Journal of Cancer,* 84, 1172–1178.

Grunfeld, E.A., Ramirez, A.J., Maher, E.J., Browne, S., Ward, P., Young, T., et al. (2005). Decision-making for palliative chemotherapy: perceptions of patients with advanced breast cancer. *British Journal of Cancer* (in press).

Hanks, G.E. (1992). The crisis in health care cost in the United States: some implications for radiation oncology. *International Journal of Radiation Oncology, Biology, Physics,* 23, 203–206.

Lawton, P.A., Maher, E.J. (1991). Treatment strategies for advanced and metastatic cancer in Europe. *Radiotherapy and Oncology,* 22, 1–6.

Lievens, Y., Kesteloot, K., Rijinders A, Kutcher, G., Van der Bogaert, W. (2000a). Differences in palliative radiotherapy for bone metastases within western European countries. *Radiotherapy and Oncology,* 56, 297–303.

Lievens, Y., Van den Bogaert, W., Rijinders, A., Kutcher, G., Kestelook, K. (2000b). Palliative radiotherapy practice within western European countries: impact of the radiotherapy financing system? *Radiotherapy and Oncology,* 56, 289–295.

Macbeth, F., Stephens, R. (2004). Palliative treatment for advanced non-small cell lung cancer. *Hematology Oncology Clinics of North America,* 18(1), 115–130.

Maher, E.J. (1991). The influence of national attitudes in the use of radiotherapy in advanced and metastatic cancer with particular reference to differences between the United Kingdom and the United States of America. *International Journal of Radiation Oncology, Biology, Physics,* 20, 1369–1373.

Maher, E.J., Jefferis, A.F. (1990). Decision-making in advanced cancer of the head and neck region: variation in the views of medical specialists. *Journal of the Royal Society of Medicine,* 83, 356–359.

Maher, E.J., Dische, S., Grosche, E., Fermont, D., Ashford, R., Saunders, M., et al. (1990). Who gets radiotherapy? *Health Trends,* 22, 78–83.

Maher, E.J., Coia, L., Duncan, G., Lawton, P.A. (1992). Treatment strategies in advanced and metastatic cancer: differences in attitude between the USA, Canada and Europe. *International Journal of Radiation Oncology, Biology, Physics,* 23, 239–244.

McQuay, H.J., Carroll, D., Moore, R.A. (1997). Radiotherapy for painful bone metastases: a systematic review. *Clinical Oncology,* 9, 150–154.

Palmer, J., O'Sullivan, B., Steele, R., Mackillop, W.J. (1990). Controversies in the management of non-small cell lung cancer: the results of an expert surrogate study. *Radiotherapy and Oncology,* 19, 17–28.

Price, P., Hoskin, P.J., Austin, A., Palmer, S.G., Yarnold, J.R. (1986). A prospective randomised trial of single and multifractionated radiotherapy schedules in the treatment of bony metastases. *Radiotherapy and Oncology,* 6, 247–255.

Priestman, T., Bullimore, J.A., Godden, T.P., Deutsche, G.P. (1989). The Royal College of Radiologists fractionation survey. *Clinical Oncology*, 1, 39–46.

Ratanatharathorn, V., Powers, W.E., Moss, W.T., Perez, C.A. (1999). Bone metastases: review and critical analysis of random allocation trials of local field treatment. *International Journal of Radiation Oncology, Biology, Physics*, 44, 1–18.

Roos, D.E. (2000). Continuing reluctance to use single fractions of radiotherapy for metastatic bone pain: an Australian and New Zealand practice survey and literature review. *Radiotherapy and Oncology*, 56, 315–322.

Roos, D.E., Fisher, R.J. (2003). Radiotherapy for painful bone metastases: an overview of the overviews. *Clinical Oncology*, 15, 342–344.

Sadler, G., Maher, E.J., Morris, T., Shah, D., Young, T. (1992). Can patients with bone metastases unsuitable for a single fraction of radiotherapy be identified? Implications for future contracting arrangements. *British Journal of Cancer* (Suppl XVII) (BOA Abstracts), 044.

Slevin, M.L., Stubbs, L., Plant, H.J., Wilson, P., Gregory, W.M., Armes, P.J., et al. (1990). Attitudes to chemotherapy: comparing views of patients with cancer with those of doctors, nurses and general public. *British Medical Journal*, 300, 1458–1460.

Tong, D., Gillick, L., Hendrickson, F.R. (1982). The palliation of symptomatic osseous metastases: final results of the study by the Radiation Therapy Oncology Group. *Cancer* 50, 893–899.

Van der Linden, Y.M., Leer, J.W.H. (2000). Impact of randomised trial-outcome in the treatment of painful bone metastases; patterns of practice among radiation oncologists: a matter of believers versus non-believers? *Radiotherapy and Oncology*, 56, 279–281.

Wu, J.S., Wong, R., Johnston, M., Bezjak, A., Whelan, T., and the Cancer Care Ontario Practice Guidelines Initiative Supportive Care Group (2003). Meta-analysis of dose-fractionation radiotherapy trials for the palliation of painful bone metastases. *International Journal of Radiation Oncology, Biology, Physics*, 55, 594–605.

# 13
## Medical Geography—Who Gets the Goods? More May Not Be Better

ROBERT M. KAPLAN

Geography can contribute to the understanding of medicine and health care. Medical geography is a research tool used to map the incidence and prevalence of diseases. It has been used by epidemiologists to identify areas where certain problems are common and other areas where these problems are absent. Although medical geography has never become a major field of study, local variations in illness rates were recognized during the fourth century BC. Hippocrates[1] stressed that the healer must understand the environment in which patients live to be effective. Between 1835 and 1855, maps were used to identify where people were at risk of contracting cholera. It was recognized that tables of numbers were ineffective in communicating important information and that visual maps more clearly identified regions where attention was necessary. During the 1970s, McGlashan and Armstrong (1972) published an entire book on techniques on medical geography.

## Geographic Distribution of Health Services

The difference in disease rates among communities is complicated by another variable. We have always assumed that if a doctor diagnoses an illness the illness exists. Furthermore, we assume that any qualified doctor presented with the same problem will come to the same diagnosis. Keen observers are aware that there is variability. Professionals make errors in diagnosis, but we assume that these errors are random. Thus, if the distribution of disease is the same in different communities, we would expect the rates of reporting to be roughly equivalent. However, physicians are quite different in the rates of illness they detect and in the services they recommend. Wennberg and his colleagues have devoted the past quarter century to the description of this problem (Wennberg, 1998; Wennberg et al., 2002). Wennberg suggested that a major factor in the use of medical services is "supplier-induced demand." This implies that providers create demand for their services by diagnosing illnesses. When new diagnostic technologies gain acceptance from physician groups, new

---

[1]Hippocrates: "father of medicine." He lived between about 460 and 377 BC in Greece.

epidemics of "disease" appear. One of the earliest documented cases of supplier-induced demand was described by Glover in the United Kingdom. Glover (cited in Wennberg, 1990) recorded the rates of tonsillectomy in the Hornse Burrough school district. In 1928, a total of 186 children in the district had their tonsils surgically removed. The next year the doctor who enthusiastically supported tonsillectomy was replaced by another physician who was less attracted to the procedure. In 1929, the number of tonsillectomies had been reduced to only 12.

In most surgical subspecialties, surgeons agree on the need to perform surgery in some well defined cases, which might include amputation of a toe with gangrene, removal of some well defined tumors, or intervention to repair a compound fracture. However, for most surgical procedures there is substantial discretion when determining the need for surgery.

## Boston Versus New Haven: A Case Example

Boston, Massachusetts and New Haven, Connecticut in the United States are similar in a variety of ways. Both are traditional New England cities that have multiethnic populations. The two cities have approximately the same climate and are both home to prestigious Ivy League universities. Because the cities are near one another, we would expect their costs of medical care to be approximately the same. Using data from the mid-1970s, Wennberg (1990) demonstrated that, in fact, medical care in Boston cost nearly twice as much as in New Haven.

Figure 13.1 shows the distribution of costs in cities in Connecticut and in Massachusetts during the 1970s. In 1975, Medicare paid $324 per recipient per month for people in Boston and only $155 per month for residents of New Haven. The situation has not changed much. In 1989, per-capita hospital expenditures for acute care were $1524 for residents of Boston and $777 for those living in New Haven. By 2000, medical care in the United States had changed, but most differences between practice in Boston and New Haven remained. Figure 13.2 shows the comparison between Boston and New Haven in 2000. Medicare still spends $1.64 in Boston for each dollar spent in New Haven.

Further study by Wennberg (1990) showed that Boston has more hospital capacity than New Haven. In Boston, there are 4.3 hospital beds for every 1000 residents, whereas in New Haven there are fewer than 2.3 beds per 1000 residents. Residents of Boston are more likely to be hospitalized for a wide variety of acute medical conditions than are residents of New Haven. For a variety of medical conditions, such as pneumonia or congestive heart failure, Bostonians are more likely to be cared for as hospital inpatients, whereas residents of New Haven are treated outside the hospital.

Boston is rich with medical institutions. New Haven has only one major medical school (Yale), whereas Boston has three medical schools. Furthermore, the Harvard Medical School is associated with a variety of teaching hospitals. Boston has four hospitals associated with various religious establishments, whereas there is only one religiously affiliated hospital in New Haven.

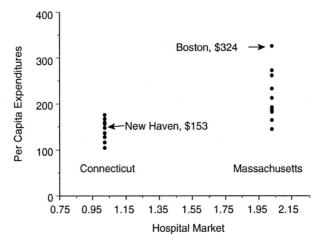

FIGURE 13.1. Hospital expenditures in Connecticut and Massachusetts in 1975.

The Boston versus New Haven comparison is particularly interesting from a public policy perspective. U.S. Medicare is a federal program meant to provide equal benefit to all of its recipients. Yet, on average, Medicare spends twice as much in Boston as it does in New Haven (Fisher et al., 1994). Are New Haven residents getting a bad deal? Because the government is spending less on New Haven residents, it might be argued that their health should suffer. However, evidence does not show that residents of Boston are any healthier than residents of New Haven. In fact, some evidence implies that Boston residents may be worse off. For example, people in Boston are more likely to be rehospitalized for the same condition than people in New Haven (Fisher et al., 1994). Residents of Boston appear to have more complications from medical treatment. More may not necessarily be better. Indeed, there is some suggested evidence that more may be worse (Fisher et al., 1994, 2003).

## Medical-Use Maps

In 2003, an estimated $1.7 trillion was spent for hospital care in the United States. According to data from the U.S. Center for Health Statistics, more than $5670 per person was spent on hospital care (Smith et al., 2005). Of course, that amount was not spent on each individual. You may not have been hospitalized in 2003, but some people were hospitalized for extended periods or for services that were very expensive. Averages do not tell us much about individual cases.

Health care spending in the United States is considerably higher than in other developed countries. Reinhart and colleagues (2004) created an index of expenditures that was concerted to purchasing power parity and then compared health care

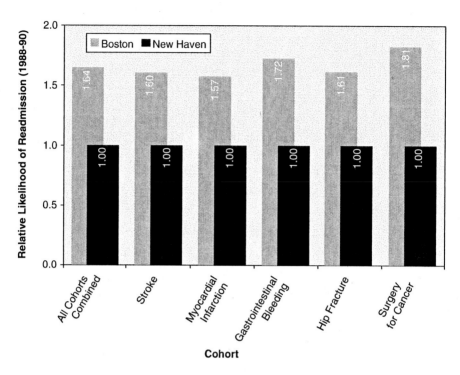

FIGURE 13.2. Medicare expenditures, Boston versus New Haven. (From Wennberg, 1998.)

spending across countries. In comparison to the United States, the next highest country, Switzerland, spent only 68% of the U.S. level. Belgium and Denmark spend about half as much, and Portugal and Spain spend about one-third as much. Turkey spends about 6% of the U.S. rate. Despite these large variations in investment, there is remarkably little evidence for differences in health outcomes, particularly among the most developed countries. The United Kingdom, for example, spends about $4 per capita on health care for every $10 spent in the United States. However, life expectancy in the United Kingdom (80.4 years for women and 74.4 years for men) is slightly longer than it is in the United States (79.5 years for women and 73.9 years for men), and infant mortality is slightly lower (5.6/1000 vs. 6.9/1000, respectively; http://www.OECD.org [2003]). Among 13 countries in one recent comparison, the United States ranked 12th when compared on 16 health indicators (Starfield, 2000).

We would expect the average costs to be similar in regions serving an equal number of people. Yet that is not the case. For example, per-capita costs in Chicago were nearly $1500, whereas they were closer to $750 in San Diego. A map summarizing hospital expenditures by hospital service area is shown in Figure 13.3. The map shows expenditures in 3436 geographic hospital service areas. These areas are grouped into 306 hospital referral regions. The maps are

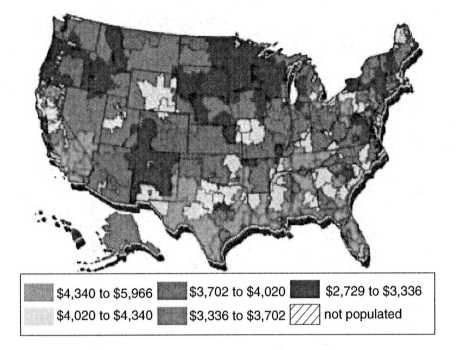

| | | |
|---|---|---|
| $4,340 to $5,966 | $3,702 to $4,020 | $2,729 to $3,336 |
| $4,020 to $4,340 | $3,336 to $3,702 | not populated |

FIGURE 13.3. Medicare reimbursements for all services. (From Wennberg, 1998.)

based on the analysis of Medicare claims. Analysis of Medicare claims has an important methodological advantage over virtually any other database. Medicare pays for health care for essentially all individuals 65 years or older. The analyses use essentially the entire claims database or a representative 5% sample. Usual sources of sampling error are essentially absent from these analyses.

To build the maps, hospital service areas and referral regions must be defined. To create hospital service areas, three steps are required. First, all acute care hospitals in the 50 states and in the District of Columbia were identified. This was accomplished using American Hospital Association and Medicare provider files. The names of these locations are then entered into a database. In the second step, each hospitalization record submitted to Medicare is broken down by zip code. Detailed analysis is used to align zip codes with the hospital that serves the area. In cities where there are multiple hospitals, rules are used to assign claims to particular service areas. There are approximately 42,000 zip codes in the United States, and these zip codes can be aggregated into 3436 hospital service areas. In 1993, most Americans lived in an area served by three or fewer local hospitals.

Although there are 3436 hospital service areas, not all of these areas have a facility offering advanced, tertiary medical care. The service areas can be aggregated into 306 hospital referral regions. Referral hospitals are those that perform both major cardiovascular surgery and neurosurgery. Most Americans (91%) live within hospital referral regions where more than 80% of the hospitalizations occur locally. The study of these referral regions is important because the referral centers should be capable of most advanced care. Although the regions vary in geographic size and population, it is still reasonable to expect that the rates at which procedures are required are roughly comparable.

Using information on rates by referral region, Wennberg and colleagues (1987) were able to analyze the Medicare claims data and to present the results in graphic form using maps. Contrary to expectation, the maps reveal wide variation in the use of various medical services.

The *Dartmouth Atlas of Health Care* systematically reviews variations in the use of a wide variety of medical services. One example is the use of techniques for the diagnosis and treatment of breast cancer. There is controversy about the age for initiating screening for breast cancer using mammography. The analyses consistently show that screening women older than 50 years of age produces health benefit. Among women between the ages of 50 and 74, periodic screening results in significantly lower rates of death from breast cancer (Navarro & Kaplan, 1996). Thus, screening women of Medicare age is commonly advocated. Nevertheless, there is substantial variation in the percentage of female Medicare recipients who have undergone mammography one or more times. For example, in Michigan and Florida, mammography is performed routinely. In Lansing, Michigan, nearly 35% of all women in Medicare had undergone mammography, and similarly high rates were observed in Fort Lauderdale and Sarasota, Florida. However, only 13% of the women in Oklahoma City had obtained mammograms, and a variety of other cities had similar rates. Salt Lake City, for example, had a rate of 13.4%.

For women diagnosed with breast cancer, there is substantial variation in the treatments delivered. During 1992–1993, more than 100,000 women in the Medicare program had surgery for breast cancer. For women who have breast cancer, the surgeon has several major options: lumpectomy, which involves removal of the tumor; partial mastectomy or quadrantectomy, which requires the removal of surrounding tissue; or total mastectomy, which involves complete removal of the breast. Clinical trials have shown little or no difference in survival rates between women who undergo lumpectomy followed by irradiation or chemotherapy and women who undergo total mastectomy. Because the outcomes are likely to be similar, the woman's own preference should play an important role in the decision-making process. However, the *Dartmouth Health Care Atlas* shows that there are some regions in the country where mastectomy is typically performed and other regions where lumpectomy is the operation of choice. Considering the proportion of women who had breast-sparing (lumpectomy) surgery, women were 33 times more likely to have lumpectomy if they lived in Toledo, Ohio than they were if they lived in Rapid City, South Dakota (48.0% vs. 1.4%). Figure 13.4 shows the variation map for breast-sparing surgery. The proportions of women having breast-sparing surgery in Patterson and Ridgewood, New Jersey, were 37.8% and 34.8%, respectively. At the other extreme, only 1.9% had breast-

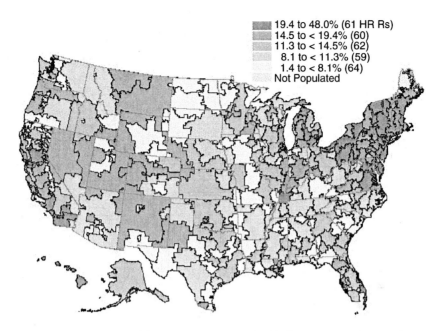

19.4 to 48.0% (61 HR Rs)
14.5 to < 19.4% (60)
11.3 to < 14.5% (62)
 8.1 to < 11.3% (59)
 1.4 to < 8.1% (64)
Not Populated

FIGURE 13.4. Percentage of breast cancer surgery in Medicare women that was breast-sparing (by hospital region 1992–1993). (From Wennberg, 1998.)

sparing surgery in Ogden, Utah and 3.8% in Yakima, Washington. In general, breast-sparing surgery is more widely used in the Northeast than anywhere else in the United States.

The *Dartmouth Atlas* also shows remarkable variability in the distribution of general physicians and specialists. Figures 13.5 and 13.6 show the maps for psychiatrists and orthopedic surgeons, respectively. The map of psychiatrists reveals an interesting pattern. There is remarkable variability in the number of psychiatrists per 1000 persons in hospital service areas. There are 43.9 psychiatrists per 1000 persons in White Plains, New York, 38.4 in San Francisco, and 35.5 in Manhattan. There are, however, only 2.8 psychiatrists per 1000 persons in Oxford, Mississippi and 3.0 per 1000 in Fort Smith, Arkansas. The map shows that psychiatrists tend to live in major metropolitan areas and to be focused on the West or East coast. They are at a high concentration in New England. There is also a substantial concentration near the ski areas of Colorado and in southeastern Arizona. Orthopedic surgeons are much more common in the western half of the country than the eastern half. There are some pockets in the eastern United States that have more orthopedic surgeons, such as the New England states and western Florida. However, the number of orthopedic surgeons per 100,000 residents tends to be low in Tennessee, Kentucky, Illinois, and other midwestern states. Analysis tends to show that there are more operations performed in areas where there are more orthopedic surgeons. However, the correlation is not absolute.

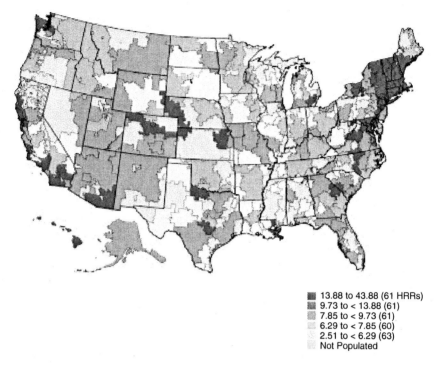

13.88 to 43.88 (61 HRRs)
9.73 to < 13.88 (61)
7.85 to < 9.73 (61)
6.29 to < 7.85 (60)
2.51 to < 6.29 (63)
Not Populated

FIGURE 13.5. Psychiatrists per 100,000 residents by referral region (1993). In 1993, most major metropolitan areas and the East and West Coasts had much higher numbers of psychiatrists per 100,000 residents than the Plains states, the Ohio Valley, and the South.

## Variation and Cost

Many medical conditions are associated with higher prevalence and treatment than others, as shown on the maps. For example, there is not a large variation in treatment options for problems such as fracture of the hip. Patients who fracture their hips are likely to be admitted to the hospital wherever they live. However, the Dartmouth group estimated that 80% of patients who are admitted to hospitals have been diagnosed with a high variation of medical conditions, such as pneumonia, chronic obstructive pulmonary disease, gastroenteritis, and congestive heart failure. They argued that hospital capacity has a major influence on the likelihood that a patient will be hospitalized.

This relation is illustrated in Figure 13.7. The figure shows the relation between hospital beds per 1000 residents and hospitalization for high variation medical conditions. The correlation between hospital beds and admissions is a remarkable 0.76. In hospital referral regions where there are fewer than 2.5 beds per 1000 residents, the hospital discharge rate for high variation condi-

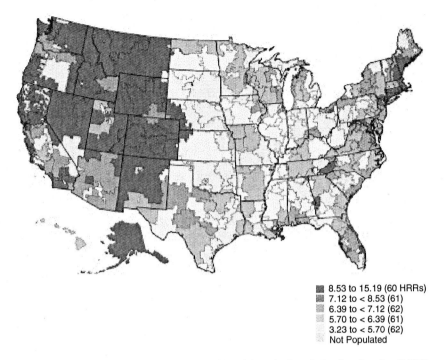

8.53 to 15.19 (60 HRRs)
7.12 to < 8.53 (61)
6.39 to < 7.12 (62)
5.70 to < 6.39 (61)
3.23 to < 5.70 (62)
Not Populated

FIGURE 13.6. Orthopedic surgeons per 100,000 residents by hospital referral region (1993). In 1993, the numbers of orthopedic surgeons per 100,000 residents in the United States tended to be far higher in the West, in Florida, and in parts of the Northeast. The numbers in the Midwest and South tended to be low.

tions was 145 per 1000. Among regions that had more than 4.5 beds per 1000 residents, the rate was 219.8. More beds mean more hospitalizations. These data argue that the decision to admit patients to the hospital is influenced by factors other than the patients' medical conditions. When beds are available, they are more likely to be used. When more hospital beds are used, health care costs go up.

It seems plausible that communities with greater hospital resources are better able to care for their populations. More health care should lead to more health. However, several analyses have shown that people are slightly more likely to die in communities where more acute hospital care is used (Fisher et al., 2003). The obvious explanation is that these communities have people who are older, sicker, or poorer. Careful analyses controlled for age, sex, race, income, and a variety of variables related to illness and the need for care have been carried out. None of these variables was able to explain the relationship. In other words, the analysis suggests that more is not better. In fact, it implies that more may be worse (Fisher & Welch, 1999; Fisher et al., 2003).

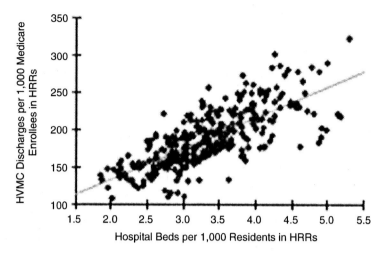

FIGURE 13.7. Association between allocated hospital beds and Medicare hospitalizations for a high variation of medical conditions (HVMC) (1992–1993). HRR = hospital referral region.

## Summary

In the language of CLINECS, this chapter considers inputs. Inputs are investments in health care and are reflected in the number of health care providers and the number of services they provide. There are remarkable differences between developed countries in the number of services offered. In the United States, for example, we spend well more than twice as much per capita than in countries such as Sweden, Italy, or Japan. More inputs may lead to more outputs in terms of cases diagnosed and treated. However, we have little evidence that there is value to patients. Surprisingly little evidence shows that patients in the United States obtain better outcomes than those in other developed countries.

Even within the United States; there is substantial variation in inputs as defined by health services uses. The *Dartmouth Health Care Atlas* shows remarkable variation in health service inputs across demographically similar regions. This raises important questions. It challenges many of our basic assumptions about health care. For example, most consumers assume that if they see a competent doctor the correct diagnosis will be made and the proper treatment offered. We assume that the distribution of disease is roughly equal in different areas. It appears that different providers, confronted with the same burden of illness, may have vastly different rates of diagnosis and treatment. Epidemiological studies that depend on physician diagnosis may be severely biased by the different approaches to illness in geographically different areas.

The *Atlas* also raises important questions for health policy. Areas that have greater capacity to provide care indeed do offer more services. This, in turn, results in greater expense. The Medicare program pays nearly twice as much for service in some communities as it does in others. Providing more hospital beds may lead to more services without necessarily improving the population's health status.

Finally, the *Atlas* suggests that decisions about health care are influenced by factors beyond the patient's health state. When providers have greater capacity, they offer more services. These decisions are primarily made by providers, and it is not clear that patients are consulted. In later chapters we consider methods for involving patients in the decision-making process.

To understand the best pathways to good health outcomes, we need new models to quantify health outcomes and quality of life. We review these models in other chapters and then describe methods by which to analyze the cost-effectiveness of medical procedures. Methods for shared medical decision-making are also reviewed.

## *References*

Fisher, E.S., Welch, H.G. (1999). Could more health care lead to worse health? *Hospital Practice (Off Ed)*, 34(12), 15–16, 21–22, 25 passim.

Fisher, E.S., Wennberg, J.E., Stukel, T.A., Sharp, S. (1994). Hospital readmissions rates for cohorts of Medicare beneficiaries in Boston and New Haven. *New England Journal of Medicine*, 331, 989–995.

Fisher, E.S., Wennberg, D.E., Stukel, T.A., Gottlieb, D.J., Lucas, F.L., Pinder, E.L. (2003). The implications of regional variations in Medicare spending. Part 1. The content, quality, and accessibility of care. *Annals of Internal Medicine*, 138, 273–287.

McGlashan, N.D., Armstrong, R.W. (1972). *Medical geography; techniques and field studies*. London: Methuen.

Navarro, A.M., Kaplan, R.M. (1996). Mammography screening: prospects and opportunity costs. *Womens Health*, 2, 209–233.

Reinhardt, U.E., Hussey, P.S., Anderson, G.F. (2004). U.S. health care spending in an international context. *Health Affairs (Millwood)*, 23(3), 10–25.

Smith, C., Cowan, C., Sensenig, A., Catlin, A. (2005). Health spending growth slows in 2003. *Health Affairs (Millwood)*, 24(1), 185–194.

Starfield, B. (2000). Is US health really the best in the world? *Journal of the American Medical Association*, 284, 483–485.

Wennberg, J.E. (1990). *Small area analysis and the medical care outcome problem*. Paper presented at the Research Methodology: Strengthening Causal Interpretations of Nonexperimental Data, Rockville MD.

Wennberg, J.E. (1998). *The Dartmouth atlas of health care in the United States*. Hanover, NH: Trustees of Dartmouth College.

Wennberg, J.E., Freeman, J.L., Culp, W.J. (1987). Are hospital services rationed in New Haven or over-utilised in Boston? *Lancet*, 1, 1185–1189.

Wennberg, J.E., Fisher, E.S., Skinner, J.S. (2002). Geography and the debate over Medicare reform. *Health Affairs (Millwood)*, Supp Web Exclusives, W96–114.

# 14
# Cancer Survival in Europe and the United States

GEMMA GATTA

For most major cancers, there is evidence that patients from affluent neighborhoods have better survival than patients from deprived neighborhoods, and that this is not simply due to chance (Kogevinas, 1990; Kogevinas et al., 1991; Carnon et al., 1994; Sharp et al., 1995; Pollock & Vickers, 1997; Coleman et al., 1999) or extent of disease at the time of diagnosis (Schrijvers et al., 1995a,b). The underlying mechanisms are complex and difficult to address (Tomatis, 1995).

A pioneering effort to compare cancer survival of cancer patients in the United States and Europe was carried out during the early 1960s (Cutler, 1964). The study indicated that survival was considerably better for Americans than Europeans for most cancer sites. At that time, few cancer registries had been in existence long enough to provide survival data, so the analysis was limited to a comparison between some northern European countries and the state of Connecticut in the United States, which is covered by the Connecticut Cancer Registry.

The opportunity to compare cancer survival in European and U.S. populations again arose when the results of the EUROCARE (EUROpean Cancer Registry based study on cancer patients' survival and CARE) project (Coleman et al., 2003), and the Surveillance and Epidemiology End Results (SEER) program became available (U.S. Department of Health and Human Services, 1973–1995). Both data sets derive from population-based cancer registries. Population-based survival studies are essential for evaluating the effectiveness of health provision and the availability of effective therapies for cancer among populations and countries. Such investigations differ substantially from those based on clinical series, as they avoid problems due to the inevitable selection of patients that occurs in single-hospital or multicentric studies.

The purpose of this chapter was to compare survival in European and U.S. populations for the major cancers in adults and children and to offer an interpretation of any differences.

# Cancer Survival in Adults

Five-year relative survival rates for major cancers in adult patients in Europe and the United States are shown in Table 14.1. European patients had significantly lower survival rates than American patients for all cancer sites considered except stomach cancer. Survival differences were extremely large for prostate cancer (relative survival 56% vs. 81%) and melanoma (relative survival 76% vs. 86%). Differences were large for colon, rectum, breast, and uterine cancer. For lung, cervical, and ovarian cancer and lymphomas, survival differences between the continents were small.

Because the European data refer to 17 countries at various stages of economic development and with differing social structures and health care systems, an overview of survival for each European country in comparison to the United States is given in Table 14.2. For most cancer sites and most countries, survival was lower in Europe than in the United States. For stomach cancer, several countries had significantly higher survival than in the United States. Survival was significantly higher for cervical cancer patients in Iceland and for non-Hodgkin's lymphoma patients in Austria than in the United States. For a few other cancers and for countries that contributed small numbers of cases (Austria, Iceland, France, The Netherlands, Switzerland), survival was higher than in the United States, but the differences were not significant. All of the European countries considered, including the most affluent (Sweden, The Netherlands, Switzerland), had significantly lower survival rates than the United States for colon, rectum, breast, and prostate cancers (Gatta et al., 2000).

TABLE 14.1. Standardized 5-year relative survival for 12 cancers in adult patients diagnosed in the United States and Europe between 1985 and 1989

| Cancer | Europe (EUROCARE) | | United States (SEER) | |
|---|---|---|---|---|
| | Survival (%) | 95% CI | Survival (%) | 95% CI |
| Stomach | 21.1 | 20.3–21.8 | 19.4 | 17.4–21.6 |
| Colon | 46.8 | 45.8–47.7 | 60.2 | 58.8–61.6 |
| Rectum | 42.7 | 41.7–43.8 | 57.3 | 55.2–59.5 |
| Lung | 9.1 | 8.7–9.5 | 13.0 | 12.4–13.6 |
| Breast, women only | 72.5 | 71.9–73.1 | 82.4 | 81.5–83.3 |
| Skin, melanoma | 76.0 | 74.5–77.5 | 86.1 | 84.1–88.1 |
| Cervix uteri | 61.8 | 60.4–63.1 | 66.1 | 63.3–69.1 |
| Corpus uteri | 73.2 | 71.9–74.6 | 83.2 | 81.4–85.0 |
| Ovary | 32.9 | 31.7–34.1 | 39.5 | 37.3–41.8 |
| Prostate | 55.7 | 54.3–57.1 | 81.4 | 80.0–82.8 |
| Hodgkin's disease | 71.7 | 69.7–73.8 | 74.9 | 71.6–78.4 |
| Non-Hodgkin's lymphoma | 46.7 | 45.3–48.1 | 50.3 | 48.4–52.3 |

EUROCARE = EUROpean Cancer Registry-based study on cancer patients' survival and CARE; SEER = Surveillance and Epidemiology End Results; CI = confidence interval.

TABLE 14.2. Five-year relative survival for 12 cancers diagnosed in the United States (SEER) and Europe (EUROCARE) between 1985 and 1989

| Cancer | Survival in the United States (%) | European countries with higher survival than the United States |
|---|---|---|
| Stomach | 19 | Austria (27%),* Spain (26%),* Germany (26%),* France (25%),* Iceland (24%), Italy (23%),* Switzerland (23%), Finland (20%) |
| Colon | 60 | None |
| Rectum | 57 | None |
| Lung | 13 | None |
| Breast, women | 82 | None |
| Melanoma of skin | 86 | Austria (89%), Switzerland (89%), Sweden (88%) |
| Cervix uteri | 66 | Iceland (85%),* Austria (69%), Sweden (68%), The Netherlands (68%), Switzerland (67%) |
| Corpus uteri | 83 | The Netherlands (84%) |
| Ovary | 40 | Sweden (45%), Austria (44%), Spain (41%), Switzerland (40%) |
| Prostate | 81 | None |
| Hodgkin's disease | 75 | France (76%), Switzerland (76%) |
| Non-Hodgkin's lymphoma | 50 | Austria (63%),* France (53%), Iceland (54%) |

*The differences in survival are significant (the 95% confidence intervals do not overlap).

## Cancer Survival of Children

Five-year survival rates for childhood cancers are shown in Table 14.3. Survival for acute nonlymphocytic leukemia was 40% in Europe and 34% in the United States (not significant), but survival rates for other hemopoietic malignancies were similar in the two places.

Among tumors of the central nervous system (CNS), survival was 4% to 7% lower in Europe than in the United States for ependymoma and medulloblastoma (not significant), but survival rates for astrocytoma were similar. Among other solid tumors, survival was 7% to 9% lower in Europe than in the United States for neuroblastoma, Wilms' tumor, and osteosarcoma and 8% higher in Europe for retinoblastoma. For neuroblastoma and Wilms' tumor, the 95% confidence intervals (CI) overlap very little.

Five-year survival rates for all malignancies combined and lymphoid leukemia are shown in Table 14.4 by geographic region. Finland, Iceland, and southern Sweden had the highest survival at 75%, and eastern European countries had the lowest survival at 55%. Among other populations, survival was 72% in the southern European countries, 66% in the United Kingdom, 65% in Denmark, 55% in the eastern European countries and 67% for the other western European countries. For the United States it was 70%, which is roughly comparable to that in Italy, West Germany, and other western European countries.

Five-year survival was also calculated for the same geographic groups for lymphoid leukemias [International Classification of Childhood Cancer (ICCC) Ia]

TABLE 14.3. Five-year survival for European and United States children (0–14 years) diagnosed with cancer from 1985 to 1989

| Diagnostic group | ICCC group[a] | No. of cases | | 5-Year survival (95% CI) | | EU (excluding eastern Europe)[b] |
|---|---|---|---|---|---|---|
| | | EU | USA | EU | USA | |
| Lymphoid leukemia | Ia | 4663 | 878 | 75 (74–76) | 77 (74–80) | 76 (74–80) |
| Acute nonlymphocytic leukemia | Ib | 915 | 146 | 40 (37–43) | 34 (27–43) | 42 (27–43) |
| Hodgkin's disease | IIa | 704 | 145 | 92 (90–94) | 90 (86–95) | 93 (86–95) |
| Non-Hodgkin's lymphoma | IIb | 860 | 141 | 75 (72–78) | 73 (66–81) | 77 (66–81) |
| Ependymoma | IIIa | 300 | 79 | 48 (42–54) | 55 (45–68) | 49 (45–68) |
| Astrocytoma | IIIb | 1265 | 375 | 73 (70–75) | 72 (67–77) | 74 (67–77) |
| PNET/medulloblastoma | IIIc | 759 | 153 | 48 (44–51) | 52 (45–61) | 49 (45–61) |
| Neuroblastoma | IVa | 1094 | 265 | 48 (45–51) | 57 (51–63)[*] | 48 (51–63)[*] |
| Retinoblastoma[c] | V | 470 | 92 | 95 (92–96) | 87 (85–90)[*] | 96 (85–90)[*] |
| Wilms' tumor | VIa | 951 | 221 | 83 (80–85) | 90 (86–94)[*] | 85 (86–94)[*] |
| Osteosarcoma[c] | VIIIa | 288 | 62 | 61 (55–66) | 68 (56–80) | 62 (56–80) |
| Ewing's sarcoma | VIIIc | 305 | 56 | 60 (55–66) | 61 (49–76) | 62 (49–76) |
| Rhabdomyosarcoma | IXa | 624 | 124 | 62 (58–66) | 60 (52–69) | 64 (52–69) |
| Germ cell: testis[c] | Xc | 106 | 20 | 95 (89–98) | 100 (89–100) | 98 (89–100) |
| Germ cell: ovary[c] | Xc | 78 | 21 | 87 (78–93) | 90 (77–100) | 92 (77–100) |

EU = Europe; USA = United States; PNET = primitive neuroectodermal tumors; Germ cell = germ cell carcinoma.
[a]ICCC group: International Classification of Childhood Cancer (Kramárová and Stiller, 1996).
[b]EUROCARE population excluding children from eastern European countries.
[c]Retinoblastoma and testicular germ cell tumors in children aged 0–4 only; osteosarcoma and ovarian germ cell tumors in children aged 10–14 only.
[*]The differences in survival are significant ($p < 0.05$) between the United States and Europe.

TABLE 14.4. Age and site standardized 5-year survival for all cancers combined and for lymphoid leukemia; children diagnosed 1985–1989 in Europe and the United States

| Region | No. of cases | | 5-Year survival (%) and 95% CI | |
|---|---|---|---|---|
| | All cancers | Lymphoid leukemia | All cancers | Lymphoid leukemia |
| Nordic countries[a] | 904 | 240 | 75 (72–78) | 83 (78–88) |
| Western Germany | 5364 | 1603 | 72 (71–73) | 78 (76–80) |
| Italy | 833 | 203 | 71 (68–74) | 76 (70–82) |
| Other western European countries[b] | 1187 | 528 | 67 (64–70) | 77 (73–81) |
| UK | 5880 | 1613 | 66 (65–67)[*] | 73 (71–75) |
| Denmark | 640 | 171 | 65 (62–68)[*] | 74 (67–81) |
| Eastern European countries[c] | 1340 | 305 | 55 (52–58)[*] | 62 (56–68)[*] |
| United States | 3476 | 878 | 70 (68–72) | 77 (74–80) |

European data are from EUROCARE, U.S. data are from SEER.
[a]Finland, Iceland, and southern Sweden.
[b]Austria, France, The Netherlands, Spain, and Switzerland.
[c]Estonia, Poland, Slovakia, and Slovenia.
[*]The differences in survival are significant ($p < 0.05$) between European regions and the United States.

(Kramárová & Stiller, 1996), which represented about one-fourth of all the malignancies. The Nordic countries again had the highest survival (83%), and Germany, Italy, and the other Western countries had survival figures similar to the average for the United States (77%). Eastern European countries had the lowest survival (62%) (Gatta et al., 2002).

## Interpretation of Cancer Survival Differences

Colorectal, prostate, stomach cancers, and Hodgkin's disease were selected for a discussion of results. The first pair of diseases were chosen for the large variation we found between cancer patients in the United States and Europe. Stomach cancer and Hodgkin's disease had similar survival in the two populations.

Before attempting to interpret these differences, it is important to consider whether the two data sets are comparable and to discuss a number of methodological issues. Differences in the age and sex distribution of cancer patients in the United States and Europe were accounted for using standardization procedures.

Mortality from other causes of death can bias survival comparisons, especially among older patients, because general mortality varies from region to region and country to country. This problem was addressed by calculating relative survival as the ratio of the survival observed for the cancer patients to that of the age-matched population (of which the patients formed part). Relative survival was calculated in slightly different ways for the U.S. data (Ederer I method) (Ederer et al., 1961) and European data (Hakulinen method) (Hakulinen & Abeywickrama, 1985). However, the 5-year relative survival calculated by the two methods never differed by more than 0.1%. Distribution by race was not considered in this study. However, the proportion of nonwhites is lower in the EUROCARE than the SEER population (about 10% of the U.S. cancer cases occurred among Blacks (U.S. Department of Health and Human Services, 1973–1995). It has been shown that black patients in the United States have lower survival than the average (Mayberry et al., 1995). If the analysis had been restricted to Caucasians (this does not include Mexicans and Asians) in the United States, the survival differences between the United States and Europe would have been slightly enhanced.

Other possible biasing factors are the quality and comparability of the data from the cancer registries. For example, the definition of cancer, the quality of registration, and the completeness of follow-up may not be the same in all registries. The magnitudes of the effects introduced by these differences can be estimated, although they cannot always be controlled for in the analysis.

In the present study, although we considered only malignant tumors, we compared broad cancer categories defined on the basis of the anatomical site of the malignancy as defined by the third digit of the International Classification of Diseases (ICD) code (World Health Organization, 1977). Variations between registries and countries in case mix, subsite, and histological characteristics can render survival comparisons less valid because survival is known to vary by subsite and histotype. This was the case for stomach cancer, for which the proportion of tumors in the cardia (proximal subsite of stomach with unfavorable prognosis compared to other gastric cancers) was higher in the SEER than in the EURO-CARE series (U.S. Department of Health and Human Services, 1973–1995; Gatta et al., 2000). There are large differences in the stomach cancer incidence: it was lower in the United States (5.9/100,000/year) than in Europe (12/100.000/year) (Parkin et al., 1997). Incidence rates are higher for distal stomach cancers than for proximal stomach cancers, the latter being quite constant among populations and over time. The declining incidence of gastric carcinomas has been observed throughout the world, although with different patterns, as the decline has generally been confined to the distal subsite and not to cardia cancer (Verdecchia et al., 2003). The survival difference between the two continents may be almost totally due to the different case mix of stomach cancer patients.

The above considerations suggest that the survival differences we have found between cancer patients in the United States and Europe are unlikely to be due principally to statistical or registration artifacts (Gatta et al., 2000, 2002).

Real survival differences may be explained in terms of three basic factors: lead time bias due to earlier tumor detection; better prognosis due to better response to treatment at an earlier disease stage; and more aggressive (or effective) treatment protocols. The latter two factors lead to a genuine survival advantage. It is possible that all three of these factors may be more prevalent in the United States than in Europe, although currently available data do not allow any firm conclusions at this point.

The specific EUROCARE (high-resolution) study on colorectal cases—whose objective was to examine the extent to which the disease stage, staging procedures (number of lymph nodes examined), and treatment explain the differences in cancer survival (Ciccolallo et al., 2005)—supports the above speculation. For colorectal cancer (Table 14.5), survival differences between Europe and the

TABLE 14.5. Three-year relative survival and distribution of cases by various parameters: EUROCARE and SEER study on colorectal cancer for patients with cancer diagnosed during 1990–1991

| Registry (no. of cases) | 3-Year survival | Distribution (%) | | | | | | |
| | | Dukes' stage[a] | | | | | Stage determinant | Surgical resection |
| | | A | B | C | D | Unstaged | Twelve or more nodes examined[b] | Resected |
| --- | --- | --- | --- | --- | --- | --- | --- | --- |
| United States (n = 11,191) | 69 | 24 | 30 | 23 | 18 | 5 | 28 | 92 |
| Europe (n = 2492) | 57 | 14 | 34 | 21 | 21 | 9 | 13 | 85 |

[a]A = localized within bowel wall; B = penetrates the bowel wall; C = spread to the regional lymph nodes; D = distant metastases.
[b]In patients who underwent resection.

United States appeared mostly attributable to differences in stage at diagnosis. There were also wide variations in diagnostic and surgical practice between Europe and the United States.

For both colorectal and prostate cancer, the inclusion of small or clinically silent lesions identified by screening and preclinical diagnostic activity boosts overall survival in one area compared to an area where such activity is less widespread. One indicator for early diagnosis of colorectal cancer is the proportion of all colorectal cancers that are adenocarcinomas in polyps; this figure was much higher among cases in the United States than in Europe (13% vs. 2%, respectively) (Gatta et al., 2003). Endoscopy and the fecal occult blood test (FOBT) have been actively recommended by the American Cancer Society. A survey showed that in 1987 a total of 24% of people over 50 years of age had undergone endoscopy at some time in the past; this proportion increased to 38% in 1992. The percentage of people older than 50 years of age who reported undergoing the FOBT within the previous year increased from 15% in 1987 to 18% in 1992 (Breen & Kessler, 1995; U.S. Department of Health and Human Services, 2000). We do not have equivalent information for Europe. The European Union delivered recommendations to member states to implement screening for colorectal cancer only in 2000 (Advisory Committee on Cancer Prevention, 2000).

Nevertheless, it is likely that earlier diagnosis may be responsible for lead time bias for some cancers. The recent dramatic increase in identification of prostate cancer in the United States (Merril et al., 1996) is in part due to the increasing frequency of surgery for adenoma of the prostate (with a concomitant increase in the incidental finding of asymptomatic prostate cancer), as well as the rapid implementation of new diagnostic procedures, including transrectal, ultrasound-guided needle biopsy and, above all, serum assay for prostate-specific antigen (PSA) (Potosky et al., 1995). The incidence of prostate cancer in the United States is more than double that detected in Europe (Parkin et al., 1997).

The relative excess risk of death reported for prostate cancer shows impressive differences between the United States and Europe during the first year after diagnosis, which suggests a marked effect of early diagnosis in the United States (Gatta et al., 2000). We cannot state that the proportion of patients cured in the United States did not increase at all over time and was higher in the United States than Europe because of the high access to early detection in the United States. Owing to the effect of earlier tumor diagnosis, we cannot exclude that lead time bias would affect the observed survival differences. The estimation of cured patients is not an easy task.

In contrast to cancer in adults, childhood cancer survival in Europe (except eastern Europe) is similar to that in the United States. This is probably partially due to the fact that childhood cancers are generally more responsive to therapy than adult cancers, but it must also reflect accessibility to these treatments. Survival was low in eastern European countries. In western Europe, survival from all childhood cancers combined ranged from 65% to 75%. Differences in the availability of effective treatments and in access to up-to-date therapeutic protocols probably explain the international differences in childhood cancer survival.

The findings of the childhood cancer survival analysis also have some relevance for the interpretation of differences in adult cancer survival. In most countries, the data for both adult and childhood cancers are collected in the same way by the same cancer registries. The overall similarity of childhood cancer survival estimates reported here for Europe and the United States suggests that the trans-Atlantic differences seen for almost all adult cancers are unlikely to be due mainly to bias.

Hodgkin's disease in adults is responsive to therapy at all stages of presentation, and agreed protocols have been available for decades. As with childhood cancers, the availability and access to therapeutic protocols for Hodgkin's disease offer likely explanations for the survival similarity between the two populations.

Geographical variation in cancer survival was much greater in Europe than in the United States. For colorectal cancer patients, for instance, 5-year survival was low in eastern Europe (less than 25% in Poland and no more than 35% in Estonia and Slovenia), whereas in western Europe survival varied from 41% to 54% for colon cancer and from 38% to 53% for rectal cancer (Gatta et al., 1998). Among patients diagnosed in the nine SEER registry areas during the same period (1985–1989), survival of colorectal cancer ranged from 56% to 65% (U.S. Department of Health and Human Services, 1973–1995). In Europe, the national health care systems are almost entirely public (Micheli et al., 2003). The health system in the United States is completely private, with a small federal contribution to health costs through the Medicaid and Medicare programs. In the United States up to 1998 (Hoffman & Schlobohm, 2000), one in six Americans did not have health insurance, so one would expect cancer survival inequalities to be higher in the private sector (McDavid et al., 2003) than in the public health system.

High survival rates in the United States with little geographical variation between the SEER registries could arise from the fact that the SEER registries are not fully representative of the entire population of the United States, as they cover only the more affluent areas (Mariotto et al., 2002). Broadening the comparison to include a wider range of U.S. populations would be an interesting future step. A large trans-Atlantic collaborative study called CONCORD (related to the history of the Battle of Lexington and Concord) is ongoing (McDavid et al., 2004) with the objective to measure and explain these differences in cancer survival.

## Summary

Cancer survival in the United States is higher than in Europe for many (but not all) adult cancers. No systematic differences are seen for childhood cancers. Methodological differences in collection, quality, and analysis of data have been explored and seem likely to play a relatively minor role in the differences in cancer survival between Europe and the United States. The differences in cancer survival for European and the U.S. populations may stem at least in part from differences in clinical practice. Biological and health care system factors are both likely to be involved, but their relative importance is unknown.

Today we cannot clearly explain the existing cancer survival variation between patients in the United States and Europe. The CONCORD study aims to obtain reliable estimates of cancer survival differences from large populations on both sides of the Atlantic and to determine the extent to which any differences are due to artifacts and/or differences in tumor biology, definition of disease, stage at diagnosis, and health care systems between contributing countries.

The CONCORD study has three phases.

• Phase 1 involves estimating population-based cancer survival rates in each country or region. The American cancer registries cover a larger population than that of the SEER regions. Furthermore, centralized data quality checks and analyses can increase the quality and comparability of the data.
• Phase 2 involves specialized studies to explore survival differences in detail. Clinical information will be obtained from the medical records of 500 representative patients diagnosed with cancer of the breast, bowel, or prostate in each contributing state, province, or country. Data will cover the diagnostic workup, tumor stage, treatment, tumor pathology, and health care system. The main innovation in CONCORD is the inclusion of data on clinical follow-up, particularly recurrence, metastasis, and the appearance of a new primary tumor.
• Phase 3 will obtain tumor pathology material from a random sample of patients included in the phase 2 studies. This material will be reviewed by independent expert pathologists who do not know the original diagnosis. This review will enable assessment of the impact of any international differences in disease definition on international differences in cancer survival.

The results of the CONCORD study will provide a firm scientific basis for formulating policy on health education and on the organization of cancer treatment and care. The CONCORD study will therefore help governments achieve its strategic objectives on cancer (Department of Health, 2000).

What should we do until these questions are solved? Cancer survival differences in Europe must be understand to remove disparities. The EUROCARE high-resolution studies (studies on samples of patients collecting specific clinical information not routinely collected by cancer registries) have this specific aim, and the results from the pilot studies have provided suggestions for health planners. The EUROCARE study has had an impact on national plans in the United Kingdom (National Board of Health Plan, 2000) and Denmark (Berrino et al., 1997), where survival rates for patients diagnosed with several of the most common cancers were lower than in comparable western European countries and in Italy, where the aim has been to reduce geographic disparities in cancer survival (Coleman et al., 2000).

## References

Advisory Committee on Cancer Prevention (2000). Recommendations on cancer screening in the European union. *European Journal of Cancer*, 36, 1473–1478.
Berrino, F., Micheli, A., Sant, M., Capocaccia, R. (1997). Interpreting survival differences and trends. *Tumori*, 83, 9–16.

Breen, N., Kessler, L. (1995). Trends in cancer screening—United States, 1987 and 1992. *MMWR Morbidity and Mortality Weekly Report*, 45, 57–61.

Carnon, A.G., Ssemwogerere, A., Lamont, D.W., Hole, D.J., Mallon, E., Gorge, W.D., et al. (1994). Relation between socio-economic deprivation and pathological prognostic factors in women with breast cancer. *British Medical Journal*, 309, 1054–1057.

Ciccolallo, L., Capocaccia, R., Coleman, M.P., Berrino, F., Coebergh, J.W.W., Damhuis, R.A.M., et al. (2005). Survival differences between European and US patients with colorectal cancer: role of stage at diagnosis and surgery. *Gut*, 54, 268–273.

Coleman, M.P., Babb, P., Damiecki, P., Grosclaude, P., Honjo, S., Jones, J., et al. (1999). *Cancer survival trends in England and Wales, 1971–1995: deprivation and NHS region; studies in medical and population subjects*. London: The Stationary Office.

Coleman, M.P., Gatta, G., Verdecchia, A., Esteve, J., Sant, M., Storm, H., et al. (2003). EUROCARE Working Group EUROCARE-3 summary: cancer survival in Europe at the end of the 20th century. *Annals of Oncology*, 2003, 14 (Suppl 5), v128–v149.

Cutler, S. J. (Ed.) (1964). *International symposium on end result of cancer therapy*. National Cancer Institute Monograph No. 15. Bethesda, MD: US Government Printing Office.

Department of Health. (2000). *The NHS cancer plan*. London: Department of Health.

Ederer, F., Axtell, L.M., Cutler, S.J. (1961). The relative survival rate: a statistical methodology. *Monograph of the National Cancer Institute*, 6, 101–121.

Gatta, G., Faivre, J., Capocaccia, R., Ponz de Leon, M. (1998). Survival of colorectal cancer patients in Europe during the period 1978–1989. *European Journal of Cancer*, 34, 2176–2183.

Gatta, G., Capocaccia, R., Coleman, M.P., Ries, L.A.G., Hakulinen, T., Micheli, A., et al. (2000). Toward a comparison of survival in American and European cancer patients. *Cancer*, 89, 893–900.

Gatta, G., Capocaccia, R., Coleman, M.P., Ries, L.A., Berrino, F. (2002). Childhood cancer survival in Europe and the United States. *Cancer*, 95, 1767–1772.

Gatta, G., Ciccolallo, L., Capocaccia, R., Coleman, M.P., Hakulinen, T., Møller, H., et al. and the EUROCARE Working Group (2003). Differences in colorectal cancer survival between European and US populations: the importance of sub-site and morphology. *European Journal of Cancer*, 39, 2214–2222.

Hakulinen, T., Abeywickrama, K.H.A. (1985). Computer program package for relative survival analysis. *Computer Programs in Biomedicine*, 19, 197–207.

Hoffman, C., Schlobohm, A. (Eds.). (2000). *Uninsured in America: a chart book*. (2nd ed.). Washington, DC: The Kaiser Commission on Medicaid and the Uninsured. pp. 3–7. Kogevinas, M. (1990). *Longitudinal study: socio-economic differences in cancer survival*. Series LS, No. 5. London: Office of Population, Census and Surveys.

Kogevinas, M. (1990). *Longitudinal study. Socio-economic differences in cancer survival.* Series LS No. 5 London: Office of Population, Census and Surveys.

Kogevinas, M., Marmot, M.G., Fox, A.J., Goldblatt, P.O. (1991). Socio-economic differences in cancer survival. *Journal of Epidemiology and Community Health*, 45, 216–219.

Kramárová, E., Stiller, C. A. (1996). The international classification of childhood cancer. *International Journal of Cancer*, 68, 759–765.

Mariotto, A., Capocaccia, R., Verdecchia, A., Micheli, A., Feuer, E.J., Pickle, L., et al. (2002). Projecting SEER cancer survival rates to the US: an ecological regression approach. *Cancer Causes Control,* 13(2), 101–111.

Mayberry, R.M., Coates, R.J., Hill, H.A., Click, L.A., Chen, V.W., Austin, D.F., et al. (1995). Determinants of black/white differences in colon cancer survival. *Journal of the National Cancer Institute*, 87, 1686–1693.

McDavid, K., Tucker, T., Sloggett, A., Coleman, M.P. (2003). Cancer survival in Kentucky and health insurance coverage. *Archives of Internal Medicine,* 163, 2135–2144.

McDavid, K., Schymura, M.J., Armstrong, L., Santilli, L., Schmidt, B., Byers, T., et al. (2004). Rationale and design of the National Program of Cancer Registries' Breast, Colon, and Prostate Cancer Patterns of Care Study. *Cancer Causes Control,* 15, 1057–1066.

Merril, R.M., Potosky, A.L., Feuer, E.J. (1996). Changing trends in US prostate cancer incidence rates. *Journal of the National Cancer Institute,* 88, 1683–1685.

Micheli, A., Coebergh, J.W., Mugno, E., Massimiliani, E., Sant, M., Oberaigner, W., et al. (2003). European health systems and cancer care. *Annals of Oncology,* 14(Suppl 5), v41–v60.

National Board of Health Plan (2000). *Report 2: epidemiology.* Copenhagen: National Board of Health.

Parkin, D.M., Muir, C.S., Whelan, S.L., Ferlay, J., Raymond, L., Young, J. (Eds). (1997). *Cancer incidence in five continents,* Vol. VII. IARC Scientific Publication No. 120. Lyon: International Agency for Research on Cancer.

Pollock, A.M., Vickers, N. (1997). Breast, lung and colorectal cancer incidence and survival in South Thames region, 1987-1992: the effect of social deprivation. *Journal of Epidemiology and Community Health,* 19, 288–294.

Potosky, A.L., Miller, B.A., Albertsen, P.C., Kramer, B.S. (1995). The role of increasing detection in the rising incidence of prostate cancer. *Journal of the American Medical Association,* 273, 548–552.

Schrijvers, C.T.M., Mackenbach, J., Lutz, J-M., Quinn, M.J., Coleman, M.P. (1995a). Deprivation, stage at diagnosis and cancer survival. *International Journal of Cancer,* 63, 324–329.

Schrijvers, C.T.M., Mackenbach, J., Lutz, J-M., Quinn, M.J., Coleman, M.P. (1995b). Deprivation and survival from breast cancer. *British Journal of Cancer,* 72, 738–743.

Sharp, L., Finlayson, A.R., Black, R.J. (1995). Cancer survival and deprivation in Scotland [abstract]. *Journal of Epidemiology and Community Health,* 49, s79.

Tomatis, L. (1995). Socioeconomic factors and human cancer. *International Journal of Cancer,* 62, 121–125.

U.S. Department of Health and Human Services. (1973–1995). National Cancer Institute, Surveillance and Epidemiology End Results Program (SEER). *Cancer Statistics Review* [Dataset on CD ROM].

U.S. Department of Health and Human Services. (2000). *Healthy People 2010.* Conference edition, section 3-12 (http://www.health.gov/healthypeople). Accessed January 2000.

Verdecchia, A., Mariotto, A., Gatta, G., Bustamante-Teixeira, A., Jiki, W. (2003). Comparison of stomach cancer incidence and survival in four continents. *European Journal of Cancer,* 39, 1603–1609.

World Health Organisation. (1977) *International classification of diseases* (9th ed.). Geneva: WHO.

# 15
# Patient Safety: What Does It Mean in the United States?

JOSEPH E. SCHERGER

Mistakes are at the very base of human thoughts, embedded there, feeding the structure like root nodules. If we were not provided with the knack of being wrong, we could never get anything useful done. We think our way along by choosing between right and wrong alternatives, and the wrong choices are made as frequently as the right ones. We get along in life this way. We are built to make mistakes, coded for error. The capacity to leap across mountains of information and land lightly on the wrong side represents the highest of human endowments (Thomas, 1974).

Patient safety in the United States was jumpstarted by the publication of *To Err Is Human: Building a Safer Health System* by the Institute of Medicine in 2000. This report was written as part of the work of the IOM Committee on the Quality of Health Care in America. With a companion report, *Crossing the Quality Chasm: A New Health System for the 21st Century* (Institute of Medicine, 2001), this committee has had a major impact on health care in the United States, shifting the focus of policy and action from finance and cost containment to safety and quality. This chapter surveys the patient safety movement in the United States. It is difficult to separate patient safety from the overall issue of quality of care, so this chapter partially addresses the broad issue of quality with an emphasis on safety. The research behind *To Err is Human* was all hospital-based, and most of the patient safety actions in the United States are in the hospital sector. Studies suggest that medical errors are at least as common in office practice with serious consequences, and parallel efforts at safety in office practice are getting started and are also discussed here.

The bottom line is this: As stated so eloquently by Lewis Thomas (1974) and as embodied in the title *To Err Is Human*, it is natural for humans to make mistakes. The patient safety effort is not about making people better or safer; it is necessarily focused on the development and application of safer technologies and systems of care.

## Origins of Safety and Quality in Health Care

Concerns about safety and quality in health care are as old as antiquity. Alexander the Great is quoted as saying, "I die by the help of too many physicians!" (Lewis, 1974). In 18th and 19th century America, health care was a disorganized trade of highly questionable quality, with many "snake-oil salesmen" roaming the country. During the early 20th century, with the reform of medical education, health care quality started to receive attention, especially in teaching hospitals (Lewis, 1974). During the 1950s, Osler Peterson led an observational study of general practice in North Carolina that was highly critical and fueled an academic bias against community general practice that lasted for decades until the specialty of family medicine was born (Peterson et al., 1956).

During the 1960s, Avedis Donabedian (1966) at the University of Michigan developed a framework for measuring the quality of care that is largely used to this day, distinguishing technical and interpersonal quality and addressing structural, process, and outcome quality as complementary measures. Contrary to the current "outcomes movement," Donabedian (1968) emphasized process quality as the most important.

Safety and quality remained largely academic concerns until the managed care movement swept the United States during the 1990s. The main focus of managed care became cost containment, and the concept of managed care as appropriate care raised questions about consistency in health care and whether evidence-based clinical guidelines should be followed regularly in the care of patients. Perceiving a large gap between the best care known through clinical evidence and the care being delivered to the masses through a fragmented cottage industry of medical practices, the IOM launched its quality initiatives in 1994 (Council of the Institute of Medicine, 1994.).

## Overuse, Underuse, and Misuse of Care

1998 was a watershed year in the quest for quality improvement of health care in the United States. Three major reports were issued detailing serious quality of care concerns. The most widely noted was the IOM National Roundtable on Health Care Quality published in the *Journal of the American Medical Association* (Chassin & Galvin, 1998). This report cited three types of quality problems: overuse, underuse, and misuse. Numerous examples of each type were presented, such as overuse of hysterectomy and other elective surgeries, underuse of lifesaving therapies, such as beta-blockers after myocardial infarction, and misuse of antibiotics for viral infections. Conclusions such as the following led to the formation of the IOM Committee on the Quality of Health Care in America in 1998 (Chassin & Galvin, 1998).

The burden of harm conveyed by the collective impact of all of our health care quality problems is staggering. It requires the urgent attention of all the stakeholders: the health care professions, health care policymakers, consumer advocates and purchasers of care. The challenge is to bring the full potential benefit of effective health care to all Americans while avoiding unneeded and harmful interventions and eliminating preventable complications of care. Meeting this challenge demands a readiness to think in radically new ways about how to deliver health care services and how to assess and improve their quality. Our present efforts resemble a team of engineers trying to break the sound barrier by tinkering with a Model T Ford. We need a new vehicle or perhaps, many new vehicles. The only unacceptable alternative is not to change.

A second national panel, The Advisory Commission on Consumer Protection and Quality, called for a national commitment to improve health care quality, concluding the following (Advisory Commission on Consumer Protection, 1998).

Exhaustive research documents the fact that today, in America, there is no guarantee that any individual will receive high-quality care for any particular health problem. The health care industry is plagued with overutilization of services, underutilization of services, and errors in health care practice.

Finally, the RAND Corporation conducted an extensive literature review of peer-review publications between 1993 and 1997 and substantiated that serious and pervasive quality-of-care problems occurred for acute, chronic, and preventive care in all medical settings in the United States (Schuster et al., 1998). By the end of 1998, the concern for the quality of health care in the United States was out in the open, setting the stage for the dramatic reaction to the publication of *To Err Is Human*.

## Medical Errors in Hospitals

Headlines across the United States in November 1999 reported that between 44,000 and 98,000 deaths per year occur in American hospitals due to medical errors. Even at the lower number, this was more than breast cancer, human immunodeficiency virus (HIV) infection/acquired immunodeficiency syndrome (AIDS), or automobile accidents. At the higher number, it was more than all three combined! Medical errors were between the fourth and eighth leading causes of death! Where did these numbers come from?

The major research behind *To Err Is Human* came from two studies conducted many years before the landmark report. Both studies were conducted by a Harvard team led by Lucian Leape and Troyen Brennan, using a retrospective review process looking for evidence of adverse events caused by medical care, not by the disease process. The first study was conducted in 1984 at New York hospitals and found adverse events in 3.7% of hospitalizations (Brennan et al., 1991; Leape et al., 1991). The second study was conducted in 1992 at hospitals in Colorado and Utah and found adverse events in 2.9% of hospitalizations (Thomas et al., 2000). In both of these studies, more than half of the adverse events resulted from medical errors that could have been prevented. In the New York study 13.6% of adverse events led to death, whereas in the Colorado and Utah study 6.6% of adverse events led to death. The 98,000 deaths per year in the United States is an extrapolation of the New York study, and the 44,000 deaths per year is an extrapolation of the Colorado and Utah study (Institute of Medicine, 2000).

Medication-related errors occur frequently in hospitals and received special attention in the IOM report. One study conducted at two prestigious teaching hospitals found that 2 of every 100 admissions experienced a preventable adverse drug event, resulting in average increased hospital costs of $4700 per admission, or about $2.8 million annually for a 700-bed teaching hospital (Bates et al., 1997).

*To Err Is Human* offers a series of recommendations that have largely been carried out. There was a call for leadership and greater knowledge in medical errors and prevention by funding a Center for Patient Safety in the U.S. Agency for Healthcare Research and Quality (AHRQ). Patient Safety Centers have sprung up throughout the United States funded by this AHRQ initiative. The report called for a combination of mandatory reporting of serious events and voluntary reporting of near-misses, which has since been implemented. The accreditation process of U.S. hospitals conducted by a Joint Commission on Accreditation of Healthcare Organizations (JCAHO) has increasingly used patient safety measures in its reviews since the IOM report. Hospitals across the United States have placed a priority on developing systems for ensuring patient safety, and public attention has not waned. Much progress is being made with information technology to guide care and prevent human errors. Five years after publication of *To Err Is Human*, there is consensus that many promising efforts have been launched, but the task is far from complete. Efforts to improve patient safety need to expand and accelerate to achieve the results called for in the IOM reports (Altman et al., 2004).

## Save 100,000 Lives

A major force in the United States for improving the safety and quality of health care is the Institute for Healthcare Improvement (IHI) in Boston led by Donald Berwick. At its annual quality forum in December 2004, IHI launched a campaign in U.S. hospitals to save 100,000 lives through six evidence-based practices.

Many other U.S. health organizations and health systems have signed on to this campaign. Evidence was presented that if U.S. hospitals adopted six straightforward practices with 90% consistency, 100,000 lives would be saved. This effort moves patient safety beyond avoiding medical errors to promoting best medical practices. Each of these practices is described briefly here; further details and references are available on the IHI website "Save 100k Lives Campaign" (http://www.ihi.org/IHI/Programs/Campaign).

## Rapid Response Teams

Pioneered in Australia and applied successfully in the United States, rapid response teams are physicians, nurses, and other critical care workers who may be called by anyone in the hospital when a patient begins to deteriorate. Patients are assessed and interventions started at the earliest sign of a serious decline. This strategy has been used successfully to reduce greatly the frequency of cardiac arrests and hospital mortality.

## Improved Care for Acute Myocardial Infarction

Evidence shows that when eligible patients receive prompt administration of aspirin and early use of beta-blockers, mortality from acute myocardial infarction (AMI) is reduced. Yet these medications have not been consistently used owing to a lack of standardized order sets and inconsistent implementation.

## Prevention of Adverse Drug Events

Adverse drug events (ADEs) occur frequently when patients are transferred from home to hospital, from the intensive care unit (ICU) to the floor, from the hospital to a skilled nursing facility, or back home. Across these transitions, information about medications is usually hand-written from sources that may not be accurate or complete. Adverse side effects of medication, some serious, are often missed, and the medication is repeated.

## Prevention of Central Line-Associated Bloodstream Infection

Forty-eight percent of ICU patients have central venous catheters, and there are about 5.3 bloodstream infections per 1000 catheter-days in the ICU. A bundle of best practices that may prevent many of these are hand hygiene, maximal barrier precautions, chlorhexidine skin antisepsis, appropriate catheter site, administration system care, and no routine replacement. Knowing these precautions are not enough, they still must be applied consistently.

## Prevention of Surgical-Site Infection

Many hospital-acquired infections are related to surgery, and most are preventable. A bundle of services that greatly reduce surgical-site infections include guideline-based use of prophylactic antibiotics, appropriate hair removal, and perioperative glucose control.

## Prevention of Ventilator-Associated Pneumonia

Nosocomial pneumonia occurs in up to 15% of patients undergoing mechanical ventilation. A bundle of best practices to prevent many of these pneumonias includes five components: elevating the head of the bed to at least 30 degrees, daily "sedation vacations," daily assessment of readiness to extubate, prophylaxis of peptic ulcer disease, and prophylaxis of deep vein thrombosis.

## Medical Errors in Office Practice

Office practice in the United States remains largely a cottage industry of independent private practices of various size. For this reason, the diffusion of innovations, such as electronic health records, is slow and now lags behind other, more organized countries such as the United Kingdom. Medical errors are common in office practice and include improper diagnosis, lack of patient information, prescription errors, failure to follow up on test results, and improper patient management (Sanders & Esmail, 2003). A prospective study of primary care practices in the Boston (USA) area found that 25% of patients had had an adverse drug event, and 11% of them were preventable (Gandhi et al., 2003). Another widely cited study of office practice revealed that only about half of the patients received the recommended care (McGlynn et al., 2003).

Preventing medical errors in office practice is a large task in a culture that values the autonomy of independent private practice. Most of the leverage for change comes from policies adopted by health insurance plans and government regulations. Because medical errors drive up costs, those that pay for care have the greatest incentive to improve safety. A decade of health information technology has been declared in the United States to improve patient information, provide clinical decision support, and improve communication through the use of online methods (Brailer, 2004). Technology alone cannot solve the problem without improving the human factors. The greater use of health care teams working in integrated practices is seen as an important step in improving office practice (Lawrence, 2002; Grumbach & Bodenheimer, 2004).

## How U.S. Consumers View Medical Errors

A recent survey of adult Americans on the safety and quality of health care was conducted by the Henry J. Kaiser Family Foundation. They found that nearly half of all consumers worry about the safety of their health care. One-third report that they or a family member have been a victim of medical errors, and one in five victims says the error resulted in serious harm. Only 28% of patients and family members who experienced an error were told about it by the physicians involved. What do consumers think are the leading causes of medical errors? The survey found overwork, stress or fatigue of health professionals (74%), doctors not having enough time with patients (70%), not enough nurses in hospitals (69%), and health professionals not working together or not communicating as a team (68%) as the most common responses (Henry J. Kaiser Family Foundation, 2004). American consumers are well tuned to the problems of safety and quality in health care and can play a pivotal role in demanding change.

# Summary

The IOM report *Crossing the Quality Chasm* identifies six aims for any health system: safe, effective, patient-centered, timely, efficient, and equitable care (Institute of Medicine, 2001). Safety is given first priority as a prerequisite for quality. In the United States, the patient safety effort has remained primary and overshadows the others. The media and the public remain focused on medical errors as a scandal that should not occur. New health information technology is seen as the panacea, but technology alone cannot solve problems and is likely to create new ones. Patient safety comes from creating a culture of safety in which everyone participates *and* systems are in place to ensure that the current best practices of safe care are consistently being employed. Other industries, such as manufacturing and electronics, have achieved near perfection, or six-sigma quality, through investing and implementing safety systems. Health care in the United States has a long way to go but is moving in the right direction with tools and methods that override human error and with strong leadership necessary to achieve organizational change.

## *References*

Advisory Commission on Consumer Protection and Quality in the Health Care Industry (1998). *Quality first: better health care for all Americans* (http://www.hcquality commission.gov/final).

Altman, D.E., Clancy, C., Blendon, R.J. (2004). Improving patient safety: five years after the IOM report. *New England Journal of Medicine, 351,* 2041–2043.

Bates, D.W., Spell, N., Cullen, D.J., Burdick, E., Laird, N., Petersen, L.A., et al. (1997). The costs of adverse drug events in hospitalized patients. *Journal of the American Medical Association, 277,* 307–311.

Brailer, D.J. (2004). *The decade of health information technology: delivering consumer-centric and evidence-rich health care.* U.S. Department of Health and Human Services. (http://www.hhs.gov/onchit/index.html).

Brennan, T.A., Leape, L.L., Laird, N.M., Hebert, l., Localio, A.R., Lawthers, A.G., et al. (1991). Incidence of adverse events and negligence in hospitalized patients: results of the Harvard Medical Practice Study I. *New England Journal of Medicine, 324,* 370–376.

Chassin, M.R., Galvin, R.W., The National Roundtable on Health Care Quality (1998). The urgent need to improve health care quality. *Journal of the American Medical Association, 280,* 1000–1005.

Council of the Institute of Medicine (1994). *America's health in transition: protecting and improving quality.* Washington, DC: Institute of Medicine.

Donabedian, A. (1966). Evaluating the quality of medical care. *Milbank Memorial Fund Quarterly, 44,* 166–203.

Donabedian, A. (1968). Promoting quality through evaluating the process of patient care. *Medical Care, 16,* 181–202.

Gandhi, T.K., Weingart, S.N., Borus, J., Seger, A.C., Peterson, J., Burdick, E., et al. (2003). Adverse drug events in ambulatory care. *New England Journal of Medicine, 348,* 1556–1564.

Grumbach, K., Bodenheimer, T. (2004). Can health care teams improve primary care practice? *Journal of the American Medical Association*, 291, 1246–1251.

Institute for Healthcare Improvement. Save 100k Lives Campaign. Revised continuously (http://www.ihi.org/IHI/Programs/Campaign).

Institute of Medicine. (2000). *To err is human: building a safer health system*. Washington, DC: National Academy Press.

Institute of Medicine. (2001). *Crossing the quality chasm: a new health system for the 21st century*. Washington, DC: National Academy Press.

Henry J. Kaiser Family Foundation (2004). *National survey on consumers' experiences with patient safety and quality information* (http://www.kff.org/kaiserpolls/7210.cfm).

Lawrence, D. (2002). *From chaos to care: the promise of team-based medicine*. Cambridge, MA: Perseus.

Leape, L.L., Brennan, T.A., Laird, N.M., Lawthers, A.G., Localio, A.R., Barnes, B.A., et al. (1991). The nature of adverse events in hospitalized patients: results of the Harvard Medical Practice Study II. *New England Journal of Medicine*, 324, 377–384.

Lewis, C.E. (1974). The state of the art of quality assessment—1973. *Medical Care*, 12, 799–806.

McGlynn, E.A., Asch, S.M., Adams, J., Keesey, J., Hicks, J., DeCristofaro, A., et al. (2003). The quality of health care delivered to adults in the United States. *New England Journal of Medicine*, 348, 2635–2645.

Peterson, O.L., Andrews, L.P., Spain, R.S., Greenberg, B.G. (1956). An analytical study of North Carolina general practice 1953–1954. *Journal of Medical Education* Pt. 2:1–165.

Sanders, J., Esmail, A. (2003). The frequency and nature of medical error in primary care: understanding the diversity across studies. *Family Practice*, 20, 231–236.

Schuster, M.A., McGlynn, E.A., Brook, R.H. (1998). How good is the quality of health care in the United States? *The Milbank Quarterly*, 76, 517–563.

Thomas, E.J., Studdert, D.M., Burstin, H.R., Orav, E.J., Zeena, T., Williams, E.J., et al. (2000). Incidence and types of adverse events and negligent care in Utah and Colorado. *Medical Care*, 38, 261–271.

Thomas, L. (1974). *The medusa and the snail: more notes of a biology watcher*. New York: Viking. pp. 37–39.

# 16
# Increasing Safety by Implementing Optimized Team Interaction: Experience from the Aviation Industry

MANFRED MÜLLER

In times of increasing cost constraints, there is increasing tension between economic efficiency and safety. In numerous economic sectors, product quality is deliberately reduced to save costs. The expenses resulting from complaints are set off against the saving potential offered by cheaper production methods. This approach can be optimized by defining specific error or rejection rates (for example, production of cheap textiles). So long as this approach is used for products with no or few safety requirements, there is no reason to object to the concept, as customers themselves define the desired quality level by purchasing. In some areas, however, this type of cost optimization cannot be accepted. When human lives and health are at stake, management following cost-cutting principles can—as soon as the public takes notice—trigger the ruin of the respective company.

## Common Goal of the Medical and the Aviation Industry: Risk Minimization

For this reason, industries sensitive to safety, such as medicine or aviation, must follow a different principle when defining their quality requirements. Maximum safety and minimum risk must be the topmost corporate objectives, even if only for ethical reasons; but there are also economic reasons for this target. The total loss of a large airplane costs an average of approximately half a billion euros. One single accident ("complete loss of production") can mean the end of an airline (for example, Birgen Air). If, on top of this, an airline is charged with negligence, which is mainly attempted by lawyers in the American legal system, there is virtually no upper limit to the possible claims of the damaged parties. (If, for example, it is proven that the crash of an Egypt Air plane after departure from the United States was caused by the suicide of one of the pilots, Egypt Air is fully liable. In this case, the insurance company is released from any indemnification, and the claims of the victims' relatives would certainly add up to several billion euros, a sum that would mean the ruin of the airline).

The phenomenon having started in America, doctors and medical institutions are also increasingly exposed to extremely high financial claims from damaged parties. In the medical field as well, a single human error can trigger a human and a financial catastrophe. Therefore, there are also substantial economic interests in avoiding complications and accidents in the health care system.

## Why Do Catastrophes Happen? A Philosophical Question

Why do disasters and catastrophes happen? Are we inevitably left unprotected to an unfavorable fate? In the past, efforts to find an answer to these questions inevitably led into the world of metaphysics. Evil spirits, magic, and witchcraft were considered the causes of "negative events." Rather unspecific means were used to "get rid of" possible "catastrophe triggers," including exorcism and the burning of witches. In those days, humans and their actions were hardly considered responsible for, and had little influence on, avoiding catastrophes. The power of destiny was the dominating factor. When the ideas of the Enlightenment pushed human beings' own personal responsibility into the foreground, safety could be enormously increased in many fields of human life (the plague, for example, was known to be transmitted not by the evil eye, but by fleas).

## Acceptance of Self-Determined Risks and Risks Determined by Others

The personal acceptance of risk, however, is not an objective variable but highly dependent on the subjectively perceived question of how far the actual risk potential is personally determined. A motorcyclist, for example, readily and voluntarily accepts an extremely high risk when exceeding the speed limit on a winding road on his Sunday joyride (self-determined). After an accident caused by the described driving behavior, the motorcyclist's readiness to accept a risk involved in the treatment of a polytrauma drops toward zero (determined by others). For the medical and the aviation industry, this means that the "customer" has extremely high expectations with regard to safety. In addition, it is normally difficult to assess personal risk because this assessment is influenced by emotions (fear of a meteorite impact but no fear of driving a car when under the influence of alcohol).

## A Definition of Safety

In the past, any airline flight included a high risk. Detailed investigations of accidents—mainly conducted in the United States after World War II—made it possible to identify their most important causes. Especially when the financial resources for risk minimization are limited, optimal use of the limited resources is paramount. The return on investment is highest when investments are made in exactly those fields where the highest risk is encountered. Reacting in this sense to the main risk areas resulted in an increase in flight safety to approximately 1.2 million flight-hours per total loss. Here, the following "equation" applies.

$$\text{Safety} = \text{prevention strategy/threat}$$

A serious threat requires a powerful defense strategy to increase the "value" of safety. To identify the respective risk areas, a detailed error analysis is required. Because aviation catastrophes are of high public interest, the pressure to identify root causes of accidents is much higher in aviation than in many other fields. The detailed investigation of more than 500 total losses of large jetliners (takeoff weight of more than 20 tons) since 1960 has made it possible to create an extensive database that reveals weak points and system deficits with the greatest possible objectivity.

## Humans: At Risk and Rescuer

A detailed investigation of the work environment combined with the analysis of the flight-recorder data and the voice recorder in the cockpit provides a clear picture of the working conditions and errors that lead to a catastrophe. Accident statistics suggest that the human being in the cockpit causes about three-fourths of all accidents. The large share of human errors suggested the initially considered brilliant solution of replacing the fallible human by an "infallible" digitally operating computer. This measure was meant to eliminate all human insufficiencies from the human/machine control loop. A computer never gets tired, is not emotional, does not need a holiday, has a constant level of motivation, and so on. (A considerable share of human work has been taken over by robots. In many cases, this measure has increased productivity and guarantees consistent product quality.)

## Automation and Safety

In aviation, an increased degree of automation has not changed the share of human errors as the cause of accidents. Even after the introduction of the so-called high-technology (HITEC) airplanes, the factor "human error" still accounts for 75% of all accidents. Up to now, the assumption that an increased degree of automation would necessarily lead to an increase in safety has not proved true. In some cases, the human error was simply replaced by a computer error. Experience has shown that the digital computer increases or guarantees safety only in "trivial" cases. Because even the best programmer is not able to anticipate all possible situations, the computer frequently fails when unconventional decisions are required or when influencing variables that have not been planned to occur in the respective context by the programmer must be weighed and assessed. Plainly speaking, the machine is an aid so long as support is not necessary but can fail when a demanding decision is required.

# Is Artificial Intelligence the Ultimate Solution?

Extensive and comprehensive research projects have made us recognize that so-called artificial intelligence (AI) has narrow limits. Even such a trivial phenomenon such as healthy common sense can be imitated by a computer only to a limited degree. The artificial generation of intuition or of ingenious new ideas by digital technology is miles away.

## Risk Factor Software

The problems resulting from the use of a complex calculating program can be demonstrated with a small intellectual experiment. Imagine a high-capacity computer whose task is to control an operation or a flight fully automatically. Before using the computer for the first time, a software test must be carried out for reasons of safety. Assuming that 100 parameters have an impact on a flight (which is a highly conservative approach if you take into consideration that more than 30,000 parameters are constantly monitored in a modern airplane), then $2^{100}$ or $1.27 \times 10^{30}$ system conditions result from those 100 parameters.

Even if a still-to-be-designed megacomputer were able to check 100 million ($10^8$) system conditions per second, the test run would take $1.27 \times 10^{30}$ divided by $10^8$ years, that is, $4 \times 10^{15}$ years. The dimension of this figure becomes clear when compared to the age of our earth, which is "only" approximately $5 \times 10^9$ years. This arithmetic example shows that complex software is most likely to be faulty and that there is no possibility to prove freedom from fault. A software test must therefore always be limited to a more or less comprehensive random sampling.

How easily minor errors can have serious consequences was demonstrated by the U.S. National Air and Space Administration (NASA) Mars mission of 1999. An unmanned spacecraft crashed on the red planet because entry into the Mars orbit had been calculated incorrectly. One department had used nautical miles to measure the distance, and the other department had used kilometers. When exchanging the data, the units of measurement were, by mistake, not matched (programming error). Because complete control of a complex calculating program is impossible, operations that decide the life or death of a person committed to our care must always be subjected to a plausibility check carried out by a specialist as the last control instance.

## Optimized Team Interaction

If the computer is ruled out as the ultimate safety system, how else can complex operations involving quick and difficult decisions be controlled? We must seek new answers in fields of activity that depend on the smooth, safest possible interactions between human and machine. In this context, findings in biology, psychology, and social sciences are gaining importance.

To be able to utilize the capacities of the human brain optimally and to correct potential errors, we have to create operating structures that can identify and correct possible errors. The interdisciplinary exchange of ideas and experience has shown that an optimal interaction between humans (team) and machine(s) in solving complex tasks under time pressure requires the use and observance of rules and standards that are applicable to all systems. In this context, it is of minor importance whether operating procedures in the operating theater, in the cockpit of an airplane, or in the control stand of a power station are considered.

## Parallel Connection of Thought Machines

Because a single person is always highly prone to error, the solution of the problem is to have him or her supported and controlled by a second person with the best possible and most suitable qualification.

The probability that two persons working independently of each other will make exactly the same mistake at the same point during an operating process is relatively low so long as the two "thinking machines" collect and evaluate the available facts independently from each other before discussing and clarifying the further steps (parallel connection of several independent thinking machines). If they have different opinions, the reasons for a decision, as well as its advantages and disadvantages, must be discussed. The independent thought processes of those individuals influencing or controlling the processes results in a safety network that can cushion human errors. The "mesh size" is determined by the qualifications of the respective individuals and the quality of cooperation.

## Error Omission in the Legal Sense

To develop effective defensive strategies, information on the actually occurring problems must be available. Unfortunately, the legal treatment of human errors according to the principle "errors must be punished and errors with severe consequences must be punished severely" has caused much harm. The legislator assumes that threatening with or inflicting a severe penalty can keep people from acting against the rules. This approach might be true with regard to the planning of crimes (bank robbery, shoplifting), but an accidental human error cannot be avoided by the threat of punishment. Possible sanctions prevent an objective investigation and follow-up of an incident and impede the development of effective defensive strategies to avoid similar problems in the future. The fear of punishment leads to hushing up and incorrect assignment of guilt.

## Zero Defect Strategy?

Quality management, too, is only partially suitable for error omission. The complete and continual documentation of production steps and operating procedures is performed to guarantee constant high quality. However valuable these measures may be, there remains one serious weakness. Dynamic processes in which flexible reactions to unexpected problems are required cannot be recorded without a gap; and, despite all efforts, the fact remains that humans do not work without ever failing. *"Errare humanum est"* As a consequence, the aim cannot be human action without error but the creation of structures that ease unavoidable human errors or that eliminate the unintended effects of errors before they can develop their undesired effects.

## Nonpunitive Error Management

To be able to tackle the problems, we must create an environment characterized by an atmosphere of mutual trust. The open discussion of errors made must not be endangered by the threat of punishment or the fear of a possible career interruption. It should be made clear that the "real professional" distinguishes himself or herself by the fact that he or she addresses errors openly and discusses them. This concept is based on the conviction that even the best expert can make nearly any serious mistake under unfavorable conditions. It is not the mistake itself that is "reprehensible" but the hiding of valuable information from colleagues. It has been shown in the past that progress is primarily achieved by investigating and following up mistakes, failures, and catastrophes (that nearly happened).

Every pilot has experienced elements of accident scenarios of others. If we succeed in identifying and eliminating single links in a possibly fatal chain of errors before a catastrophe happens, the system works. If the relevant knowledge is acquired only after a catastrophe, the system has failed.

## Limits of Confidentiality

To gain colleagues' confidence in a nonpunitive reporting system, certain prerequisites are required. The reporting system must be operated independent of the disciplinarian. The relevant incidents must be collected and analyzed by an independent organizational unit. Protection of the reporting person must have top priority. Analogous to confession in church, the confessing person must be protected under all circumstances. Serious incidents are reported only if the staff fully trusts the reporting system. If we do not succeed in building up a basis of confidence, only minor incidents are reported, which frequently result in the assignment of guilt to others. Experience with nonpunitive reporting systems has shown that it is usually single persons, not abstract organizations, who enjoy the trust of the staff members. An accepted confidant is prerequisite for the system's success. Of course the required basis of confidence cannot be built up over night; rather, it is a time-consuming process. A suitable confidant is an experienced colleague who is appreciated by everybody and who has already reached his or her own professional goals. This person should be supported by younger colleagues as well as contact persons for staff members his or her own age.

# Human Factor Research Project

The analysis of accident statistics involves the dilemma that, owing to the fortunately low number of catastrophes, it is difficult to make valid statistical statements. Reference to the number of incidents that have actually occurred is often missing. A comprehensive survey is therefore essential to obtain an objective picture of the safety situation: A well structured analysis of as many catastrophes that have almost occurred as possible demonstrates the hidden part of the "incident iceberg," in other words, that which is outside the immediate access of the event analysts. The question of how large this normally invisible part is also arises.

To get a better idea of situations that are potentially critical for safety, the aviation industry has conducted a Human Factor Research Program. It has been the most comprehensive study of its kind. A 120-page questionnaire was filled in by 2070 pilots. The survey asked for explanations and descriptions of the critical incident that was last experienced. The answers added up to 3,200,000 data records. Evaluation of the data took more than 2 years. Table 16.1 shows the six risk classes that resulted from this evaluation.

The mean risk value in the above survey is 3.4, that is, an incident in which the safety critical impacts could be almost entirely controlled by the pilots. It is striking that the higher risk classes 4, 5, and 6 together make up for more than 40% of all critical incidents. A large portion of the reported events represent significant danger potential. In contrast to a collection of reports on safety critical incidents, the questionnaires do not reveal how the event developed in detail (no scandalous stories); they deal only with possible influencing and disturbance variables (this is done also for reasons of anonymity).

TABLE 16.1. Risk classes

| Risk class | Example |
| --- | --- |
| 1 | There was an irregular incident. But there was *no need to act*. It was clear that there would be no safety-relevant effects. ("No problem.") |
| 2 | There was an incident relevant to safety. Appropriate actions of the crew made it possible to *avoid the building up* of any effects that would have impaired safety. ("Routine.") |
| 3 | There was an incident relevant to safety. The crew was able to *control all the effects* of the incident *completely*. ("Well done") |
| 4 | There was an incident relevant to safety. The *effects* of the incident could be *controlled only partially* by the crew (cockpit, cabin). ("Things turned out all right in the end.") |
| 5 | There was an incident relevant to safety. The *effects* of the incident *could not be controlled* by the crew (cockpit, cabin). In the end, it was possible to manage the situation only because no further aggravating factors occurred. The last link in the error chain was missing. ("By a hair's breadth....") |
| 6 | There was an incident relevant to safety. The situation *got completely out of control*, and we survived only by chance. ("Oh, shit!") |

Based on the survey data, four main categories were established that cover the major aspects of the problems.

TEC: technical problems, failure of systems
HUM: human errors
OPS: operational problems, complications
SOC: aggravating social factors

The OPS category refers to influences complicating the operating procedure beyond the standard rate. SOC refers to the team situation in the cockpit, such as communication deficits, bad crew resource management (CRM; a strategy for optimal utilization of all resources and information available to a team), conflicts (which quite often are not openly expressed), a too steep or too flat hierarchy, psychological problems, and so forth.

For evaluation, the different risk categories were first considered separately. If the above factors occur alone, the following percentages result (percentage of the total number of incidents).

| | |
|---|---|
| Technical problems, failure of system | 7.7% |
| Human errors | 4.9% |
| Operational problems, complications | 1.2% |
| Aggravating social factors | 0.7% |

It shows that when considering individual incidences technical problems are at the top of the scale (7.7% of all events) followed by human factors (4.9%). At first sight, this is surprising. How does this figure explain the fact that 75% of all accidents worldwide are human factor accidents? The analysis shows that cockpit crews are normally well able to manage a *single* error. The safety network of "structured cockpit work" eases solitary human errors.

## Effect of Simultaneously Occurring Risk Factors

In a second step, the analysis comes closer to the actual risk potential. Two categories are combined (for example, TEC + HUM or OPS + SOC, and so forth). Here we see that the dangerous impact of the human factor increases when it is combined with other factors. If operational problems (complications) and a human error occur simultaneously, the portion of safety critical incidents increases to 8.3%. Statistics show that a well organized working environment has considerable risk-reducing influence. The largest risk group with two combined factors is the combination of human factor (HUM) and problematic social climate (SOC). This combination is responsible for 13.7% of all incidents. This reveals that the working atmosphere has a much larger influence on risk than complications.

All three categories (HUM, HUM + OPS, HUM + SOC) together, however, account for only 26.9% of all safety critical incidents. What makes up the most important share of the often potentially fatal human factor?

# Social Factors: "Turbofactor" with Regard to Human Error

The next evaluation step considers combinations of three risk factors (for example, TEC + OPS + SOC). By far the most frequent safety critical situation (37.8% of all events) consists of the following combination.

1. A complication develops (OPS).
2. In this situation of increased stress a human error occurs (HUM).
3. The negative effects of the error cannot be corrected or eased because the working climate (SOC) is not optimal.

This means that a negative social climate has the effect of a "turbocharger" when a human error occurs: In many cases, tense human relationships turn a "harmless" error into a potentially life-threatening situation. A tense atmosphere is usually not identical with a dispute. In many cases, the working climate is burdened without the person responsible for the bad climate noticing it. The others involved in the situation frequently only sense an "undefined feeling of unease." A first negative impression, too much or too little respect, contempt, misunderstandings, a bad mood brought from home, lack of motivation, and so on can reduce the efficiency of a team considerably.

A first and important step to ease the problem is to express clearly one's own feeling of unease or other personal feelings. Normally, a considerable inner reluctance needs to be overcome to be able to do this. However, statements such as: "I do not feel comfortable with our teamwork" or "I have the feeling that there are problems nobody addresses" can be a first step to improving cooperation.

Especially in professions characterized by the image of brilliant experts who solve any problem without difficulties, it is a real challenge to address "soft" psychosocial factors. Nonetheless, this area must not be neglected or repressed, as this risk potential was not discovered, articulated, and put into the foreground by psychologists ignorant of aviation problems but by the people responsible for the problems.

# Working Climate and Safety

Everyone knows that the working climate has an influence on the quality of work and on safety. It is surprising, however, that the impact of "atmospheric disturbances" is so high. According to the above findings, the fact that colleagues do not get along well with each other ranges highest on the scale of safety problems. Social tensions in the team increase the risk of a safety critical incident by fivefold: in other words: *an optimal working atmosphere could mitigate or ease 80% of all safety critical human errors.*

The study has thus proven a quantitative connection between the social climate and the risk of dangerous incidents. Not only the number of incidents increases but also the risk class. (The mean risk of incidents caused by the human factor amounts to 3.57.)

## Training for Optimized Teamwork

What does this statement imply for our work organization and for training? The efforts to achieve optimal CRM and optimal team structures must be intensified. In the past, bad team behavior and a miserable atmosphere in the work environment were frequently tolerated with the argument, "But she (or he) is technically quite competent!" This statement should no longer be accepted. Survey evaluations show that bad team behavior triggers a major share of safety-critical incidents, and they are frequently not eased by excellent abilities but simply by good luck.

This implies that deficits in team behavior must be addressed by individual colleagues as well as by trainers and superiors. As already mentioned, this is more easily said than done, as the subject often requires more far-reaching discussions. A first reaction to this result of the survey could be to ask not to assign any "unpleasant" colleagues to the job who do not immediately create a "great atmosphere" in the team. In general, however, this measure would not ease the problem, as everyone occasionally (often unconsciously) burdens the work climate for colleagues by his or her behavior. Therefore, providing all colleagues with tools that ensure optimal handling of social problems is probably a more successful plan (in a wider sense).

Social competence obviously is also important for managing safety problems in technically oriented fields of endeavor, a fact that has been seriously underestimated in the past.

## Risk Categories

Figure 16.1 shows the percentages for the individual risk groups. The figures reveal that the survey made it possible to break down the fine structure of the safety-relevant human factors. When adding up all categories in which the factor HUM appears, the total is 79.1%, and this is the figure that corresponds more or less with the 75% of the International Air Transport Association (IATA) accident statistics.

## Social Problems in the Team

What does the term SOC mean if you look at it more closely? The structure of the questionnaire deliberately addressed possible impairments. Approximately 32% of these unfavorable CRM events are triggered by a single-handed action of one pilot. This figure shows that a behavior that is not jointly coordinated and agreed upon poses a safety problem. There is normally no ill will behind such an approach. Time pressure, target fixation, or unexpected complications shortly before the expected completion of a task can turn a good team player into a "Rambo" in no time.

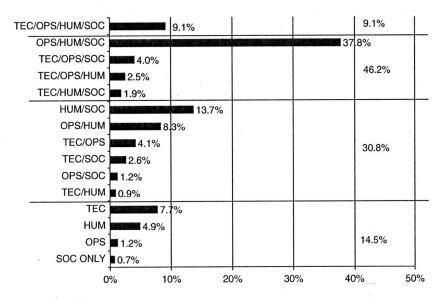

FIGURE 16.1. Possible combinations of the various risk categories. The uppermost line shows the combination of all four groups. Technology (TEC), operational problems (OPS), human error (HUM), and social problems (SOC) account for 9.1% of all incidents. The second data block shows the combinations of three factors. By far the largest block (37.8%) consists of OPS, HUM, and SOC. As to the combinations of two factors, the mixture of HUM and SOC is at the top of the list. The smallest group (in the lowest data block) comprises social problems, with only 0.7%.

A single-handed attempt by one team member is usually triggered by the captain. Because of the hierarchical structure and the overall responsibility, it is normally a simple matter for the boss to stop a single-handed action by a team member. For a hierarchically subordinate employee, it is much more difficult to convince the boss of the problematical nature of a decision that was made alone because he or she must overcome a huge emotional hurdle before expressing criticism from a subordinate position. The larger the difference in age or in hierarchy between the team members, the more difficult it can be for the employee to express criticism.

The fact that approximately one-third of all CRM problems is due to "lone wolfing" shows that there is an urgent need for action in this field and that repeated efforts are needed to create a common work basis. To avoid any rush is an important preventive measure in this context.

The graph in Figure 16.1 shows that the factor SOC ONLY is at the end of the list, with only 0.7%. This clearly demonstrates that social problems, as an isolated factor, are practically irrelevant as the cause of a safety-critical event. Great efforts are being made to create a positive working atmosphere. Existing difficulties become obvious only when additional burdening factors occur.

## Who Is Going to Teach Optimized Teamwork?

Who should carry out the relevant training? The basics of CRM should certainly be taught by psychologists. However, this method of teaching can be applied to only a relatively limited extent, as the actual knowledge transfer takes place in the working situation and must therefore be explained and accompanied by colleagues in the same professional field. To be efficient and accepted, the training must be implemented in the specific environment and can therefore be rendered only by specialists (pilots, medical doctors) as trainers and multipliers. The results of the survey give additional support to these efforts. More training in this field, however, must never make cutbacks in basic technical training tolerable. CRM training is no substitute for technical knowledge; it is only a necessary supplement.

## Communication Deficits

The following figures should illustrate the problems assigned to the field of SOC. It has already been mentioned that "additional aggravating factors in the field of social interaction" were found in 68.4% of all events. That this rarely means a dispute in the common sense of the word or an openly fought conflict has already been explained. In 77.4% of the cases with aggravating factors in the area of social interaction, communication problems were reported—in 48% of all incidents.

• Necessary statements were not made, and corresponding hints were not given.
• Unclear concerns were not expressed.
• Important statements were incomplete, insufficient, or were not heard.

In the above cases, the sender of the message is the one who was negligent, as the quality of communication is entirely determined by whatever arrives at the other end. For this reason, the sender of a message has the obligation to check what information the receiver has perceived.

The problem, therefore, is not the captain's lack of readiness to put a hint received into the according action, but the missing courage of the first officer to address deviations consequently and clearly.

No corresponding reaction followed a clearly understood hint in only 23% of all communication problems. There is a strategy to deal with this type of situation, too. If there is no reaction to a correcting hint, the concern must be repeated.

If the first officer does not speak up and the captain is exclusively fixed on the target, this can result in the noncorrection of an error. (The worst accident in civil aviation with 583 casualties happened because a young copilot did not have the courage to correct the experienced trainer captain a second time.)

## Violation of Rules

So-called violation of rules constitutes a large share of human errors by the cockpit crew. A few years ago, a Boeing taskforce dealt with this phenomenon. The study analyzed accidents. When investigating cases of total loss, the investigating team did not ask what caused the accident but searched for means that could have prevented it. The survey shows that about 80% of all accidents could have been prevented by strictly observing the rules and regulations. For this reason, the area "working in accordance with rules" is of special interest to us in the evaluation of the cockpit study because the findings of the Boeing study mean that the number of accidents (at present about 18 per year on average) could be reduced by 80% (or approximately 14 total losses per year) at once if the pilots observed the rules strictly.

Seventy-seven percent ($n = 940$) of all human errors that trigger a safety critical incident are nonobservances of rules (omission/violation). The total number of reported violations of rules is 1513, which is much higher owing to the fact that multiple violations (nonobservance of at least two rules) were reported in 573 cases. The usefulness and protective effect of the rules is not questioned in principle. Nonetheless, violations of fundamental rules obviously occur repeatedly as a result of time pressure, immense routine, complacency, and the feeling of being invulnerable.

## Standard Operating Procedure

There are generally several procedures to fulfill a task, all of which offer the same level of safety. For this reason, it does not necessarily become clear at first glance why they should be limited to a few strictly defined standard procedures. There are, however, several reasons for making and observing binding agreements.

To be able to control each other and to address deviations from the rules, all cockpit members must be able to refer to commonly accepted procedures. When applying "personal procedures," the controlling person can no longer determine if the working step is desired in the way it is implemented or if an unintentional human error has crept in. If a crew works in this gray zone, it must rely on its feelings, which are bad or even fatal advisors, as has been documented by many flight accidents.

## Failure and Readiness to Take a Risk

Behaviorism presents another important argument for disciplined work. After a tolerated rule violation, the threshold for further, often more serious violations is reduced. For this reason, deviations from rules must be addressed as soon as they occur to prevent a cascade of violations.

The captain is responsible for the observance of binding rules. He or she is assisted by a responsible first officer as a means of support and an additional "control and redundancy organ." Thus, a violation of defined rules always means that the redundancy structure in the cockpit has failed. The tolerance threshold accepted by the first officer determines the mesh size of the safety network.

## Experience and Adherence to Rules

A high level of self-discipline is required to observe rules that are considered inflexible after years of successful work. Training and management personnel are particularly endangered in this respect. A person who has participated in working out the rules and constantly remembers the often controversial discussion resulting in their implementation sometimes has great difficulty adhering to these rules. However, because of the trainer's model function, a violation of rules by the trainer has an especially strong negative effect because human errors occurring in this context most probably are not corrected by the inexperienced colleague because he or she does not expect this type of rule violation.

## Risk and Motivation

In this context, motivation also plays a major role. An investigation by the U.S. Navy has shown that 90% of the pilots who get involved in a human-error accident have serious motivation problems. With fading motivation, the readiness to violate a rule and to accept a higher risk increases. Only those who are highly motivated work carefully and with foresight. The more reluctantly one performs his or her job, the more difficult it is to anticipate possible consequences.

Apart from discipline and motivation, the readiness to accept one's own imperfection is an imperative prerequisite for good teamwork. Only a person who accepts his or her own weaknesses is convincing when asking for and expressing criticism (passive and active ability to criticize).

## Morals and Values

The personal system of values also plays a decisive role. If we do not show empathy and a certain principal generosity toward our team members, they will not point out incongruities and possible mistakes with the necessary clarity in a complex critical situation.

## Summary

The factor "human error" still accounts for 75% of all accidents, even after the introduction of the so-called high-technology (HITEC) airplanes. Because the computer cannot provide the ultimate safety system, how else can complex operations involving quick and difficult decisions be controlled? To guarantee the highest possible human performance level, the following steps should be observed.

- Select the right people.
- Training should include real-life scenarios that are likely to create time pressure and stress (simulation).
- Implement recurrent training.

Optimized team interaction involves support and control by a second person, as well as structures and training to enable individuals to recognize impending errors and verbalize them and to accept such information when received and to act accordingly.

Known errors or risks cannot be analyzed and eliminated if they are not first openly discussed. The threat of punishment, however, curtails such discussion.

Because nearly 40% of all dangerous situations result from poor team interaction in the face of human error caused by the duress of an unexpected complication, far more research and training must be devoted to the complexities of human interaction.

It is almost a paradox of human history that man's efforts to develop machines to compensate human weaknesses have led to the present situation where the inherently human abilities of social competence are of utmost importance when dealing with high technology.

# 17
# Evidence-Based Information Technology: Concept for Rational Information Processing in the Health Care System

Horst Kunhardt

The application of information technology (IT) in all health care organizations has become a complex process. For a long time, IT was only used in administration, but hospitals with modern management recognized the potential of the optimal use of IT in all forms of service provision and established hospital information systems early.

Because of the long-term effects of IT in health care organizations, it is difficult to provide evidence of its usefulness. Confirming the benefits of IT requires sophisticated IT controlling and continuous feedback with the users. Management often only considers IT as an additional cost factor. Lack of transparency in the field of IT, lack of knowledge about IT processes in management, problems with acceptance among users due to obligatory tasks, and the perceived increased amount of work required from medical and nursing personnel for documentation on personal computers have worsened these problems.

Well organized IT solutions, such as those that minimize transportation times by avoiding paper documents or the parallel use of data by different users, can cut costs. High quality relevant treatment information is also instantly available. In the United States, for example, 522,000 incorrect prescriptions for medication could be avoided by consistent IT printout and/or transmission of physicians' orders, as the supply and administration of medication in a clinical setting undergoes many clinical and administrative steps (Birkmeyer et al., 2000).

According to a study sponsored by Microsoft (Rainzer, 2003), approximately 70% of the transactions in the North American health care system are based on paper forms. In other words, 20 cents of every dollar spent on administrative costs is for paper forms. The economic feasibility of many institutions in the health care system today depends directly on the quality of their documentation and the availability of information—and thereby on the optimal application of IT. These problems provided the incentive for David Sackett to develop methods in the field of medicine to solve the problem of floods of worthless information with the concept of evidence-based medicine more than a decade and a half ago.

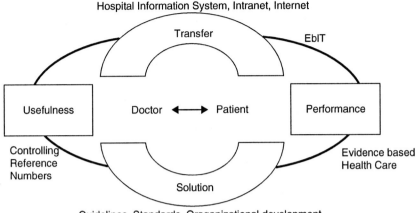

FIGURE 17.1. Evidence-based information technology (EbIT) as a concept for transfer, service, solutions, and usefulness for the dissemination of evidence in IT systems. HIS = hospital information system; EbHC = evidence-based health care.

As a holistic approach, evidence-based information technology (EbIT[1]) combines evidence-based information from different specialties, such as evidence-based health care (EbHC), and implements these solutions in the IT structure of the respective organization. The integration of these principles into hospital information systems, intranets, or evidence-based guidelines brings added value to the organization that can be measured with reference numbers and can contribute to the development of the organization and its long-term success. Figure 17.1 shows EbIT as a concept for the transfer of solutions into practice with simultaneous assessment of its usefulness.

This chapter shows how application of the methods of evidence-based medicine in IT processes can improve access to information in a hospital, improve the quality of the information, and reduce costs.

## Concept of Evidence-Based Information Technology

The conception and implementation of EbIT proceed from the following assumptions.

1. Information processing is a key technology for organizations in the health care system that has hitherto received too little attention.

---

[1]The term "evidence-based information technology" was introduced by Dr. Jeremy C. Wyatt of the University College in London. He investigated the fundamental possibilities for applying information technology (IT) in the field of medicine.

- Applying this key technology could reveal additional potentials for cost reduction and improve the quality of service.
- An effective and efficient use of IT requires a modern form of organization.
- Standardizing information processes can improve their quality and reduce IT costs.

2. Implementation of EbIT requires a "learning" organization.

- Continuous online requests for feedback provide a good assessment of the acceptance of IT solutions among the users and management.
- Documentation of suggested solutions helps create a knowledge base and promotes accumulation of useful information.

Because information constitutes an indispensable factor in the production and supply of medical services, it is only logical to organize the process of information provision according to the rules of evidence-based medicine (EbM). The supply of information for treatment procedures must fulfill certain requirements. The user of an IT system evaluates the usefulness of the provided information according to its relevance (R) and validity (V) and the time and effort (E) required to receive the information. If the user has to wait too long for the information, the acceptance and usefulness of the information decrease because the situation demanding information might have changed. Figure 17.2 shows the relations among relevance, validity, and effort in obtaining information.

Many communicating partners are involved in patient treatment, all of whom require information. It is not uncommon that, together with physicians, nursing staff, therapists, relatives, administration, health insurance providers, and other stakeholders in the treatment process, a large number of communicating partners must be included in the IT solution quickly. Managing the interfaces presents a large problem because IT systems from the various manufacturers and suppliers must be coordinated. Figure 17.3 shows a rapidly growing communication network with a number of communicating partners. The example shows 28 directly communicating relationships with eight communicating partners. This could represent, for example, eight medical subsystems, such as the laboratory, radiology department, and so on, all of which must exchange data. Interface problems arise not only because of technical reasons but also the different terminology used by the various specialist groups.

$U$ sefulness of the information
$R$ elevance of the information
$V$ alidity of the information
$E$ ffort to access the information

$$U = \frac{R \times V}{E}$$

FIGURE 17.2. Benefit of information for the user (Slawson & Shaughnessy, 1997).

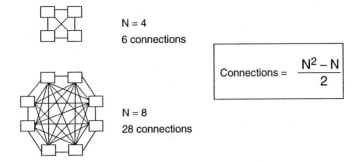

$$\text{Connections} = \frac{N^2 - N}{2}$$

FIGURE 17.3. Number of connections depending on the number of communicating partners (Comer, 2002).

Evidence-based medicine, together with evidence-based nursing (EbN) or other disciplines that combine internal and external evidence, are like parts of a building whose roof is EbIT. Without this edifice of valid and relevant information that reaches the right service provider in the health care system in the right place at the right time, it would be difficult to achieve safe, effective, patient-oriented treatment. The concept EbIT therefore provides a holistic approach to supplying information during the treatment process and the related secondary processes, as shown in Figure 17.4.

Information plays an essential role in all evidence-based concepts. It is the task of IT to transport information in an appropriate manner, that is, at the correct time

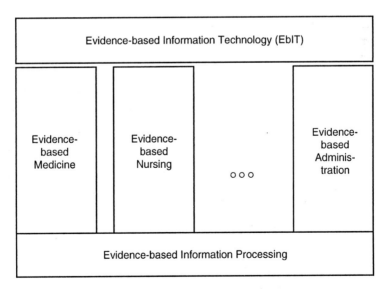

FIGURE 17.4. Evidence-based information technology in the context of evidence-based medicine, evidence-based nursing, and other evidence-based applications.

to the correct place and to the correct user securely and reliably. The solution of an IT-related user problem should itself be fashioned on evidence-based rules. That this is not always the case is demonstrated by dissatisfied users, overspent IT budgets, and problems with the quality of information provision.

Figure 17.5 illustrates the structured procedure used in EbM applied to solve an IT user problem. First, an answerable question is formulated and then answered according to internal evidence. In the next step, external evidence for this specific problem is sought, and the identified information is examined for validity and relevance. If this external evidence is sufficient to justify changing an established method of operation, the new solution is applied and documented. In the final step, after application of the IT solution the user is included in a feedback process, and the solution is evaluated from his or her point of view. This final step integrates the user in the solution and promotes a learning organization. Documentation of evidence-based solutions builds up a knowledge base in the organization.

The following problematical areas arise from the EbIT problem-solving concept consisting of the six steps shown in Figure 17.5.

- According to which assessment criteria can internal and external evidence be evaluated?
- How can the outcome of an IT solution be assessed from the user's point of view; that is, how useful is the solution to the user.

Evaluating the quality of information from different knowledge sources in the field of IT is confronted with the same problems as when evaluating the quality, validity, and relevance of medical information. EbM has solved the problem of

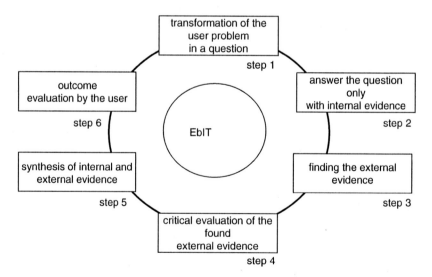

FIGURE 17.5. Solving problems in information technology according to the evidence-based information technology (EbIT) concept.

evaluating the scientific validity of medical information according to the well known classes of evidence Ia through V (Classes of Evidence according to the FDA, 1998; Sackett, 1999). The classes of evidence from the field of medicine can be compared with external evidence from the field of IT.

Systematic studies about the effectiveness and usefulness of IT solutions, if existent, are available only at hardware and software manufacturers. Professional associations and user groups in the field of IT represent independent sources of information; but because of the intimate connection of an IT solution with the respective organizational form and the difficulty of determining its long-term effects, transference of knowledge from one organization to another must be critically tested. Table 17.1 presents a summary of step 4, "critical evaluation of external evidence," to show how external information from the IT can be compared with grades of external evidence from the field of medicine. This is necessary because IT information can directly affect the validity and relevance of medical information processed in a hospital IT system.

The outcomes of an IT service or an IT solution can only be measured in the context of the organization using the EbIT, that is, the IT user(s). Aside from established reference numbers used for the assessment of IT service, such as fulfillment of service-level agreements (SLA) or the availability of IT systems, so-called soft factors such as user satisfaction and faith in the competence of the solution must also be taken into consideration. This is referred to as *IT*

TABLE 17.1. Comparison of classes of evidence from evidence-based medicine with external sources in the field of information technology

| Grade of external evidence | Class of evidence in medicine (based on) | Information technology evidence (based on) | Source |
|---|---|---|---|
| Ia | Meta-analyses of randomized controlled trials (RCTs) in systematic reviews | Handbooks with installation instructions | Standardizing agencies Manufacturers', professional, and users' organizations |
| Ib | At least one RCT | | |
| IIa | At least one controlled study without randomization | Documentation of IT solutions with comparable IT system | System handbooks Best practice |
| IIb | At least one quasi-experimental study | environment and type of organization | Specialist journals Specialist textbooks Internet pages of the manufacturer FaQ |
| III | Nonexperimental, descriptive studies | Reported experience and recommendations from expert groups | Discussions and reports in expert groups |
| IV | Reports and opinions from expert groups without transparent documentation | | Discussions and reports in user groups |

FaQ = frequently asked questions; IT = information technology *governance*. IT concepts that holistically emphasize the key role IT plays in organizational processes are needed today. IT controlling requires the prior existence of an IT strategy, such as the balanced scorecard, calculation of services, and standard processes according to the Infrastructure Library (http://www.itil.org), which are available but have been practically implemented by only a few organizations. Service orientation requires a process model for application. Owing to the enormous speed at which changes are taking place and their complexity, many organizations in the health care system have not taken full advantage of these potentials.

# Results

Results of the consistent application of the EbIT concept are demonstrated in the example of a user–help desk system,[2] which has been utilized at a hospital for psychiatry, forensic medicine, neurology, and rehabilitation for 3 years. A form was developed for the systematic recording of IT problems so all entries can be stored in a central database and categories of problems, causes of problems, and user feedback or the status of the reported problem can be called up at any time from the IT network by the hospital management.

The application of EbIT in a hospital with 800 beds improved the quality of information and increased user satisfaction. The time saved when searching for information can be devoted to improving the quality of treatment. The rising quality of IT procedures and results also produces a learning effect and an increase in patient volume and thereby a reduction in costs.

The consistent application of EbIT can result in a larger number of users being served by fewer IT specialists. Three members of the IT support staff in the district hospital in Mainkofen serve 650 client personal computers (PCs) and about 1100 IT users. Comparable data from industry assume the need for one IT support person for about 60 to 80 PCs.[3] We achieved an obvious reduction in the necessary number of IT support staff with the same high quality results.

Figure 17.6 shows an evaluation of the distribution of causes of about 4500 IT problems that were documented from 650 users in one hospital during 1 year. This helps the IT management react quickly to IT problems, which increases the acceptance among IT users. Consistent recording and solving of IT problems according to an established EbIT pathway makes it possible to analyze the data from a multitude of perspectives and to carry out preventive maintenance of the IT system. If the satisfaction level of the IT users in a certain area changes, the IT management can react quickly (for example, by offering training sessions for the user group involved, or systems with frequent errors can be

---

[2]At a user help desk, the reported IT user problems are recorded, handed over to an IT specialist, and the solution of the problem is documented. User–help desk systems are stored in databanks and in the local network of an organization.

[3]According to Compaq, 60 to 80 PCs can be supported by one member of the IT staff.

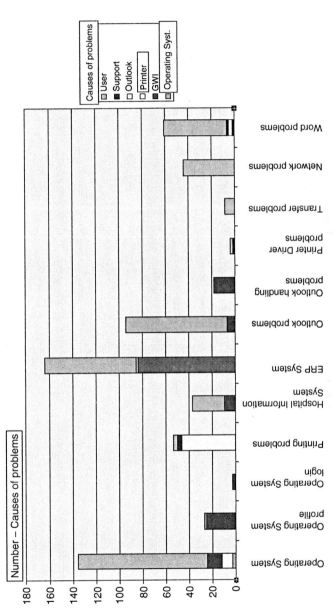

FIGURE 17.6. Evaluation of the distribution of causes of different IT problems from 650 users in the Mainkofen District Hospital during 1 year. ERP = enterprise resource planning.

exchanged). This increases the quality of the data processed in the hospital information system.

Documentation of each IT problem and its solution enables the causes of problems to be classified. The cause of a specific problem can thereby be defined, and the cost of the solution can be reduced. IT problems caused by the users themselves also become obvious and can be reduced by tailored training.

A balanced scorecard can be produced from these online data that supplies management with a continuous overview of the IT provision, acceptance among IT users, and important parameters of system security, such as unauthorized use of files.

Figure 17.7 shows the time required to solve IT problems and illustrates that most IT problems can be solved within an hour. This is especially important for IT users in a hospital, as IT systems should be available 24 hours a day.

The time saved by avoiding duplication of documentation, transport, and waiting time can be transferred from pure data recording to strategically more important tasks, such as quality management. In the Mainkofen District Hospital, 87% of the time previously required to record sociodemographic data was saved by changing from paper forms to digital recording systems. For 7500 annual hospital admittances, the time saved by using a digital form to fill out basic documentation was 13 minutes per case compared to using paper forms. When the basic documentation has been filled out at admission and discharge, this adds up to a total savings of 195,000 minutes, or 406 working days. This saved time can be dedicated to patient care.

Before the introduction of digital forms in the hospital information system, 12 tons of paper forms were printed in the hospital printing shop. EbIT cut the amount of paper forms by 30%. Avoidance of duplication increased the quality of the data as well as the time required for transport and filing of the paper forms.

Clinics that have already achieved the change from paper to digital documentation and can illustrate a resulting workflow with the digital forms can certainly report similar experiences. Considering the huge amounts of circulating paper documents, IT departments have a considerable task cut out for them. Analogous savings could be achieved by switching from paper forms to digital forms for recording meals.

## Discussion

The introduction of EbIT, exemplified by the transfer from paper to digital documentation forms, requires a long process in a hospital in which many professional groups are involved. It, however, presents the opportunity to discuss and restructure established procedures that have long remained static. In the Mainkofen District Hospital, we have already digitalized about 150 processes in the fields of medicine and nursing. Changing these processes is now achieved with relatively little effort. When presenting a new process to the hospital information system, discussions arose concerning critical evaluation or the measurement of outcomes of interventions in the fields of medicine, nursing, and informatics. The solution or the presentation of a process was structured on the reality in the hospital infor-

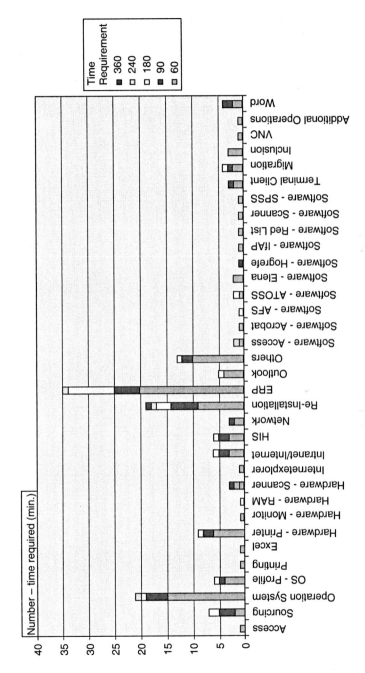

FIGURE 17.7. Time (in minutes) required to solve different IT problems from 650 users in the Mainkofen District Hospital during 1 year.

mation system according to EbM or EbIT methods. Training the users and hospital management to practice disciplined, structured problem-solving was in itself a success. This type of problem-solving strategy led to faster, longer lasting, higher quality solutions, even among professional groups that were previously unfamiliar with the concept of EbM or EbIT.

Continuous measurement of progress in IT user support by regularly requesting user feedback helps identify problematical areas quickly and introduce strategies to rectify them. The evidence-based user–help desk system provides a good basis for the construction of a balanced scorecard solution and, thereby, for management of the complex IT process.

By elevating the quality of problem-solving regarding the supply of information in medical service provision, the incidence of errors can be reduced and the processes further optimized. The quality of information is improved by the digital service requirements because plausibility controls and input assistance are provided in the form of context-related, helpful instructions on the digital forms. In Mainkofen District hospital, for example, a so-called service tree was developed that provides documentation of service reference numbers for invoicing and cost calculations along with the demands for services.

The entire health care system can increase the quality of processes and cut costs through consistent and optimal use of IT by avoiding redundancy and inconsistency. A combination of procedural optimization and integrated IT application can change IT structures that are segmented and fragmented into a cooperative structure characterized by agreement, functionality, and transparency. If the fundamental IT processes already function according to the rules of EbIT, a transparent data-driven IT system ensuring high satisfaction among those who run and use the system can be achieved through continuous optimization.

Personal experience in a clinic that consistently applies EbIT confirms the robustness of this concept. The next step is to develop evidence-based clinical treatment pathways under consideration of economic criteria and to implement them in the hospital information system.

## References

Birkmeyer, J.D., Birkmeyer, C.M., Wenberg, D.E., Young, M. (2000). Leapfrog patient safety standards: the potential benefit of universal adoption. The LeapFrog Group for Patient Safety, p. 1 (http://www.leapfroggroup.org/PressEvent/Birkmeyer_ExecSum.pdf).

Comer, D.E. (2002). *Computernetzwerke und Internets.* [Computer Networks and Internets.] Munich: Pearson Studium. p. 121.

Classes of Evidence (http://www.hon.ch).

Infrastructure library (http://www.itil.org).

Rainzer, W. (2003). Mit IT-Einsatz könnten fünf bis acht Prozent Kosten gespart werden. [The use of IT could save 5–8% of costs.] *Krankenhaus-IT-Journal*, 64.

Sackett, D.L. (1999) *Evidenzbasierte Medizin.* [Evidence-based medicine.] Munich: Zuckschwerdt. p. 9.

Slawson, D.C., Shaughnessy, A.F. (1997). Obtaining useful information from expert based sources. *British Medical Journal*, 314(7085), 947–949.

# 18
# Cost-Effectiveness Analysis: Measuring the Value of Health Care Services

ROBERT M. KAPLAN

Linking inputs, outputs, and outcomes requires systematic analysis. In previous chapters we have discussed the measurement of all three of these components. In this chapter, we consider linkages between the inputs and costs to patient outcomes. The goal is to show that systematic analysis can lead to efficiency in health care.

Health care costs in most countries have grown exponentially since 1940. However, the United States provides the best example of the inability to contain health care expenditures. Although there was a temporary slowdown during the early 1990s, the rate of increase began to accelerate again after the turn of the century. Health care in the United States now consumes about 15.3% of the gross domestic product (GDP), whereas few other countries in the world spend more than 10% of their GDP on health care (Smith et al., 2005). Although the rate of growth has slowed, annual increases in health care costs increased by 7% to 8% percent each year following the turn of the century. Despite high expenditures, the U.S. system may not be producing exceptional health outcomes. Among 13 countries in one recent comparison, the United States ranked 12th when compared on 16 health indicators (Starfield, 2000).

## Opportunity Cost Problem

Health care resources are limited, and there is constant pressure to spend more on attractive new treatments or diagnostic procedures. Without containment, it is likely that the health care bill will dominate the economies of developed countries and limit the opportunity to develop other sectors, such as education, energy, or national defense (Reinhardt et al., Hussey, 2004). Although most provider groups understand that health care costs must be contained, few acknowledge that their own expenditures should be subject to evaluation. Successful lobbying to obtain reimbursement for a specific service may necessarily mean that another service is excluded. Suppose, for example, that the amount that can be spent on health care is fixed, and $3 of each $100 (3%) is devoted to prevention. If preventive medicine advocates are able to get $10 of each $100 spent on their services, there will be less to spend on other health services. This is called the opportunity cost problem. Opportunity costs are the foregone opportunities that are surrendered as a result of using resources to support a particular decision. If we spend a lot of money in one sector of health care, we necessarily spend less money elsewhere (Kaplan, 2000). How do we decide which services should get more and which should get fewer resources?

When confronted with the choice between two good programs, it is always tempting to support both. The difficulty is that it costs more to offer multiple programs. The cost of programs is represented in the fees for health insurance or the cost of health care to taxpayers. A society can choose to offer as many health programs as it wants. However, more programs require more funding. Employees do not want the fees for their health insurance to rise, and taxpayers do not want tax increases. The goal of formal decision models is to obtain higher quality health care at a lower cost. Although it has been possible to control health care costs in some European countries (such as The Netherlands), no public policy has ever been shown to control costs effectively in the American health care system (Reinhardt et al., 2004; Eddy, 2005). The development of effective health policy may require the application of generic methods to assess cost effectiveness and cost utility. These terms are often misunderstood, so we briefly introduce them.

## Cost Effectiveness, Cost Utility, and Cost Benefit

The terms cost utility, cost effectiveness, and cost benefit are used inconsistently in the medical literature (Doubilet et al., 1986). The key concepts are summarized in Table 18.1. Some economists favor the assessment of cost-benefit analyses. These approaches measure both program costs and treatment outcomes in dollar units. For example, treatment outcomes are evaluated in relation to changes in the use of medical services or the economic productivity of patients. Treatments are cost beneficial if the economic return exceeds treatment costs. Patients with cancer who are aggressively treated with surgery, for example, may need fewer emergency medical services. The savings associated with decreased services might exceed treatment costs. Sometimes investment in a service results in more general economic returns. For example, investment in a psychotherapy program may reduce overall use of health services. The bottom line for those paying for health services is improved because there has been a cost offset.

Although there are many reports of cost offsets, in fact, few are well documented using strict accounting principles (Kaplan & Groessl, 2001). Typically,

TABLE 18.1. Comparison of cost-effectiveness, cost-utility, and cost-benefit analyses

| Type of analysis | Definition |
| --- | --- |
| Cost/effectiveness | $ Value of resources used/clinical effects |
| Cost/utility | $ Value of resources used/quality of life produced |
| Cost/benefit | $ Value of resources used/$ value of resources saved or created |

health services produce a benefit, and resources are used to obtain desired outcomes. However, a requirement of a good cost-benefit analysis is that all outcomes have a dollar value attached. Therefore, side effects of a drug or functional limitations from a surgical procedure must have a dollar value placed on them. This poses a variety of problems, as people attach different values to health, and many people have a difficult time placing monetary values on it. Estimating costs for these variables can compound the measurement error already introduced by the tradeoff between mortality and morbidity.

The requirement that health care treatments reduce costs may be unrealistic (Russell, 1986, 1987). Patients are willing to pay for improvements in health status, just as they are willing to pay for other desirable goods and services. We do not treat cancer to save money. Allowing patients to die would certainly be less expensive. Treatments are given to achieve better health outcomes. In other words, treatments should be evaluated in terms of their effectiveness, not just their financial benefit.

The term cost-effectiveness is rarely used as intended. In many professional articles, services are described as cost-effective if they are inexpensive. Cost-effectiveness analysis is an alternative approach in which the unit of outcome is a reflection of the treatment effect. In recent years, cost-effectiveness analysis has gained considerable attention. Some approaches emphasize simple, treatment specific outcomes. For example, Curry and colleagues (1998) evaluated the effects of various types of health insurance coverage on smoking cessation rates in a health management organization. They found that people are more likely to use the services if there is no co-payment. Even though programs with co-payments may be more effective in getting participants to quit smoking, the programs with full coverage attract more people and result in the best overall rate of smoking cessation in the population. However, the program is expensive.

The major difficulty with cost-effectiveness methodologies is that they do not allow comparison across very different treatment interventions. Health care administrators often need to choose between investments in different alternatives. Should the money be used to support tobacco cessation programs for all enrollees, or should it be devoted to supporting organ transplantation for a few patients? For the same cost, they may achieve a large effect for a few people or a small effect for a large number of people. The treatment-specific outcomes used in cost-effectiveness studies do not permit these comparisons.

## Features of Cost-Effectiveness Analysis

The purpose of cost-effectiveness analysis is to evaluate the comparative potential of expenditures on various health care interventions. Typically, the analysis starts with the assumption that some resources are available to spend on health care. The purpose of the analysis is to identify decisions that maximize the amount of health gained for the expenditure of these resources. For example, an administrator may need to decide between supporting a program on smoking cessation or a program to screen for prostate cancer. The question is whether using the resources to support smoking cessation will produce more or less health benefit than spending the same amount of money on a screening project for prostate cancer. There is not enough money to support both programs, and a decision between the alternatives must be made.

Cost-effectiveness analysis typically considers cost-per-unit benefit. A measure of outcome is often years of life gained, but it can also be cost per tumor identified, cost per successful smoking cessation, and so on.

Cost-utility approaches use the expressed preference or utility of a treatment effect as the unit of outcome. The goals of health care are designed to make people live longer (decrease mortality) and help them have a higher quality of life (decrease morbidity) (Kaplan, 2005). Cost-utility studies use outcome measures that combine mortality outcomes with quality of life measurements. The utilities are the quality of life ratings or preferences for observable health states on a continuum between 0 for death to 1.0 for asymptomatic, optimal function (Kaplan et al., 1993; Kaplan, 1994, 1997, 2005). A state rated as 0.70, for example, is judged to be 70% of the way between death and perfect health. A year in that state is scored as 0.70 quality-adjusted life years (QALYs). We return to the discussion of QALYs later in the chapter. In recent years, cost-utility approaches have gained increasing acceptance as methods for comparing many diverse options in health care (Gold et al., 1996; Kaplan, 2005).

Although once thought to be the exclusive domain of economists, the terms cost-effectiveness, cost-utility, and cost-benefit analysis are now a common part of the vocabulary of health services researchers and health care providers. The *New England Journal of Medicine* requires the consistent use of these terms for all reports on cost-effectiveness analyses (Kassirer & Angell, 1994).

## Standards for Cost-Effectiveness Analysis

Contrary to the portrayal of cost-effectiveness analysis in the popular media, the purpose of the analysis is not to cut costs but to identify which interventions produce the greatest amount of health that can be produced using the resources that are available. Because of the confusion about cost-effectiveness analysis, the U.S. Office of Disease Prevention and Health Promotion in the Public Health Service developed standards for cost-effectiveness analysis. In 1993, they appointed a 13-member panel co-chaired by Louise Russell and Milton Weinstein. The panel was co-sponsored by a variety of agencies, including the Agency for Health Care Policy and Research (now known as the Agency for Healthcare Research and Quality), the National Institutes of Health, the Healthcare Financing Administration, the Centers for Disease Control, and several others. The panel was created to develop recommendations for the consistent practice of cost-effectiveness analysis in preventive medicine, medical therapy, rehabilitation, and public health. Ultimately, the goal was to create common standards. The work of the panel appeared as a book (Gold et al., 1996) and in a series of papers published in the *Journal of the*

*American Medical Association* (Russell et al., 1996; Weinstein et al., 1996). In the following sections, we review some of the major elements of cost-effectiveness analysis as defined by this panel.

## Perspective

The results of cost-effectiveness analysis may depend on the perspective applied. From the societal perspective, all health care benefits and costs are considered, regardless of who uses them or pays for them. The administrative perspective evaluates the problem through the eyes of a specific agency. Individual perspectives consider costs and benefits from the viewpoint of an individual citizen or patient. There may be occasions in which results differ dramatically as a function of perspective. A health care organization, for example, may save money by denying a particular mental health service. From an administrative perspective costs may be reduced, but from a societal perspective costs may increase because other agencies may be required to pay for this service or for the consequences of conditions being left untreated. After much deliberation, the panel decided to apply a societal perspective. They concluded that fair decisions must take all parties into consideration. Decision makers must wrestle with who gains and who loses, and they must consider the broad consequences of their decisions.

## Comparators

It makes little sense to say that a program is cost effective. Cost effective in comparison to what? Virtually all decisions involve evaluation in comparison to some alternative. For example, physical therapy for back pain could be compared to no treatment at all, surgery, or medical management. The choice of the comparator is of critical importance in the analysis. Evaluations of innovative new therapies should compare the new approach to care that was usual before the new intervention was available. The panel recommended that new approaches should be compared to the best available alternative. In addition, other comparators might be the low cost alternative, different intensities of treatment, or care provided by alternative providers.

Many studies compare a treatment group to a control group and report the difference in outcomes. In such cases, cost effectiveness for the treatment is evaluated considering only the costs of the treatment. The standards for cost-effectiveness analysis suggest that costs and effects be evaluated for both the treatment and the comparator and the difference in cost effectiveness be reported.

## Measure of Effectiveness

The purpose of health care is to improve health. Remarkably, many cost-effectiveness analyses never measure health outcomes. The task force suggested that outcomes be measured using quality-adjusted life years (QALYs), which are measures of life expectancy with adjustments for quality of life (Russell, 1986, 1987). QALYs integrate mortality and morbidity to express health status in terms of equivalents of healthy years of life. If a woman dies of breast cancer at age 50 and one would have expected her to live to age 75, the disease was associated with 25 lost life-years. If 100 women died at age 50 (and also had life expectancies of 75 years), 2500 ($100 \times 25$ years) life-years would be lost.

Death is not the only outcome of concern in cancer. Many adults continue to suffer from the disease, leaving them somewhat disabled over long periods of time. Although still alive, the quality of their lives has diminished. QALYs take into consideration the quality of life consequences of these illnesses. For example, a disease that reduces quality of life by one-half takes away 0.5 QALYs over the course of 1 year. If it affects two people, it takes away 1.0 QALY ($2 \times 0.5$) over a 1-year period. A pharmaceutical treatment that improves quality of life by 0.2 for each of five individuals results in the equivalent of 1 QALY if the benefit is maintained over a 1-year period. The basic assumption is that life-years can be adjusted for quality of life by multiplying the time spent in each health state by its quality of life preference weight to estimate QALYs. QALYs can be added together and estimated over multiple patients and multiple years. This system has the advantage of considering both benefits and side effects of treatment programs in terms of the common QALY units.

Although QALYs are typically used to assess patients, they can also be measured for others, including caregivers who are placed at risk because they experience stressful life events. In their report *Summarizing Population Health*, the U.S. Institute of Medicine (IOM) of the National academies of Science recommended that population health metrics be used to evaluate public programs and to assist the decision-making process (Field & Gold, 1998).

In summary, QALYs combine measures of morbidity and mortality and do not require medical diagnoses. The measures include time or prognosis and incorporate preferences for health outcomes.

## Accounting for Costs

Costs are an important component of cost-effectiveness analysis. From the societal perspective, the cost component considers all resources required for the intervention and for the comparator. An evaluation of a preventive intervention, for example, must consider all costs required to deliver the intervention or the comparison program. They include all costs for all people exposed to the program, regardless of whether they eventually developed a health problem. From an administrative perspective, direct-cost estimates include all costs of treatment and any costs associated with caring for side effects of the treatment. Direct costs may be the only ones recognized by the administrative perspective. However, from the perspective of the patient or from a societal perspective, several indirect costs must be taken into consideration. Indirect costs include patient time required for therapy, income lost because a family member offers home care, and morbidity and mortality costs associated with reduced productivity due to disability or premature death. A thorough analysis must also include the intangible costs associated with pain and suffering.

In the cost-benefit analysis, the cost savings in reduced health care are subtracted from the cost of an intervention period. For example, an intervention to manage anxiety may reduce the number of visits to health care providers. If the resources saved by reduced visits exceed the costs of the programs, a cost offset has been achieved. Although there are bold claims that programs produce cost offsets, careful analysis rarely shows that intervention programs actually save money (Russell, 1986). Some cost-effectiveness analyses examine how changes in utilization as a result of a treatment or program affect health care costs. A related approach involves estimates of productivity gains. These gains may occur because healthy people who live longer are able to contribute more to the economy and pay more taxes. These approaches have been seriously criticized because they value only the portion of life used for paid work. The models exclude or devalue activity, such as child care, school work, or volunteer efforts. Furthermore, these methods place greater weight on wealthy individuals and may favor programs that care for the rich.

## Discounting Costs and Outcomes

It is commonly acknowledged in economic theory that future gains (or losses) should be discounted because people have time preferences for outcomes that are both monetary and otherwise (Berwick et al., 1981). Although there is considerable variation among individuals, most people prefer positive events or rewards sooner and negative events or punishments later in time (Redelmeier et al., 1996). For example, even if inflation were held constant, most people would choose to receive $100 today versus $100 one year later. Why? Because they have an extra year to either invest that money or spend it on things they can enjoy sooner.

Theoretically, health is expected to be valued and preferred earlier in life in the same manner as money and should therefore be discounted in a similar manner (Gold, 1996). However, there is still considerable debate about whether this is correct (Parsonage & Neuburger, 1992). The Cost/Effectiveness Task Force reviewed the issue and found it to be extremely complex (Gold et al., 1996). They concluded that until a different consensus is reached and for the purposes of standardization health outcomes should be discounted at the same rate as monetary costs. They recommend a discount rate of 3% per year.

## Time Horizon and Modeling

The concept of time horizon simply refers to how long after the intervention the costs and outcomes are evaluated. Preventive interventions may change outcomes over a lifetime, or longer, if subsequent generations are affected by the intervention.

Obviously, the longer the follow-up period the better because there is the potential for unintended side effects or benefits in the distant future. However, it is not possible to measure health outcome data accurately or costs indefinitely.

An increasingly popular technique for extending the time horizon of a cost-effectiveness analysis is modeling of future outcomes. Modeling uses estimates of the probability of each possible health outcome to calculate future costs and health consequences of the intervention by computer. Probability estimates for some health problems have been fairly well established through epidemiological research. However, there are also concerns about how much of the future should be estimated from past data. Sensitivity analysis is one way to address some of this uncertainty, but it is not a complete remedy for these concerns.

## Sensitivity Analysis

Sensitivity analysis is a statistical technique that is not specific to cost-effectiveness analysis, but it is usually included in a quality study. Almost every study on cost effectiveness involves estimating certain costs or rates of outcomes. For example, actual health care costs are often difficult to identify because these costs vary widely and often contain sensitive or confidential information. Health care utilization rates are easier to obtain, but they require an estimate of the cost per type of utilization. Likewise, effect sizes from multiple studies of a similar intervention may vary widely, so an estimate of the average effect size is used. Sensitivity analysis examines how the results of the cost-effectiveness analysis would change if these estimated values were allowed to vary between a realistic upper and lower limit. In other words, researchers examine and report how sensitive their results are to the estimates contained in their analysis.

Utility-based measures of quality of life are often used to evaluate the cost effectiveness of health care programs (Kaplan et al., 2004). For example, one study using the Quality of Well-Being Index (QWB) showed that a new medication for patients with arthritis produced an average of 0.023 QALY per year, whereas a new medication for acquired immunodeficiency syndrome (AIDS) produced nearly 0.46 QALY per year. However, the benefit of the arthritis medication may last as long as 20 years, ultimately producing $0.023 \times 20$ years $= 0.46$ year. The AIDS treatment produced a benefit for only 1 year, so its total effect was $0.46 \times 1$ year $= 0.46$ year. In other words, the general system allows the full potential benefits of these two very different treatments to be compared (Kaplan & Frosch, 2005).

Quality-adjusted life-years are generic measures of life expectancy with adjustments for quality of life (Russell, 1986). QALYs include both benefits and side effects of regimens in terms of common outcome units.

In addition to health benefits, programs also have costs. Resources are limited, and good policy requires allocation to maximize life expectancy and health-related quality of life. Thus, in addition to measuring health outcomes, costs must also be considered. Methodologies for estimating costs have now become standardized (Gold et al., 1996). From an administrative perspective, cost estimates include all costs of treatment and costs associated with caring for any side effects of treatment. From a social perspective, costs are broader and may include costs of family members staying off work to provide care. Comparing programs for a given population with a given medical condition, cost effectiveness is measured as the change in costs of care for the program compared to the existing therapy or program relative to the change in health measured in a standardized unit, such as the QALY. The difference in costs over the difference in effectiveness is the incremental cost effectiveness and is usually expressed as the cost/QALY. Because the objective of all programs is to produce QALYs, the cost/QALY ratio can be used to show the relative efficiency of different programs (Gold et al., 1996).

Randomized clinical trials of treatment efficacy are the most compelling studies in which quality of life measures and cost-effectiveness analysis have been used. Although several authors have used quality of life measures to estimate the effectiveness of clinical interventions, most of these analyses use subjective estimates of clinical outcomes because the studies did not incorporate quality of life measures. Two excellent examples of policy analysis associated with prospective randomized clinical trials have been published. In each case, the quality of life measurement was incorporated into the study protocol and the cost-effectiveness analysis was part of the study planning. These studies were the Diabetes Prevention Program (DPP) and the National Emphysema Treatment Trial (NETT).

In the diabetes prevention program (Diabetes Prevention Program Research Group, 2003), patients at risk for type II diabetes were randomly assigned to one of three conditions: intensive lifestyle modification, metformin, or placebo. The DPP included 3234 adults with impaired glucose tolerance. The intensive lifestyle intervention was designed to reduce the initial body weight by 7% through regular physical activity and diet. The metformin group took one 850 mg tablet each day. The placebo group also took one tablet per day. The patients were evaluated prior to randomization and at yearly intervals over the course of 3 years.

Quality of life was measured using the Quality of Well-Being Scale (QWB). The measure was chosen because it can be used to estimate QALYs. Over the course of 3 years, those randomly assigned to the lifestyle intervention accrued 0.050 more QALY than those assigned a regular dose of metformin. Among the three interventions, the lifestyle approach was the most expensive (total cost $27,065 US in 2001). Metformin was less expensive ($25,937), and the placebo was the least expensive option ($23,525). Figure 18.1 summarizes the cost/QALY ratios for the lifestyle and the metformin conditions from a health care system prospective. It shows the cost/QALY ratios attributable to the interventions in comparison to placebo and in comparison to doing nothing. Although both interventions offer significant benefits over placebo or doing nothing, the cost/QALY for the lifestyle invention was significantly lower than that for metformin. In other words, even though the lifestyle intervention was more expensive, it offers significantly better value for money.

The second example is an evaluation of surgery for emphysema. Emphysema is the dominant cause of chronic obstructive pulmonary disease (COPD), which is the fourth leading cause of death and a major cause of disability in the United

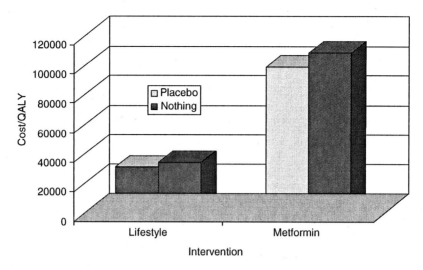

FIGURE 18.1. Cost per quality-adjusted life-year (QALY) of lifestyle and metformin.

States (National Vital Statistics Report, 2004). COPD is caused by a loss of elastic recoil of lung tissue in addition to chronic inflammation in the airways. Lungs often become hyperinflated, and there is an increase in the functional residual capacity. Hyperinflation may place greater strain on the muscles of respiration, increasing the effort required to breathe and reducing the capacity for exercise. This disease is associated with activity limitations, premature death, and reduced quality of life (Pauwels & Rabe, 2004). Despite major advances in diagnosis and medical therapeutics, standard medical therapy often has little effect on life quality (Sutherland & Cherniack, 2004). Thus, many patients seek surgical treatments that may produce more dramatic improvements.

Lung volume reduction surgery (LVRS) is an intervention designed to reduce the volume of the hyperinflated lung. The procedure was introduced during the 1950s, but one in six patients died from the surgery. As a result, the procedure was abandoned by the late 1950s (Brantigan & Mueller, 1957; Lefrak et al., 1997). An improved procedure was reintroduced during the 1990s, and the initial results were encouraging. Shortly thereafter, patient testimonials and marketing efforts resulted in popular enthusiasm for the procedure and pressure for Medicare to pay for it (Cooper et al., 1996; Lefrak, et al., 1997). A report commissioned by the Center for Medicare and Medicaid Services (CMS) cited another article that reported that more than 1200 LVRS procedures had been performed on Medicare beneficiaries. Furthermore, the rate of growth was exponential. The technology assessment raised significant questions about the benefits of the procedure. For example, it was noted that about one-fourth of the Medicare beneficiaries who underwent LVRS died within 1 year (Huizenga et al., 1998). In response to these concerns, Medicare decided to halt payment for the procedure until it could be studied.

The National Emphysema Treatment Trial (NETT) was a multicenter, randomized clinical trial designed to evaluate LVRS. Subjects with moderate to severe emphysema were randomly assigned to usual medical therapy alone or to usual medical therapy plus LVRS. All patients in the trial participated in pulmonary rehabilitation prior to randomization.

Quality of life was one of the primary outcome measures because surgery was not expected to improve life expectancy. Health-related quality of life was measured using four methods: two generic and two disease-specific. One of the measures was chosen because it could be used to estimate QALYs in a cost-effectiveness analysis. The study was unusual because it included a prospective plan for policy analysis.

The NETT trial randomized 1218 patients to either maximum medical therapy or to the combination of maximal medical therapy plus LVRS (Fishman et al., 2003). Over the first 12 months of the study, LVRS patients had significantly more hospital days, ambulatory care days, and nursing home admissions. However, hospital utilization began to change by the 13- to 24-month interval. During the second year, those in the maximal medical arm accumulated more hospital days and had more emergency room visits. During the third year, hospital utilization was equivalent for the two groups.

The results from the NETT are very complex and we devote an entire chapter (Chapter 19) to the findings. Theoretically, there are a variety of possible results. In order to place the results in perspective, Figure 18.2 summarizes outcomes in a two-dimensional "policy space". The horizontal dimension is for the effect of treatment. The right side shows the treatment is effective, while the left side shows the treatment is ineffective. The vertical dimension is for costs. The

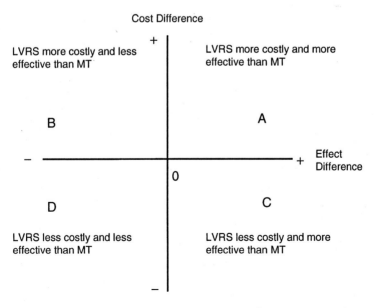

FIGURE 18.2. Mean cumulative quality-adjusted life-years (QALYs): years 1–3.

top half of the plane indicates that the procedure increases costs, while the bottom half of the plane suggests that the operation reduces costs. The two dimensions form four quadrants. In quadrant A, LVRS would be more effective and more costly than medical therapy. Quadrant B (upper left) suggests the LVRS increases costs and is less effective than medical therapy. Quadrant C (lower right) indicates that LVRS is more effective and less costly than medical therapy, while quadrant D (lower left) suggests that LVRS costs less than medical therapy but is less effective. If the outcome lands in quadrant B or C, the choice would be clear. In quadrant B, medical therapy would be the clear choice, while in quadrant C, surgery would be preferred. As we will see in chapter 19, the NETT found that surgery was both more expensive, but more effective than medical therapy (Quadrant A). However, the cost-effective analysis suggested that the additional costs were justified in terms of additional benefits.

The cost/QALY ratio was evaluated 3 years following randomization. Using best estimates for cost, mortality, and quality of life, it was estimated that LVRS was more expensive than maximal medical therapy ($98,952 vs. $62,560). However, QALYs were also greater in the LVRS arm (1.463 vs. 1.271). Thus, the incremental cost/QALY ratio was approximately $190,000.

The NETT trial demonstrated that the cost effectiveness of LVRS is comparable to several other surgical procedures. The relative cost effectiveness of LVRS is particularly impressive if benefits of the procedure are projected into the future. The NETT was a milestone study because the cost-effectiveness analysis was planned and executed as a companion to the randomized controlled trial. Furthermore, the NETT trial allowed rapid dissemination of the findings. The results of the trial were published in the *New England Journal of Medicine* in May 2003 (Ramsey et al., 2003). The trial and cost-effectiveness analysis were used as the basis of Medicare policy funding LVRS surgery. By early 2004, Medicare coverage for LVRS had been approved. The trial offers an excellent example of rapid translation from research to policy.

## Conclusions

Obtaining value for patients may require making comparisons between very different alternative expenditures. Using the CLINECS terminology, we must link inputs to outcomes. This chapter reviewed applications of cost-effectiveness analysis, a methodology that allows these broad comparisons. Figure 18.3 compares various programs that have been analyzed using the cost/QALY ratio. Some traditional interventions, such as mammographic screening for younger women, may cost as much as $240,000 to produce a QALY. Cholesterol screening programs may also require many resources (more than $100,000) to produce a QALY. By comparison, public health programs, such as tobacco access restrictions, may produce a QALY at a very low cost. Figure 18.3 shows a hypothetical "pay line." It might be argued that programs to the left of the pay line should be funded, but those with cost/QALY ratios to the right of the line should be examined more carefully.

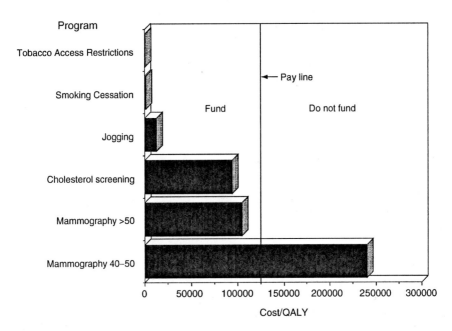

FIGURE 18.3. Cost per quality-adjusted life-year (QALY) for a variety of medical, surgical, and public health interventions. LVRS = lung volume reduction surgery; QALY = quality-adjusted life-year. (From Diabetes Prevention Program Research Group, 2003.)

## References

Berwick, D.M., Cretin, S., Keeler, E. (1981). Cholesterol, children, and heart disease: an analysis of alternatives. *Pediatrics,* 68, 721–730.

Brantigan, O.C., Mueller, E. (1957). Surgical treatment of pulmonary emphysema. *American Surgeon,* 23, 789–804.

Cooper, J.D., Gaissert, H.A, Patterson, G.A., Pohl, M.S., Yusen, R.D., Trulock, E.P. (1996). [Lung volume reduction surgery in advanced emphysema: results of the Washington University, St. Louis.] *Wien Medizinische Wochenschrift,* 146, 592–598.

Curry, S J., Grothaus, L C., McAfee, T., Pabiniak, C. (1998). Use and cost effectiveness of smoking-cessation services under four insurance plans in a health maintenance organization. *New England Journal of Medicine,* 339, 673–679.

Diabetes Prevention Program Research Group (2003). Within-trial cost-effectiveness of lifestyle intervention or metformin for the primary prevention of type 2 diabetes. *Diabetes Care,* 26, 2518–2523.

Doubilet, P., Weinstein, M.C., McNeil, B.J. (1986). Use and misuse of the term "cost effective" in medicine. *New England Journal of Medicine,* 314, 253–256.

Eddy, D.M. (2005). Evidence-based medicine: a unified approach. *Health Affairs (Millwood),* 24, 9–17.

Field, M.J., Gold, M.R. (1998). *Summarizing population health.* Washington, DC: Institute of Medicine, National Academy Press.

Fishman, A., Martinez, F., Naunheim, K., Piantadosi, S, Wise, R, Ries, A. (2003). A randomized trial comparing lung-volume-reduction surgery with medical therapy for severe emphysema. *New England Journal of Medicine,* 348, 2059–2073.

Gold, M. *Cost-effectiveness in health and medicine*. New York: Oxford Press; 1996.

Gold, M., Franks, P., Erickson, P. (1996). Assessing the health of the nation: the predictive validity of a preference-based measure and self-rated health. *Medical Care*, 34, 163–177.

Huizenga, H.F., Ramsey, S.D., Albert, R.K. (1998). Estimated growth of lung volume reduction surgery among Medicare enrollees: 1994 to 1996. *Chest*, 114, 1583–1587.

Kaplan, R.M. (1994). Value judgment in the Oregon Medicaid experiment. *Med Care*, 32, 975–988.

Kaplan, R.M. (1997). Decisions about prostate cancer screening in managed care. *Current Opinion in Oncology* 9, 480–486.

Kaplan, R.M. (2000). Two pathways to prevention. *American Psychologist*, 55, 382–396.

Kaplan, R.M., Frosch, D.L. (2005). Decision making in medicine and health care. *Annual Review of Clinical Psychology*, 1, 525–556.

Kaplan, R.M., Groessl, E. (2002). Cost/effectiveness analysis in behavioral medicine. *Journal of Consulting and Clinical Psychology*, 70, 482–493.

Kaplan, R. M., Feeny, D., Revicki, D.A. (1993). Methods for assessing relative importance in preference based outcome measures. *Quality of Life Research*, 2, 467–475.

Kaplan, R.M., Ries, A.L., Reilly, J., Mohsenifar, Z. (2004). Measurement of health-related quality of life in the national emphysema treatment trial. *Chest*, 126, 781–789.

Kassirer, J.P., Angell, M. (1994). The journal's policy on cost-effectiveness analyses [editorial]. *New England Journal of Medicine*, 331, 669–670.

Lefrak, S.S., Yusen, R.D., Trulock, E.P., Pohl, M.S., Patterson, A., Cooper, J.D. (1997). Recent advances in surgery for emphysema. *Annual Review of Medicine*, 48, 387–398.

National Vital Statistics Report (2004). Available at: http://www.cdc.gov/nchs/fastats/copd.htm. Accessed October 15, 2004.

Parsonage M., Neuburger, H. (1992). Discounting and health benefits. *Health Economics*, 1(1), 71–76.

Pauwels, R.A., Rabe, K.F. (2004). Burden and clinical features of chronic obstructive pulmonary disease (COPD). *Lancet*, 364, 613–620.

Ramsey, S.D., Berry, K., Etzioni, R., Kaplan, R.M., Sullivan, S.D., Wood, D.E. (2003). Cost effectiveness of lung-volume-reduction surgery for patients with severe emphysema. *New England Journal of Medicine*, 348, 2092–2102.

Redelmeier, D.A., Guyatt, G.H., Goldstein, R.S. (1996). Assessing the minimal important difference in symptoms: a comparison of two techniques. *Journal of Clinical Epidemiology*, 49, 1215–1219.

Reinhardt, U.E., Hussey, P.S., Anderson, G.F. (2004). U.S. health care spending in an international context. *Health Affairs (Millwood)*, 23, 10–25.

Russell, L.B. (1986). *Is prevention better than cure?* Washington, DC: Brookings Institution.

Russell, L.B. (1987). *Evaluating preventive care: report on a workshop*. Washington, DC: Brookings Institution.

Russell, L.B., Gold, M.R., Siegel, J.E., Daniels, N., Weinstein, M.C. (1996). The role of cost-effectiveness analysis in health and medicine; Panel on Cost-Effectiveness in Health and Medicine. *Journal of the American Medical Association*, 276, 1172–1177.

Smith, C., Cowan, C., Sensenig, A., Catlin, A. (2005). Health spending growth slows in 2003. *Health Affairs (Millwood)*, 24, 185–194.

Starfield, B. (2000). Is US health really the best in the world? *Journal of the American Medical Association*, 284, 483–485.

Sutherland, E.R., Cherniack, R.M. (2004). Management of chronic obstructive pulmonary disease. *New England Journal of Medicine*, 350, 2689–2697.

Weinstein, M.C., Siegel, J.E., Gold, M.R., Kamlet, M.S., Russell, L.B. (1996). Recommendations of the Panel on Cost-effectiveness in Health and Medicine. *Journal of the American Medical Association*, 276, 1253–1258.

# 19
# Cost-Effectiveness of Lung Volume Reduction Surgery

ROBERT M. KAPLAN AND SCOTT D. RAMSEY

Chronic obstructive pulmonary disease (COPD) is the fourth leading cause of death and a major cause of disability in the United States (National Vital Statistics Report, 2004). It is caused by a loss of elastic recoil related to parenchymal destruction due to emphysema in addition to chronic airway inflammation. Lungs often become hyperinflated, and there is an increase in the functional residual capacity. Hyperinflation may place greater strain on the muscles of respiration, increasing the effort required to breathe and reducing exercise capacity. The physiologic abnormalities include a reduction in diffusing capacity of carbon monoxide, hypoventilation, and hypoxemia (Sutherland & Cherniack, 2004).

A number of activity limitations, premature death, and reduced quality of life are associated with COPD (Pauwels & Rabe, 2004). Despite major advances in diagnosis and medical therapeutics, many patients remain dyspneic despite standard medical therapy. Typical management of COPD includes a variety of medications. However, treatment may also include respiratory chest physiotherapy techniques, exercise, and advice to quit smoking. Most patients are confronted with complex combinations of antibiotics, bronchodilators, antiinflammatory drugs, and in some cases supplemental oxygen (Sutherland & Cherniack, 2004). However, the benefits of medical therapy are limited because therapies are not able to prevent further decline of the 1-second forced expiratory volume ($FEV_{1.0}$). Thus, many patients seek surgical treatments that may produce more dramatic improvement.

In the following sections we review the history of lung volume reduction surgery (LVRS) and describe some of the controversies associated with the procedure. In particular, we consider the cost of the procedure and its cost effectiveness. However, before discussing LVRS, it is important to review some of the conceptual background and standards used in cost-effectiveness analysis.

## Standards for Cost-Effectiveness Analysis

Contrary to the portrayal of cost-effectiveness analysis in the popular media, the purpose of the analysis is not to cut costs. Cost-effectiveness analysis is performed to identify which interventions produce the greatest amount of health using the resources that are available. Because of the confusion about cost-effectiveness analysis, the Office of Disease Prevention and Health Promotion in the Public Health Service (PHS) appointed a 13-member panel to create common standards. The work of the panel was published as a book (Gold, 1996) and in a series of articles published in the *Journal of the American Medical Association* (Russell et al., 1996; Siegel et al., 1996; Weinstein et al., 1996). The major elements of cost-effectiveness analysis as defined by this panel were reviewed in Chapter 18.

## History of Lung Volume Reduction Surgery

Lung volume reduction surgery (LVRS) is an intervention designed to reduce the volume of the hyperinflated lung. The procedure was introduced by Otto Brantigan during the 1950s. However, early use was associated with an operative mortality of nearly one of six patients. As a result, the procedure was abandoned by the late 1950s (Brantigan & Mueller, 1957; Lefrak et al., 1997). It was reintroduced by Cooper in the 1990s. Cooper's procedure was a modification of the original LVRS using access to both lungs through a median sternotomy (Cooper et al., 1995, 1996). The initial results from Cooper's procedure were encouraging. Shortly thereafter, patient testimonials and marketing efforts resulted in popular enthusiasm for the procedure (Lefrak et al., 1997). A report commissioned by the Health Care Financing Administration (HCFA), now known as the Center for Medicare and Medicaid Services (CMS), noted that 1200 LVRS procedures had been performed on Medicare beneficiaries and that the rate of increase was exponential. The technology assessment is available at http://www.ncbi.nlm.nih.gov/books/bv.fcgi?rid=hstat6.chapter.41412/. The technology assessment, however, raised significant questions about the benefits of the procedure. For example, it was noted that about one-fourth of the Medicare beneficiaries who underwent LVRS died within 1 year (Huizenga et al., 1998). In response to these concerns, HCFA decided LVRS would no longer be a procedure covered by Medicare. Furthermore, in collaboration with the National Heart, Lung, and Blood Institute (NHLBI), HCFA co-sponsored a randomized controlled clinical trial to determine the effectiveness of LVRS. The trial began in 1997, and results were reported in 2001 and 2003. We describe the results of the trial later in the chapter.

## National Emphysema Treatment Trial

The National Emphysema Treatment Trial (NETT) was a multicenter randomized clinical trial designed to evaluate LVRS. Subjects with moderate to severe emphysema were randomly assigned to the usual medical therapy alone or to the usual medical therapy plus LVRS. All patients in the trial participated in pulmonary rehabilitation prior to randomization. This chapter summarizes outcomes from the trial along with the findings of a cost-effectiveness analysis (Ramsey et al., 2003).

## Subjects

The subjects were 746 male and 472 female volunteers with an average age of 64 years. Participants were studied at one of 17 approved NETT sites. The inclusion criteria were (1) radiographic evidence of bilateral emphysema, (2) studies demonstrating severe airflow obstruction and hyperinflation, and (3) participation in pulmonary rehabilitation with the attainment of preset performance goals. Exclusion criteria were (1) a broad range of medical conditions that place patients at risk for perioperative morbidity and/or mortality, (2) emphysema thought to be unsuitable for LVRS, and (3) medical conditions or other circumstances that make it likely the patient would be unable to complete the trial. The exclusion criteria relating to cardiology issues were based on the work of Goldman and colleagues (1977). A more detailed description of the NETT methodology can be found in "Rationale and design of the National Emphysema Treatment Trial: a prospective randomized trial of lung volume reduction surgery" (National Emphysema Treatment Trial Research Group, 1999).

Following baseline evaluation, all participants completed comprehensive pulmonary rehabilitation. A second assessment was completed after rehabilitation and prior to randomization.

## Quality of Life Measures

Among several quality of life measures, the NETT used the self-administered version of the Quality of Well-Being Scale (QWB-SA) (see Chapter 7). The QWB-SA is a comprehensive measure of health-related quality of life that includes five sections: acute symptoms, chronic symptoms, self-care, mobility, and social activity (Kaplan et al., 1976, 1984, 1995, 1998). The observed level of function and the subjective symptomatic complaints are weighted by preference, or the utility for the state, on a scale ranging from 0 (for dead) to 1.0 (for optimum function). The QWB-SA has been used in a wide variety of clinical and population studies (Kaplan et al., 1995, 1996; Pyne et al., 1997; Rocco et al., 1997) to evaluate therapeutic interventions for a range of medical and surgical conditions.

## Clinical Interventions

All subjects participated in the prerandomization pulmonary rehabilitation program (10 sessions over 8 to 9 weeks) supervised by a NETT clinical center. Portions of the program could be carried out at a NETT-certified rehabilitation facility closer to the participant's home. The NETT rehabilitation program was similar to that described by Ries and colleagues (2003).

## Cost-Effectiveness in NETT

A team headed by Scott Ramsey from the Fred Hutchinson Cancer Center conducted the cost-effectiveness analysis. The group at Fred Hutchinson received guidance from an external advisory committee. The objective of the substudy was to evaluate the cost effectiveness of LVRS in comparison to maximal medical therapy for patients with severe emphysema (Gold, 1996). In the cost-utility analysis the unit of effectiveness is the quality-adjusted life-year (QALY). The analysis used a societal perspective. The time horizon for the study included observations during the trial and projections 10 years into the future.

## Measurement of Resource Utilization

Medical care utilization was based on Medicare claims for trial participants provided by the Centers for Medicare and Medicaid Services (CMS). Medicare reimbursed the trial-related medical care for study participants, including the screening evaluation, pulmonary rehabilitation prior to randomization, the surgical procedure itself, and trial-related follow-up visits after surgery. Other Medicare services included inpatient care, outpatient physician care, ambulatory laboratory, diagnostic, and radiology services, home health services, home oxygen, up to 100 days of skilled nursing facility care, and hospice care. Outpatient medications used for emphysema (not covered by Medicare) were recorded at follow-up visits. Medication doses were based on the usual adult dose recorded in the manufacturer's package insert (Physician's Desk Reference, 2002).

Several methods were used to estimate emphysema-related utilization of non-medical goods and services. Travel distances to care facilities were estimated using software that calculated distances traveled from the patient's residence zip code to NETT-affiliated facilities (Statistical Analysis Software, 2002). Enrollees gave estimates of the weekly average number of hours of unpaid caregiver time (family and friends) provided to them. Patient time spent seeking medical care was based on Medicare records for ambulatory care and hospitalizations. Table 19.1 summarizes the resourcs and valuations in the NETT.

## Valuation of Resources Used

The value of medical care was based on Medicare reimbursements for covered services adjusted to 2002 (U.S.) dollars using the medical care component of the Consumer Price Index. Costs for respiratory-related medications were based on the 2002 average wholesale price discounted 15% to adjust for typical retail acquisition costs, with a $2.50 dispensing fee added each 30 days. The lowest price for available generic versions of medications was used. Transportation costs

TABLE 19.1. Recources and Valution in NETT

| Cost element | Source |
| --- | --- |
| Medicare services | Medicare reimbursements |
| Emphysema medications | A WP less 15% acquisition + dispensing fee |
| Travel costs | Federal travel reimbursement per mile |
| Patient time | Wages for persons age 65 atleast (Bureau of Labor Statistics) |
| Caregiver time | Wages for age 65 or less (Bureau of Labor Statistics) |

to and from health care facilities were estimated by multiplying travel distances by federal government reimbursement rates per mile. The value of time spent by family and friends caring for patients was based on average wages for workers aged 20 to 64 as reported by the Bureau of Labor Statistics. The value of patients' time spent in treatment was based on wages for workers over age 65.

In accordance with guidelines for conducting cost-effectiveness studies (Gold, 1996), costs and benefits accruing after year 1 were discounted at an annual rate of 3%. A more detailed description of the methodology is available from previous publications (Ramsey et al., 2001, 2003).

## Results

The NETT trial randomized 1218 patients to either maximum medical therapy or the combination of maximal medical therapy plus LVRS. Both groups completed a rehabilitation phase. In November 2001, recruitment into the trial was halted for high risk patients. High risk was defined as $FEV_{1.0} < 20\%$ of the predicted value and either diffuse emphysema or low diffusing capacity (or both). Early results indicated that this group experienced excess mortality following LVRS. However, the Data Safety and Monitoring Board (DSMB) concluded that it was safe for other patients to continue the trial. Ultimately, 1078 patients without high risk characteristics completed the trial (National Emphysema Treatment Trial Research Group, 2001). Among them, 14 patients (7 from each arm) were excluded from the cost-effectiveness analysis. Nine of the patients were excluded because they were in a Medicare health maintenance organization (HMO), three because they were not Medicare recipients, and two because their Medicare HIC number was faulty.

Utilization of health care services is summarized in Table 19.2. During the first 12 months of the study, LVRS patients had significantly more hospital days, ambulatory care days, and nursing home admissions. However, utilization began to change by the 13- to 24-month interval. During the second year, those in the maximal medical arm required more hospital days and had more emergency

TABLE 19.2. Mean utilization per person for those alive at the start of the time period

| | 0–12 Months | | 13–24 Months | | 25–36 Months | |
|---|---|---|---|---|---|---|
| Parameter | LVRS ($n = 531$) | Medical ($n = 535$) | LVRS ($n = 407$) | Medical ($n = 424$) | LVRS ($n = 277$) | Medical ($n = 278$) |
| Hospital days | 24.9* | 4.9* | 3.2** | 6.1** | 4.0 | 5.2 |
| Ambulatory care days | 10.3** | 8.6** | 5.0 | 4.9 | 4.5 | 4.4 |
| Emergency room visits | 0.6 | 0.8 | 0.5*** | 0.7*** | 0.5 | 0.7 |
| Oxygen claims | 6.7 | 7.2 | 5.8 | 6.5 | 5.9 | 5.6 |
| Nursing home admissions | 0.08* | 0.04* | 13 | 16 | 4 | 9 |

LVRS = lung volume reduction surgery.
$p < 0.05$ ; **$p < 0.01$; ***$p < 0.001$.

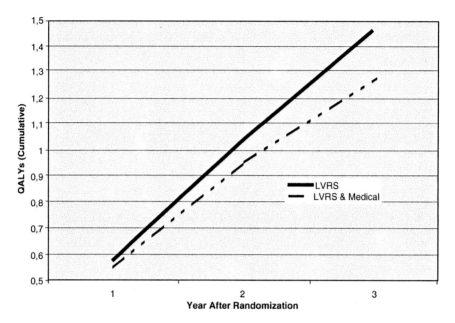

FIGURE 19.1. Mean cumulative quality-adjusted life-years (QALYs) during years 1 to 3. LVRS = lung volume reduction surgery.

room visits. During the third year, utilization was equivalent for the two groups. Figure 19.1 summarizes the cumulative QALYs per person over the first 3 years of the project. After 1 year the groups differed, but the effect was not significant. However, by year 2 the groups began separating, and this difference grew by year 3. Figure 19.2 summarizes the mean total monthly cost for each group following randomization. As the figure shows, there was a sharp increase in costs for the LVRS group during the first few months following randomization. This was expected because the surgery requires hospital recovery and there are associated hospital costs. However, by about 7 months following randomization, costs for the two groups were equivalent and remained so throughout the trial. Table 19.3 summarizes the mean total monthly cost for each group following randomization. As also noted in Figure 19.2. Costs were higher in the first year for the surgery group, but they were lower in the second year. By the third year, cost differences between the surgery and the medical therapy group were non-significant.

## Cost per Quality-Adjusted Life-Year

Cost per QALY was evaluated 3 years following randomization. Using best estimates for cost, mortality, and quality of life, it was estimated that LVRS was more expensive than maximal medical therapy ($98,952 vs. $62,560). However, QALYs were also greater in the LVRS arm (1.463 vs. 1.271). Thus, the incremental cost per QALY was approximately $190,000.

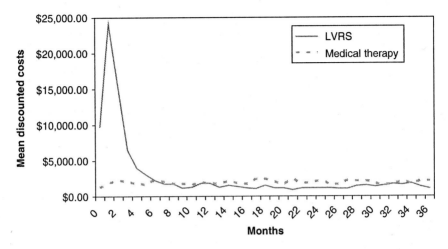

FIGURE 19.2. National Emphysema Treatment Trial (NETT) mean total monthly cost for each group following randomization.

TABLE 19.3. Mean Direct Medical Costs and Total Health Care-Related Costs According to Time after Randomization*

| | Surgery Group | | Medical-Therapy Group | | |
| Variable | No. of Patients | Mean Cost (95% CI) | No. of Patients | Mean Cost (95% CI) | P Value |
| --- | --- | --- | --- | --- | --- |
| | | S | | S | |
| 0–12 Mo after randomization | 531 | | 535 | | |
| Direct medical costs | | 61,145 (56,069–66,220) | | 15,738 (14,006–17,470) | <0.001 |
| Total costs | | 71,515 (65,921–77,109) | | 23,371 (21,056–25,686) | <0.001 |
| 13–24 Mo after randomization | 407 | | 424 | | |
| Direct medical costs | | 9,474 (8,260–10,688) | | 15,648 (12,934–18,362) | <0.001 |
| Total costs | | 13,222 (11,479–14,964) | | 21,319 (18,004–24,635) | <0.001 |
| 25–36 Mo after randomization | 277 | | 278 | | |
| Direct medical costs | | 10,199 (8,161–12,236) | | 12,303 (9,977–14,629) | 0.18 |
| Total costs | | 14,215 (11,529–16,901) | | 17,870 (14,785–20,954) | 0.08 |

*Costs are reported in 2002 dollars. Direct medical costs include Medicare reimbursements and pharmacy costs. Total costs include direct medical costs plus the value of the time spent by caregivers, the value of the time spent by the patient, and travel costs. After year 1, costs were discounted by 3 percent per year. P values were derived by two-sided t-tests for equality of means. CI denotes confidence interval.

To capture potential longer-term gains, the analysis also estimated projected benefits over an extended period of time. To conduct these analyses, the log logistic for the Kaplan-Myers survival curves was extrapolated over the course of 10 years. These analyses excluded the high risk subgroups and assumed that the relative risk of death would be 1.0 following the 3-year observation. For quality of life estimates, trends in quality of well-being scores over the first 3 years were projected up to 10 years into the future. The cost analysis projected the trends in annual costs from the first 3 years an additional 7 years into the future. The analyses suggested that at 5 years the incremental cost per QALY was $88,000 for non-high risk patients, and at 10 years it was $53,000.

An important feature of the NETT evaluation was the creation of four post hoc subgroups of patients. These subgroups were defined by combinations of two baseline characteristics: (1) upper lobe predominance in emphysema distribution [determined by computed tomography (CT) scans] or not and (2) low versus high maximal exercise capacity following pulmonary rehabilitation ($\leq 25$ watts for women, $\leq 40$ watts for men). Benefits of surgery varied by subgroup. There were significant benefits for those with upper lobe emphysema and low initial exercise capacity. For the two other groups (upper lobe/high exercise capacity, non-upper lobe/low exercise capacity) there were significant but weaker effects. For the fourth group (non-upper lobe/high exercise capacity), surgery doubled the 2-year mortality risk without symptomatic improvement compared to medical therapy.

Table 19.4 summarizes the cost effectiveness for the subgroups 3 years following randomization. In cost-utility analysis, some decisions "dominate" because they incur costs and reduce health (decision against treatment) or because they produce health and save money (decision for treatment). For the high risk group, LVRS was associated with excess mortality. Because it produces harm, the decision was dominated in favor of medical therapy. For those with upper lobe emphysema and low exercise capacity, LVRS produces a QALY for less than $100,000. For those with upper lobe emphysema and high exercise capacity, LVRS produces a QALY at nearly $250,000, and the cost per QALY is even higher for those with non-upper lobe emphysema and low exercise capacity ($330,000). For those with non-upper-lobe emphysema and high exercise capacity, LVRS does not provide benefit, and the decision is dominated in favor of medical therapy.

TABLE 19.4. Cost-effectiveness for the subgroups 3 years after randomization

| Subgroup | Cost per QALY gained at 3 years |
|---|---|
| High risk ($n = 138$) | Dominated[a] |
| Upper lobe + low exercise capacity ($n = 137$) | $98,000 |
| Upper lobe + high exercise capacity ($n = 204$) | $240,000 |
| Non-upper lobe + low exercise capacity ($n = 82$) | $330,000 |
| Non-upper lobe + high exercise capacity ($n = 108$) | Dominated[a] |

QALY = quality-adjusted life-years.
[a]Higher costs and less favorable outcomes for the group with lung volume reduction surgery.
Derived from an unpublished talk. Scott D. Ramsey is the coauthor.

Figure 19.3 shows the cost-effectiveness acceptability curves at 3 years and projected 10 years into the future. The graph estimates the probability that the procedure will be cost effective given different value ceilings for the cost per QALY ratio. For example, using the traditional cost per QALY ratio of $50,000 (Gold, 1996), the analyses suggested that the probability is greater than 0.70 that the procedure would be judged to be cost effective for those with non-upper lobe emphysema and low exercise capacity. Using a threshold of $150,000, the probability is close 0.80 that the procedure would be cost effective for all patient subgroups except those in whom medical therapy dominated.

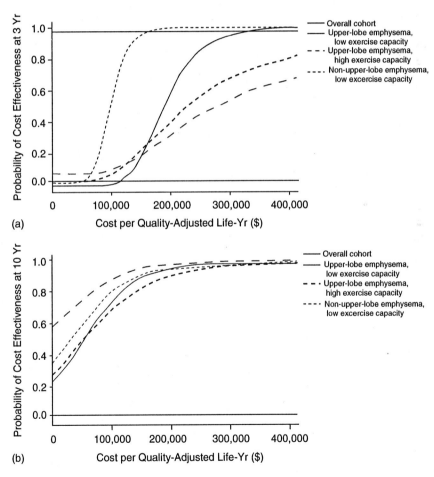

FIGURE 19.3. Cost-effectiveness acceptability curves at the 3-year observation (A) and projected 10 years into the future (B). (From Ramsey et al., 2003.)

## Discussion

In 1996 there was an increasing interest in the use of lung volume reduction surgery. However, a variety of problems faced policy makers. All of the data available were from non-controlled studies. As a result, there were serious questions as to whether the surgery was effective. A second problem was that the studies were of short duration and the long-term effects of surgery were not known. When the uncontrolled studies were compared, it was clear that many patients were lost to follow-up. Further, the criteria for selecting patients in these studies was highly variable. Overall, there was not enough evidence to decide if Medicare should cover the surgery. The NETT trial addressed these issues with a randomized clinical trial and prospective cost-effectiveness analysis.

LVRS competes for resources with a variety of other medical services. One of the advantages of cost-utility analysis is that it allows comparisons between programs that have different specific objectives. Table 19.5 compares the cost effectiveness of LVRS with other thoracic surgery procedures. LVRS compares favorably with other interventions if a 10-year horizon is used. Even considering the 3-year interval for which outcomes were observed in the NETT, LVRS is in a range comparable to that for lung transplantation. It is worth noting that the alternatives in Table 19.5 are very different from one another. Lung transplantation and LVRS patients are drawn from very different populations. Nevertheless, cost per QALY for the two procedures can be compared directly.

The ultimate economic effect of LVRS remains uncertain. Early estimates suggested that about two million American adults suffer from emphysema. If each procedure costs $20,000 and 1% of these patients receive LVRS, the cost would exceed $400,000,000. However, one of the important lessons from the NETT trial was that it is difficult to recruit patients to participate. It remains to be demonstrated if the high demand for surgery during the early years of LVRS can be sustained. For example, the NETT expected to enroll 4500 patients but was able to attract only 1218. Experience during the last few years indicates that costs may be lower than these projections because demand for the procedure has declined.

TABLE 19.5. Cost-effectiveness of LVRS in comparison to other thoracic surgery procedures

| Intervention | Cost per QALY |
|---|---|
| Coronary artery bypass graft | $8,300–$64,000 |
| Heart transplantation | $65,000 |
| Implantable defibrillator | $47,000 |
| Lung transplantation | $133,000–$216,000 |
| Lung volume reduction surgery | |
| 3 Years | $190,000 |
| 10 Years | $53,000 |

# Summary

Chronic obstructive pulmonary disease is a challenging problem. It remains the fourth leading cause of death in the United States, and medical options are of limited value. Lung volume reduction surgery is an attractive addition. However, the procedure carries the risks of operative and perioperative mortality (Meyers, 2002). Furthermore, the procedure represents an option for only a fraction of patients with emphysema. Some subgroups of patients, particularly those with upper lobe emphysema with low initial exercise capacity, are most likely to benefit from LVRS. Several minimally invasive methods for lung volume reduction are being currently studied (Brenner et al., 2004; Maxfield, 2004). Further analysis is necessary to determine if these minimally invasive techniques prove to be more cost effective than open lung volume reduction.

The NETT trial demonstrated that the cost effectiveness of LVRS is comparable to that for several other surgical procedures. The relative cost effectiveness of LVRS is particularly impressive if benefits of the procedure are projected into the future. Clinicians should consider LVRS for patients who are in a subgroup most likely to benefit. Because the procedure is relatively expensive, administrators must continue to consider the cost per QALY of LVRS in relation to other competing uses of resources. The NETT was a milestone study because the cost-effectiveness analysis was planned and executed as a companion to the randomized controlled trial. Furthermore, the NETT trial allowed rapid diffusion of the findings. Based on the NETT, Medicare has restored coverage for LVRS in qualified patients. The trial offers an excellent example of rapid translation from research to policy.

*Acknowledgments.* Some of the work reported here was supported by the National Heart, Lung, and Blood Institute (NHLBI), the Centers for Medicare and Medicaid Services, and the Agency for Healthcare Research and Quality (AHRQ).

As a postscript to the NETT trial, it appears that many patients have lost interest in the procedure. The trial showed no improvement in life expectancy and a 10% risk of operative or peri-operative mortality. Between January of 2004 and September of 2005, only 458 Medicare patients filed claims for LVRS surgery. Although the surgery was covered by Medicare, remarkable few patients have received the procedure.

# References

Brantigan, O.C., Mueller, E. (1957). Surgical treatment of pulmonary emphysema. *American Journal of Surgery 23*, 789–804.

Brenner, M., Hanna, N.M., Mina-Araghi, R., Gelb, A.F., McKenna, R.J., Jr., Colt, H. (2004). Innovative approaches to lung volume reduction for emphysema. *Chest, 126*, 238–248.

Cooper, J.D., Trulock, E.P., Triantafillou, A.N., Patterson, G.A., Pohl, M.S., Deloney, P.A., et al. (1995). Bilateral pneumectomy (volume reduction) for chronic obstructive pulmonary disease. *Journal of Thoracic and Cardiovascular Surgery, 109*, 106–119.

Cooper, J.D., Patterson, G.A., Sundaresan, R.S., Trulock, E.P., Yusen, R.D., Pohl, M.S., et al. (1996). Results of 150 consecutive bilateral lung volume reduction procedures in patients with severe emphysema. *Journal of Thoracic and Cardiovascular Surgery,* 112, 1319–1330.

Field, M.J., Gold, M.R. (1998). *Summarizing population health.* Washington, DC: Institute of Medicine, National Academy Press.

Gold, M.R. (1996). *Cost-effectiveness in health and medicine.* New York: Oxford University Press.

Goldman, L., Caldera, D.L., Nussbaum, S.R., Southwick, F.S., Krogstad, D., Murray, B., et al. (1977). Multifactorial index of cardiac risk in noncardiac surgical procedures. *New England Journal of Medicine,* 297, 845–850.

Huizenga, H.F., Ramsey, S.D., Albert, R.K. (1998). Estimated growth of lung volume reduction surgery among Medicare enrollees: 1994 to 1996. *Chest,* 114, 1583–1587.

Kaplan, R.M., Bush, J.W., Berry, C.C. (1976). Health status: types of validity for an Index of Well-being. *Health Services Research,* 11:478–507.

Kaplan, R.M., Atkins, C.J., Timms, R. (1984). Validity of a quality of well-being scale as an outcome measure in chronic obstructive pulmonary disease. *Journal of Chronic Diseases,* 37, 85–95.

Kaplan, R.M., Anderson, J.P., Patterson, T.L., McCutchan, J.A., Weinrich, J.D., Heaton, R.K., et al. (1995). Validity of the Quality of Well-Being Scale for persons with human immunodeficiency virus infection: HNRC Group, HIV Neurobehavioral Research Center. *Psychosomatic Medicine,* 57, 138–147.

Kaplan, R.M., Alcaraz, J.E., Anderson, J.P., Weisman, M. (1996). Quality-adjusted life years lost to arthritis: effects of gender, race, and social class. *Arthritis Care and Research,* 9, 473–482.

Kaplan, R.M., Ganiats, T.G., Sieber, W.J., Anderson, J.P. (1998). The Quality of Well-Being Scale: critical similarities and differences with SF-36. *International Journal for Quality in Health Care,* 10, 509–520.

Lefrak, S.S., Yusen, R.D., Trulock, E.P., Pohl, M.S., Patterson, A., Cooper, J.D. (1997). Recent advances in surgery for emphysema. *Annual Review of Medicine,* 48, 387–398.

Lenert, L., Kaplan, R.M. (2000). Validity and interpretation of preference-based measures of health-related quality of life. *Medical Care,* 38(Suppl), II138–II150.

Maxfield, R.A. (2004). New and emerging minimally invasive techniques for lung volume reduction. *Chest,* 125, 777–783.

Meyers, B.F. (2002). Complications of lung volume reduction surgery. *Seminars in Thoracic and Cardiovascular Surgery,* 14, 399–402.

National Emphysema Treatment Trial Research Group (1999). Rationale and design of the National Emphysema Treatment Trial: a prospective randomized trial of lung volume reduction surgery. *Chest,* 116, 1750–1761.

National Emphysema Treatment Trial Research Group. (2001). Patients at high risk of death after lung-volume-reduction surgery. *New England Journal of Medicine,* 345, 1075–1083.

National Vital Statistics Report. (2004). Available at: www.cdc.gov/nchs/fastats/copd.htm (accessed October 15, 2004).

Pauwels, R.A., Rabe, K.F. (2004). Burden and clinical features of chronic obstructive pulmonary disease (COPD). *Lancet,* 364, 613–620.

*Physician's Desk Reference.* (2002). (http://www.pdr.net.) (2002). Montvale, NJ: Thompson Healthcare.

Pyne, J.M., Patterson, T.L., Kaplan, R.M., Gillin, J.C., Koch, W.L., Grant, I. (1997). Assessment of the quality of life of patients with major depression. *Psychiatric Services,* 48, 224–230.

Ramsey, S.D., Sullivan, S.D., Kaplan, R.M., Wood, D.E., Chiang, Y.P., Wagner, J.L. (2001). Economic analysis of lung volume reduction surgery as part of the National Emphysema Treatment Trial; NETT Research Group. *Annals of Thoracic Surgery,* 71, 995–1002.

Ramsey, S.D., Berry, K., Etzioni, R., Kaplan, R.M., Sullivan, S.D., Wood, D.E. (2003). Cost effectiveness of lung-volume-reduction surgery for patients with severe emphysema. *New England Journal of Medicine,* 348, 2092–2102.

Ries, A.L., Kaplan, R.M., Myers, R., Prewitt, L.M. (2003). Maintenance after pulmonary rehabilitation in chronic lung disease: a randomized trial. *American Journal of Respiratory and Critical Care Medicine,* 167, 880–888.

Rocco, M.V., Gassman, J.J., Wang, S.R., Kaplan, R.M. (1997). Cross-sectional study of quality of life and symptoms in chronic renal disease patients: the Modification of Diet in Renal Disease Study. *American Journal of Kidney Diseases,* 29, 888–896.

Russell, L.B., Gold, M.R., Siegel, J.E., Daniels, N., Weinstein, M.C. (1996). The role of cost-effectiveness analysis in health and medicine; Panel on Cost-Effectiveness in Health and Medicine. *Journal of the American Medical Association,* 276, 1172–1177.

Siegel, J.E., Weinstein, M.C., Russell, L.B., Gold, M.R. (1996). Recommendations for reporting cost-effectiveness analyses; Panel on Cost-Effectiveness in Health and Medicine. *Journal of the American Medical Association,* 276, 1339–1341.

*Statistical Analysis Software, Incorporated* (2002). Cary, NC: Statistical Analysis Software.

Sutherland, E.R., Cherniack, R.M. (2004). Management of chronic obstructive pulmonary disease. *New England Journal of Medicine,* 350, 2689–2697.

Weinstein, M.C., Siegel, J.E., Gold, M.R., Kamlet, M.S., Russell, L.B. (1996). Recommendations of the Panel on Cost-effectiveness in Health and Medicine. *Journal of the American Medical Association,* 276, 1253–1258.

# 20
# Health Economic Evaluation of Adjuvant Breast Cancer Treatment

REINHOLD KILIAN AND FRANZ PORZSOLT

Breast cancer is the most common type of cancer affecting women. Currently, the worldwide annual incidence of neoplasm of the breast is more than 1 million cases, with an increasing tendency, particularly in developing countries (Love et al., 2004). Initial local treatment of breast cancer includes breast surgery and postoperative radiotherapy. However, in about 50% of the women with a confirmed diagnosis of breast cancer the disease recurs within 5 years after initial therapy. Therefore, systemic adjuvant treatment with chemotherapy or hormonal manipulation is commonly provided to reduce the likelihood of relapse and prolong disease-free survival (Gelber et al., 1996; Emens & Davidson, 2003; Love et al., 2004).

Although the general efficacy of systemic adjuvant therapy has been proved in several randomized clinical trials, it has also been shown that the efficacy of therapeutic alternatives depends on the tumor's characteristics as well as on the patient's age in relation to menopausal status (Gelber et al., 1996; Emens & Davidson, 2003). Adjuvant chemotherapy (ACT) has been found to be effective in younger, premenopausal women but not or only marginally effective in postmenopausal women (Gelber et al., 1996; Bonadonna et al., 2005); and hormonal treatment is mainly effective in women with hormone receptor-positive tumors. The standard chemotherapy regimen is a combination of cyclophosphamide, methotrexate, and fluorouracil (CMF). For the last three decades, the standard hormonal treatment has been the antiestrogen tamoxifen (TAM) (Emens & Davidson, 2003). Recently, newer types of aromatase inhibitors (ATIs), such as letrozole or anastrozole, have proven advantageous in efficacy and tolerability in comparison to tamoxifen as first-line adjuvant therapy of estrogen receptor-positive (ER+) breast cancer (Wong & Ellis, 2004). Chemotherapy and hormonal treatment are usually accompanied by serious negative side effects, and the balance between prolonging life and maintaining the quality of the saved life-years must be carefully considered in treatment decisions (Perez et al., 2001; Ganz et al., 2002; Goodwin et al., 2003 Fallowfield et al., 2004). Therefore, the health economic evaluation of adjuvant therapy commonly takes into consideration the qualitative dimension of effectiveness as well as the costs of alternative interventions.

# Health Economic Evaluation

The task of health economics is to provide the information necessary for optimal allocation of health care resources (Russel et al., 1996). The main tools of health economic evaluation are the incremental cost-effectiveness analysis (ICEA) and the incremental cost-utility analysis (ICUA) (Garber et al., 2005). Whereas ICEA considers the additional (incremental) costs of a medical intervention in relation to its additional (incremental) effect on health, ICUA considers the incremental costs in relation to the incremental utility for the patient.

Using the concept of utility instead of the sole health effect in the economic evaluation is thought to be more appropriate assuming that the subjective utility of health varies among individuals depending on their personal preferences (Garber et al., 2005). The concept of utility is of particular importance when life-prolonging treatment may have considerable negative effects on quality of life (QOL), as is the case with breast cancer treatment (Russel et al., 1996; Muening, 2002; Goodwin et al., 2003; Garber et al., 2005). Utility indicators, such as the quality-adjusted life-year (QALY), are created by combining saved life-years with preference-based, health-related quality of life (HRQOL) instruments (Gold et al., 1996; Perez et al., 2001; Muening, 2002). In contrast to the general HRQOL, preference-based HRQOL is measured by assessing the values of several health states on a continuum between optimal health and the poorest imaginable health state or death using techniques such as the visual analogue scale (VAS), time trade-off (TTO), or standard gamble (SG) (Gold et al., 1996; Perez et al., 2001). The outcome of a cost-utility analysis is the incremental cost-utility ratio (ICUR).

$$\text{ICUR} = \frac{\text{cost intervention A} - \text{cost intervention B}}{\text{utility intervention A} - \text{utility intervention B}} = \frac{\Delta \text{ Cost}}{\Delta \text{ Utility}}$$

The ICUR is defined as the ratio between the cost differences and the utility differences of two alternative treatments or of a treatment in comparison to no treatment. The interpretation of the ICUR depends on its position on the cost-effectiveness plane (CEP) (Sendi & Briggs, 2001).

On its vertical axis of Figure 20.1 the CEP shows the cost differences, and on its horizontal axis the effectiveness or utility differences between the interventions are compared. If the ICUR is located in the upper left quadrant of the CEP, the ICUR has a negative value, indicating that the alternative intervention is more expensive and less effective than the conventional treatment or nonintervention. If the ICUR is located in the upper right quadrant of the CEP, the positive value indicates that the alternative intervention is more effective but also more expensive than the conventional treatment or nonintervention. If the ICUR is located in the lower left quadrant of the CEP, the positive value indicates that the alternative intervention is less expensive but also less effective than the conventional treatment or nonintervention. If the ICUR is located in the lower right quadrant of the

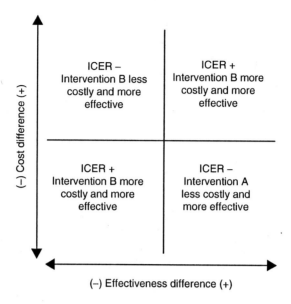

FIGURE 20.1. Cost-effectiveness plane (CEP). ICER = incremental cost-utility ratio.

CEP, the negative value indicates that the alternative intervention is less expensive and more effective than the conventional treatment or nonintervention.

Obviously, a negative ICUR provides a much more clear decision basis than a positive one. If the ICUR is located at the upper left quadrant, the conventional treatment or nonintervention is more efficient than the alternative intervention, and if the ICUR is located at the lower right, the alternative intervention is more efficient. Unfortunately, the ICUR generally appears in the upper right quadrant. In this case, an additional criterion is needed to decide whether an alternative treatment is efficient. This additional criterion is the maximum amount of money one is willing to pay for an increase of the effect—the utility by one unit—and is usually called maximum willingness to pay (MWTP).

The MWTP can be projected as a growth curve onto the CEP (Figure 20.2), and an alternative intervention is assessed as efficient if the ICUR is located below this curve (Briggs & O'Brien, 2001; Sendi & Briggs, 2001).

A methodological complication results from the fact that confidence intervals for the ICUR are difficult to estimate because its theoretical distribution is not defined (Briggs & Fenn, 1998). Because parametric statistical estimation of the standard error and the confidence interval is not possible in this case, it has become common practice to estimate the distribution of the ICUR as a confidence ellipse by simulation techniques, such as bootstrapping, and to compute the MWTP at which 95% of the estimated ICUR values are located below the MWTP curve (Figure 20.3).

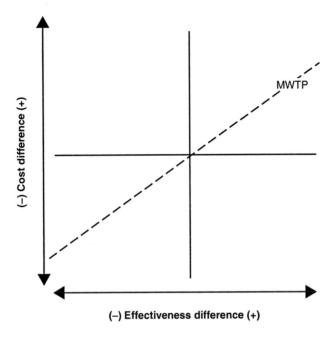

FIGURE 20.2. Maximum willingness to pay (MWTP) curve in the cost-effectiveness plane (CEP).

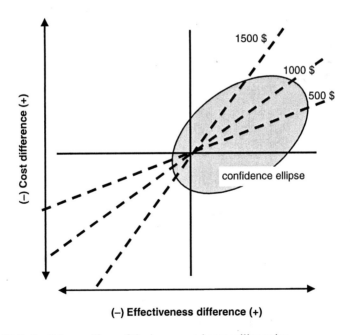

FIGURE 20.3. Confidence ellipse of the incremental cost-utility ratios.

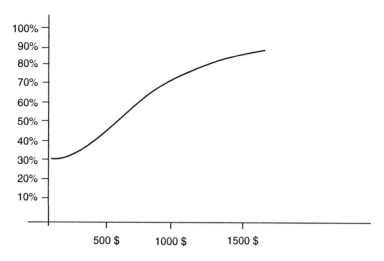

FIGURE 20.4. Cost-effectiveness acceptability curve.

The cost-effectiveness acceptability curve (CEAC) is the common technique to visualize this criterion (Briggs & Fenn, 1998). On the horizontal axis, the CEAC shows potential values for MWTP in increasing order (Figure 20.4). The vertical axis shows the percentages of the estimated ICUR values that are located below the MWTP curve. Similar to the statistical confidence interval, the CEAC indicates at which MWTP a particular percentage (90%, for instance) of the estimated ICUR falls below the MWTP curve.

Data for health economic evaluations mostly come from randomized clinical trials (RCTs). However, in most cases the time horizon of the RCT is too short for a meaningful estimation of economic effects. Therefore, most health economic analyses apply simulation modeling, such as decision tree, state transition, or Markov chain models (Muening, 2002). The advantage of these techniques is the possibility of using any meaningful time horizon. The disadvantage is that the outcomes of the analysis depend strongly on the data used and on the assumptions made if sufficient data are lacking.

Although there have been several recommendations for the publication of health economic evaluation studies (Drummond & Jefferson, 1996; Drummond et al., 1997), current publication practices show a great variety of methods. Therefore, when assessing the evidence provided by existing studies one should carefully consider to what extent the authors followed these recommendations (Drummond et al., 1997).

# Health Economic Evaluation of Adjuvant Breast Cancer Treatment

A systematic MEDLINE search without time limitations was conducted with the following search terms: breast cancer + adjuvant therapy + cost effectiveness;

breast cancer + chemotherapy + cost effectiveness; breast cancer + hormone therapy + cost effectiveness; breast cancer + adjuvant therapy + cost utility; breast cancer + chemotherapy + cost utility; breast cancer + hormone therapy + cost utility. An additional hand search based on the reference lists of articles was carried out. Only articles concerning first-line systemic adjuvant chemotherapy or hormone therapy were included in the review. If necessary, currencies have been converted to U.S. dollars and are provided in parentheses.

A total of eight articles were identified that met the criteria of the review. In four studies, the incremental cost effectiveness or cost utility of adjuvant chemotherapy compared to no adjuvant treatment was tested (Hillner & Smith, 1991; Desch et al., 1993; Messori et al., 1996; Norum, 2000); three articles compared chemotherapy with hormonal intervention (Smith & Hillner, 1993; Karnon & Brown, 2002; Naeim & Keeler, 2005); and one article compared tamoxifen with third-generation aromatase inhibitors (Hillner, 2004).

## Cost Utility of Adjuvant Chemotherapy Compared to no Adjuvant Therapy

Hillner and Smith (1991) used a Markov model to assess the cost utility of treating 45- and 60-year-old women with stage I, lymph-node negative (N–),ER– breast cancer with adjuvant CMF chemotherapy. The authors evaluated various scenarios of the benefit of therapy. For the 45-year-old women, the average lifetime benefit from chemotherapy was 5.1 quality-adjusted months at a cost of $15,400 per QALY (Table 20.1). For the 60-year-old women, the analysis revealed a survival gain of 4.0 quality-adjusted months at a cost of $18,800 per QALY. On the basis of their results, the authors concluded that adjuvant CMF chemotherapy substantially increases the quality-adjusted life expectancy of a 45-year-old woman and that of a 60-year-old woman with stage I breast cancer at a acceptable cost.

Desch et al. (1993) expanded Hillner and Smith's model by including women with N– and ER– breast cancer from the age of 60 to the age of 80 years. Results of the analysis indicated that the benefit of adjuvant CMF chemotherapy declines with increasing age from 2.8 quality-adjusted months for a 60-year-old woman to 1.4 quality-adjusted months for women at age 80. Consequently, the costs per QALY increase from $28,800 at age 60 to $57,100 at age 80 (Table 20.1). The authors concluded that adjuvant chemotherapy has an acceptable relation of costs per QALY up to the age of 70.

Messori et al. (1996) used a survival curve fitting method based on clinical trial data to estimate the lifelong cost effectiveness of adjuvant CMF chemotherapy for women with lymph node-positive (N+) breast cancer. No adjustment was made for age. Results of the analysis revealed a cost-effectiveness ratio of $447 per lifeyear gained (Table 20.1). The cost per QALY was not provided by the authors. Using the recommended range of preference weights between 0.7 and 0.9 results in an estimated cost per QALY of $496 to $638 (Table 20.1). The authors

TABLE 20.1. Cost utility of adjuvant chemotherapy versus no adjuvant therapy

| Study | Treatment | Target groups | Time horizon | Incremental cost-utility ratio | Conclusion |
|-------|-----------|---------------|--------------|-------------------------------|------------|
| Hillner & Smith (1991, USA) | Adjuvant chemotherapy vs. none | Age 45 years, 60 years; node-negative | Lifetime | 45 Years, $15,400 60 Years, $18,800 | Chemotherapy substantially increases the quality-adjusted life expectancy of an average woman at a cost comparable to that of other widely accepted therapies. |
| Desch et al. (1993, USA) | Adjuvant chemotherapy vs. none | Age 60–80 years; node-negative; estrogen receptor-negative | Lifetime | 60 Years, $28,200 65 Years, $31,300 70 Years, $36,300 75 Years, $44,400 80 Years, $57,100 | There is a small survival benefit for adjuvant chemotherapy in elderly patients. The cost of this benefit is high but within the range of commonly reimbursed procedures up to a point between ages 75 and 80 years. |
| Messori et al. (1996, Italy) | Adjuvant chemotherapy vs. none | No age range reported; node-positive | Lifetime | Cost/life-gained, $447 Cost/QALY, $496–$638 | The cost-effectiveness ratio of adjuvant chemotherapy in patients with node-positive breast cancer seems to be particularly favorable compared to estimates of cost per life-year saved previously calculated for other types of pharmacological intervention. |
| Norum (2000, Norway) | Adjuvant chemotherapy vs. none | | Lifetime | £2973–£7860 ($4,781.65–$12,641.70) | Adjuvant chemotherapy in breast cancer is cost-effective in Norway. |

QALY = quality-adjusted life-years.

concluded that CMF adjuvant chemotherapy is cost effective for the average breast cancer patient in Italy.

Norum (2000) estimated the cost utility of adjuvant CMF chemotherapy for Norwegian women on the basis of international clinical trials. No adjustments were made for age, lymph node status, or ER status. Results of the analysis indicated that adjuvant CMF chemotherapy in Norway costs between £2973 ($4781.65) and £7860 ($12,641.70) per QALY saved (Table 20.1). Based on these results the author concluded that adjuvant CMF chemotherapy is cost effective in Norway.

## Cost Utility of Adding Antiestrogen Therapy to Chemotherapy

In 1992 results of the Early Breast Cancer Trialists' Collaborating Group (EBCTCG) study suggested that endocrine therapy with tamoxifen should have an additive benefit to adjuvant chemotherapy not only for ER+ breast cancer but also for ER− breast cancer (Early Breast Cancer Trialists' Collaborative Group, 1992).

Smith and Hillner (1993) used the EBCTCG data to assess the cost utility of endocrine therapy with TAM in addition to chemotherapy for premenopausal 45-year-old women with various lymph node and ER status combinations. Chemotherapy alone versus no adjuvant therapy was found to be most cost effective for women with N+/ER− status (cost per QALY $4890) or N−/ER− status (cost per QALY $4970).

Adjuvant hormonal therapy with TAM alone versus no adjuvant therapy was most cost effective in women with N+/ER+ status (cost per QALY $4330) and in women with N−/ER+ status (cost per QALY $11,440) (Table 20.2). Combined TAM and CMF versus no adjuvant therapy was most cost effective for women with N+/ER+ status (cost per QALY $14,750) and for women with N−/ER+ status (cost per QALY $33,100) (Table 20.2). The least cost utility was found for TAM versus no adjuvant treatment in women with N−/ER− (cost per QALY $214,000) and for combined TAM and CMF versus no adjuvant therapy in women with N−/ER− status (cost per QALY $186,200) (Table 20.2). In women with ER− status, TAM was found to be slightly more cost effective than no adjuvant therapy (cost per QALY $57,800) if the patient has N+ status (Table 20.2). Based on these results the authors concluded that adjuvant hormonal therapy alone or combined therapy with TAM and CMF is cost effective only for premenopausal women with ER+ breast cancer.

Karnon and Brown (2002) used a discrete event simulation model to analyze the cost utility of adding CMF to TAM in N+ patients (ER status not provided). Results of their study revealed that, compared to patients who received only TAM, patients given additional chemotherapy gained an average of 0.56 QALY. Whereas adjuvant hormonal therapy with TAM was found to cost £615.48 ($871.51) per QALY on average, adding CMF chemotherapy to TAM resulted in additional average costs of £3483 ($4932.28) per QALY gained (Table 20.2).

The uncertainty of the average cost-utility ratio has been calculated using a Monte-Carlo simulation with 2500 runs of randomly sampled sets of input parameter values. Based on the stochastic simulation, the authors found that at an MWTP value of £4000, combined TAM + CMF was cost effective in comparison to TAM

TABLE 20.2. Cost utility of combined chemotherapy and hormonal therapy (tamoxifen) versus adjuvant chemotherapy alone

| Study | Treatment | Target group | Time horizon | Incremental cost-utility ratio | Conclusion |
|---|---|---|---|---|---|
| Smith & Hillner (1993, USA) | None vs. chemotherapy None vs. tamoxifen None vs. chemotherapy + tamoxifen None vs. tamoxifen None vs. chemotherapy + tamoxifen | 45-year-old women with premenopausal early-stage breast cancer; estrogen receptor status positive or negative; lymph node status positive or negative | Lifetime | Tamoxifen vs. none N− ER+, $11,440 N− ER−, $214,000 N+ ER+, $4,330 N+ ER−, $57,800 Chemotherapy vs. none N− ER+, $11,370 N− ER−, $ 4,970 N+ ER+, $9,230 N+ ER−, $4,890 Combined vs. none N− ER+, $33,100 N− ER−, $186,200 N+ ER+, $14,750 N+ ER−, $80,700 | In pre-menopausal women with early-stage breast cancer, chemotherapy adds substan-tial clinical benefit at a modest cost. Tamoxifen alone adds meaningful benefit only in ER-positive cancer. Combined therapy is most efficient in ER-positive cancer. |
| Karnon & Brown (2002, UK) | Tamoxifen vs. tamoxifen + chemotherapy | 65 years and older; post-menopausal; node-positive | Lifetime | TAM vs. none, £615.48 ($871.51) Combined vs. TAM, £3483 ($4932.28). | The addition of chemotherapy to tamoxifen in patients with node-positive early breast cancer is cost-effective at an MWTP of £5000 with a probability of 64% and an MWTP of £20,000 with a probability of 85%. |

TABLE 20.2. (*Continued*)

| Study | Treatment | Target group | Time horizon | Incremental cost-utility ratio | Conclusion |
|---|---|---|---|---|---|
| Naeim & Keeler (2005, USA) | None vs. chemotherapy (CHT) None vs. CHT and tamoxifen (TAM) | 5 years and older; 6 node-positive; ER-negative or ER-positive | Lifetime | ER-negative; CHT vs. none 65 years, $30,451 75 years, $75,559 85 years, $298,000 ER-positive; TAM vs. none 65 years, $ 10,194 75 years, $19,530 85 years, $58,085 ER-positive; combined vs. TAM 65 years, $22,220 75 years, $54,430 85 years, $299,517 | Adjuvant therapy is cost-effective in 65-year-old women with early breast cancer. In a 75-year-old ER-positive patient, hormone therapy, specifically tamoxifen, is cost-effective. In 75-year-old ER-negative women the use of chemotherapy (AC or CMF) or in 85-year-old ER-positive women the use of hormone therapy was only marginally cost-effective and only if efficacy was assumed to be age-insensitive (similar to 65-year-old women). |

ER+ = estrogen receptor-positive; ER− = estrogen receptor-negative; N+ = lymph-node status positive; N− = lymph-node status negative; TAM = tamoxifen; MWTP = maximum willingness to pay; AC = adriamycin/cyclophosphamide; CMF = cyclophosphamide/methotrexate/ fluorouracil.

alone with a probability of 50%. Nevertheless, results indicated a probability of 10% that TAM alone is more effective and cheaper than combined TAM + CMF.

Naeim and Keeler (2005) assessed the cost utility of CHT or TAM versus no adjuvant treatment and of CMF + TAM versus no adjuvant therapy for women 65 years or older with N−, ER−, or ER+ breast cancer. Results of the analysis revealed the best cost effectiveness for TAM in women age 65 ($10,194 per QALY) or age 75 ($19,530 per QALY) with ER+ status, followed by CMF + TAM in women age 65 with ER+ status ($22,220 per QALY) and CMF chemotherapy alone in women age 65 with ER− status ($30,451 per QALY)

(Table 20.2). Cost effectiveness of all types of adjuvant therapy, but particularly of CMF chemotherapy, decreased considerably with increasing age. The cost per QALY of CMF alone in women with ER− breast cancer increased to $75,559 at age 75 and to $298,000 at age 85 (Table 20.2). In women aged 85 with ER+ breast cancer, the cost per QALY of TAM alone increased to $58,085, and the cost per QALY of CMF + TAM increased to $299,517 (Table 20.2). The authors did not interpret the meaning of their results for resource allocation but extensively discussed the methodological limitations of their study.

## Cost Utility of Aromatase Inhibitors Compared to Tamoxifen

Hillner (2004) analyzed the incremental cost utility of anastrozole in comparison to TAM as initial adjuvant therapy in postmenopausal women at age 64 with early-stage ER+ breast cancer. The results of the analysis show that the efficiency of the aromatase inhibitor depends strongly on the time horizon of the analysis model. Although the incremental cost-utility ratio (ICUR) of anastrozole versus TAM was found to be $75,500 at a time horizon of 20 years, the additional cost per additional QALY increased to $533,000 if a shorter time horizon of only 4 years was used (Table 20.3). Given an MWTP of $100,000 per QALY gained, the author concluded that the use of anastrozole in comparison to TAM is cost effective only for patients who live longer than 12 years.

## Discussion

Results from health economic evaluation studies have become increasingly important as criteria for the allocation of health care resources. However, a great variety of methods and a lack of standardization make it difficult for the clini-

TABLE 20.3. Cost utility of first-line hormonal therapy with aromatase inhibitors versus tamoxifen

| Study | Treatment | Target group | Time horizon | Incremental cost-utility ratio | Conclusion |
|---|---|---|---|---|---|
| Hillner (2004, USA) | Anastrozole vs. tamoxifen | 64 years; postmeno-pausal; ER-positive | 4–20 years | 4-year horizon, $533,000<br>8-year horizon, $201,800<br>12-year horizon, $111,300<br>20-year horizon, $75,500 | Anastrozole would be acceptable for patients expected to live longer than 12 years. |

cian or the health policy expert to assess the validity and the substance of health economic studies. During the last decade, the incremental cost-utility analysis has been established as the gold standard of the health economic evaluation of alternative medical interventions. Nevertheless, there are several limitations that make it difficult to interpret the results of cost-utility analyses and to transform them into recommendations for medical decision making.

Drummond et al. (1997) developed 10 criteria for the quality of a health economic evaluation. These criteria include the quality of the underlying clinical data regarding the treatment effects and the utility of these effects, as well as the accurate measurement of intervention costs, the treatment of uncertainty, and an adequate discussion of results. Moreover, interpretation of health economic evaluations needs a consensus about the maximum amount of money that should be paid for a QALY gain. Since the 1970s, the cost-utility ratio of hemodialysis for a patient with end-stage renal disease, $50,000 per QALY, had been used as a threshold for the MWTP. This threshold, however, is regarded as arbitrary by health economists (Earle et al., 2000). Currently, it is common practice to compare the cost-utility ratios of several health care interventions to obtain information about the possible range of costs per QALY. In a recent review of the cost-utility ratios of 89 oncology interventions, Earle et al. (2000) identified a range between less than zero and $7,900,000 per QALY in U.S. prices in 2000. The detailed comparisons revealed that 64% of the 89 interventions had cost-utility ratios below $50,000, and 75% had cost-utility ratios below $100,000. The median cost per QALY was found to be $20,000.

According to these figures, the economic efficiency of adjuvant therapy for early-stage breast cancer is considered to be in an acceptable range. Most cost-utility ratios were found to be less than $100,000 or even less that $50,000. Nonetheless, the cost effectiveness of several therapy alternatives was found to depend on the patient's age, as well as the node and estrogen receptor status of the tumor. Chemotherapy with a combination of cyclophosphamide, methotrexate, and fluorouracil was found to be the most cost-effective treatment in premenopausal women with positive lymph node status, whereas the cost effectiveness decreased sharply after age 75. In contrast, endocrine therapy with tamoxifen or aromatase inhibitors was found to be cost effective primarily in women with ER+ breast cancer, with no strong age effects. However, analyses of these treatment alternatives are based on a single RCT that was still ongoing at the time of the health economic evaluation (Hillner, 2004). The few studies from European countries reveal better cost-utility relations than the studies from the United States. The main reason for this difference is the different drug costs among countries.

According to the criteria discussed above, the results of existing studies suggest that adjuvant therapy should generally be recommended for early breast cancer treatment from the perspective of health economy. Cost-utility ratios above $100,000 were found for endocrine therapy with TAM, combined endocrine and chemotherapy in women with ER− tumor status, and adding CMF chemotherapy to TAM in women with ER+ tumor status at age 85. With regard to the available therapy alternatives, CMF chemotherapy should be recommended particularly for premenopausal women with ER− breast cancer and for post-menopausal women less than 80 years of age. For women with ER+ breast cancer, adjuvant hormonal therapy with tamoxifen or aromatase inhibitors should be recommended without age limits. Combining TAM and chemotherapy should be recommended up to age 80 years. With regard to the ongoing status of the ATAC trial (ATAC Trialists' Group, 2005), it is too early to recommend anastrozole instead of TAM for adjuvant therapy of breast cancer in women with ER+ tumor status. Decisions about the payment for medical interventions require a broad consensus about how available health care resources should be allocated.

This consensus must be based not only on economic but also on ethical considerations, such as equity of health care access. Strictly limiting the payment for medical interventions to a particular cost-utility ratio would possibly exclude people with poor health from access to care. For example, a strict limit of $50,000 per QALY would exclude women above age 80 with ER− tumors from any adjuvant therapy. Many of these patients have additional health care problems that are more serious than the risk of recurring breast cancer. Paying for each treatment that provides a QALY gain without considering costs and gained values would quickly result in exceeding the available health care budget. Therefore, it is necessary to enable the clinician to consider the situation of the individual patient without disregarding the responsibility for economic consequences.

## References

ATAC Trialists' Group (2005). Results of the ATAC (arimidex, tamoxifen, alone or in combination) trial after completion of 5 years' adjuvant treatment for breast cancer. *Lancet*, 365, 60–62.

Bonadonna, G., Moliterni, A., Zambetti, M., Daidone, M.G., Pilotti, S., Gianni, L., et al. (2005). 30 Years' follow up of randomised studies of adjuvant CMF in operable breast cancer: cohort study. *British Medical Journal*, 330, 217.

Briggs, A., Fenn P. (1998). Confidence intervals or surfaces? Uncertainty on the cost-effectiveness plane. *Health Economics*, 7, 723–740.

Briggs, A.H., O'Brien, B. (2001). The death of cost-minimization analysis? *Health Economics*, 10, 179–184.

Desch, C.E., Hillner, B.E., Smith, T.E., Retchin, S.M. (1993). Should the elderly receive chemotherapy for node-negative breast cancer? Cost-effectiveness analysis examining total and active life-expectancy outcomes. *Journal of Clinical Oncology*, 11, 777–782.

Drummond, M.F., Jefferson, T.O. (1996). Guidelines for authors and peer reviewers of economic submissions to the BMJ. *British Medical Journal*, 313, 275–283.

Drummond, M.F., O'Brien, B., Stoddart, G.L., Torrance, G.W. (1997). *Methods for the economic evaluation of health care programmes*. Oxford: Oxford University Press.

Earle, C.C., Chapman, R.H., Baker, C.S., Bell, P.W., Stone, P.W., Sandberg, E.A., et al. (2000). Systematic overview of cost-utility assessments in oncology. *Journal of Clinical Oncology*, 18, 3302–3317.

Early Breast Cancer Trialists' Collaborative Group (EBCTCG) (1992). Systemic therapy of early breast cancer by hormonal, cytotoxic or immune therapy. *Lancet*, 339, 1–15.

Emens, L.A., Davidson, N.E. (2003). Adjuvant hormonal therapy for premenopausal women with breast cancer. *Clinical Cancer Research*, 9(Suppl), 468s–494s.

Fallowfield, L., McGurk, R., Dixon, M. (2004). Same gain, less pain: potential patient preferences for adjuvant treatment in premenopausal women with early breast cancer. *European Journal of Cancer*, 40, 2403–2410.

Ganz, P.A., Desmond, K.A., Leedham, B., Rowland, J.H., Meyerowitz, B.E., Belin, T.R. (2002). Quality of life in long-term, disease-free survivors of breast cancer: a follow-up study. *Journal of the National Cancer Institute*, 94, 39–49.

Garber, A.M., Weinstein, M.C., Torrance, G.W., Kamlet, M.S. (2005). Theoretical foundations of cost-effectiveness analysis. In: M.R. Gold, J.E. Siegel, L.B. Russel, M.C. Weinstein (Eds.), *Cost-effectiveness in health and medicine*. New York: Oxford University Press. pp. 25–53.

Gelber, R.D., Cole, B.F., Goldhirsch, A., Rose, C., Fisher, B., Osborne, C.K., et al. (1996). Adjuvant chemotherapy plus tamoxifen compared with tamoxifen alone for post-menopausal breast cancer: meta analysis of quality-adjusted survival. *Lancet*, 347, 1057–1058.

Gold, M.R., Patrick, D.L., Torrance, G.W., Fryback, D.G., Haydorn, D.C., Kamlet, M.S., et al. (1996). Identifying and valuing outcomes. In: M.R. Gold, J.E. Siegel, L.B. Russel, M.C. Weinstein (Eds.), *Cost-effectiveness in health and medicine*. New York: Oxford University Press.

Goodwin, P.J., Black, J.T., Bordeleau, L.J., Ganz, P.A. (2003). Health-related quality of life measurement in randomized clinical trials in breast cancer: taking stock. *Journal of the National Cancer Institute*, 95, 263–281.

Hillner, B.E. (2004). Benefit and projected cost-effectivness of anastrozole versus tamoxifen as inital adjuvant therapy for patients with early-stage estrogen receptor-positive breast cancer. *Cancer*, 101, 1311–1322.

Hillner, B.E., Smith, T.E. (1991). Efficacy and cost effectiveness of adjuvant chemotherapy in women with node-negative breast cancer: a decision-analysis model. *New England Journal of Medicine*, 17, 160–168.

Karnon, J., Brown, J. (2002). Adjuvant Breast Cancer (ABC) Steering Committee. tamoxifen plus chemotherapy versus tamoxifen alone as adjuvant therapies for node-positive postmenopausal women with early breast cancer: a stochastic economic evaluation. *Pharmacoecon*, 20, 119–137.

Love, R.R., Love, S.M., Laudico, A.V. (2004). Breast cancer from a public health perspective. *The Breast Journal*, 10, 136–140.

Messori, A., Becagli, P., Trippoli, S., Tendi, E. (1996). Cost-effectiveness of adjuvant chemotherapy with cyclophosphamide + methotrexate + fluorouracil in patients with node-positive breast cancer. *European Journal of Clinical Pharmacology*, 51, 111–116.

Muening, P. (2002). *Designing and conducting cost-effectiveness analyses in medicine and health care*. San Francisco: Jossey-Bass.

Naeim, A., Keeler, E.B. (2005) Is adjuvant therapy for older patients with node(−) early breast cancer cost-effective. *Critical Reviews in Oncology/Hematology*, 53, 81–89.

Norum, J. (2000). Adjuvant cyclophosphamide, methotrexate, flurouracil (CMF) in breast cancer: is it cost effective? *Acta Oncologica*; 39, 33–39.

Perez, D.J., Williams, S.M., Christensen, E.A., McGee, R.O., Campbell, A.V. (2001). A longitudinal study of health related quality of life and utility measures in patients with advanced breast cancer. *Quality of Life Research*, 10, 587–593.

Russel, L.B., Siegel, J.E., Daniels, N., Gold, M.R., Luce, B.R., Mandelblatt, J.S. (1996). Cost-effectiveness analysis as a guide to resource allocation in health: roles and limitations. In: M.R. Gold, J.E. Siegel, L.B. Russel, M.C. Weinstein (Eds.). *Cost-effectiveness in health and medicine*. New York: Oxford University Press. pp. 3–24.

Sendi, P.P., Briggs, A.H. (2001). Affordability and cost-effectiveness: decision making on the cost-effectiveness plane. *Health Economics*, 10, 675–680.

Smith, T.J., Hillner, B.E. (1993). The efficacy and cost-effectiveness of adjuvant therapy of early breast cancer in premenopausal women. *Journal of Clinical Oncology*, 11, 771–776.

Wong, Z.W., Ellis, M.J. (2004). First-line endocrine treatment of breast cancer: aromatase inhibitor or antiestrogen. *British Journal of Cancer*, 90, 20–25.

# 21
# Aims and Value of Screening: Is Perceived Safety a Value for Which to Pay?

Franz Porzsolt, Heike Leonhardt-Huober, and Robert Kaplan

In Chapter 4 on evidence-based medicine and ethics, we presented the example of breast cancer screening and reported that more than 1000 women must be screened with mammography to prevent only one death from breast cancer. In addition, screening generates several false-positive and some false-negative results. Furthermore, 13 women would be diagnosed with breast cancer and would probably be treated. However, these 13 women would not benefit from the treatment because they have a "pseudodisease" (see Chapter 11). Pseudodisease is a result of breast screening in that it cannot be diagnosed in individual patients but only concluded statistically by comparing populations of women who have or have not been screened.

These 13 women with pseudodisease would undergo surgical treatment and eventually radiotherapy as well as hormonal and/or chemotherapy because histologically confirmed breast cancer has been identified. In these 13 women, their disease would have affected neither the quality nor quantity of the patient's life. The treatment does not offer benefit and might even cause harm. The dilemma arises because at the time of diagnosis we cannot differentiate forms of breast cancer that will later behave like a benign or a malignant disease.

## Traditional View of Health Economics

Economic analysis suggests that the benefits may not justify the monetary costs of screening. The lively and emotional discussion on the mammography controversy in 1997 (see Chapter 11) reflected concerns about the appropriate use of resources for a program that benefits only 1 of 1000 patients but produces harm in a considerable proportion of screened women.

## Standpoint of Clinical Economics

From a clinician's point of view, other variables may need to be considered in the economic analysis. Clinicians would first ask about the goals of breast cancer screening. Most patients and doctors identify two goals: (1) to identify cases of breast cancer early enough to increase the chance of cure and (2) to induce "perceived safety" in most of the screened women by confirming the absence of suspicious findings.

From a scientist's point of view, the absence of evidence never constitutes evidence of absence. Nonscientists, like patients, have a different perception and rate these negative findings as absolutely valuable. This difference in the perception between scientists and the public raises the question of who is right. Should we disregard the perception of the majority, or is our scientific concept flawed?

Our answer to this question was derived from a discussion with the head of Flight Safety of Lufthansa, the German airlines. We discussed what aviation can learn from medicine and vice versa (see Chapter 16). Proud of our new strategy of evidence-based decisions in medicine, we asked for the scientific evidence that justifies expenditures for life vests in airplanes and were surprised to learn that no life has ever been saved by such life vests. As an "evidence-based" consequence, we suggested that life vests in airplanes be replaced by measures that are more efficient in saving the passengers' lives. Unfortunately, our suggestion was considered absolutely unacceptable, as about eight organizations definitely would refuse this proposal as a "nonrealistic idea." This disappointing experience led to the consideration that the utility of life vests is perceived safety rather than actual safety.

We spend billions of dollars or euros in medicine to induce perceived safety. Banking, buying and using a car, and almost every facet of our lives is governed by perceived rather than actual safety.

## Concept of Perceived Safety

Perceived safety may be a value in health care that consumers are willing to pay for. Unfortunately, the demand, as well as the offers, for perceived safety will soon become unlimited unless criteria are defined to differentiate acceptable from unacceptable forms of perceived safety. Two criteria may help to solve this problem: First, perceived safety must be quantified, as shown in Table 21.1. Second, quantified perceived safety must be compared with quantified actual safety. The smaller the difference between perceived and actual safety, the more legitimate it is to offer and to pay for services that induce perceived safety.

## Economics of Perceived Safety

Comparing the benefits and the harm associated with breast cancer screening (Table 21.1), we consider harmed the proportion of women with false-positive results ($n = 219$) because they would be extremely worried until the suspect findings have been clarified. Patients with false-negative results ($n = 10$), in whom the diagnosis of breast cancer was overseen by mammography, are also added to the harmed group. The third subgroup that must be included in this group are patients with pseudodisease ($n = 13$), as they would not benefit from the given treatment.

TABLE 21.1. Clinical economics of screening

| Parameter | Breast cancer confirmed | Breast cancer not confirmed | Patients examined | Deaths due to breast cancer |
|---|---|---|---|---|
| Breast cancer detected by mammography | 23 | 219** | 242 | |
| Breast cancer **not** detected by mammography | 10** | 748 | 758* | |
| Examination including mammography | 33 | 967 | 1000 | 5/1000 |
| Examination **without** mammography | 20Δ = 13** | 980 | 1000 | 6/1000 Δ = 1* |

Δ = difference.
The benefit of screening is described quantitatively by (*); that is, one death from breast cancer can be prevented, and perceived safety is mediated to 758 women (plus some in whom a false-positive result could be clarified). The harm of screening is described quantitatively by (**); that is, 219 (at least transiently false-positive results), 10 false-negative results, and 13 cases of pseudodisease. Data are from Zahl et al. (2004) and Barratt et al. (2005).

One of the advantages or good points of mammography is that one death from breast cancer can be avoided for each 1000 women screened. Mammography can offer other benefits to our patients. There would be 758 women who experience perceived safety and reassurance when the message of the negative result of breast cancer screening is received. This number increases when some of the false-positive cases are clarified.

To avoid abuse of the tool of perceived safety, we requested, in addition to quantification, a comparison of perceived safety with actual safety. In the case of breast cancer screening, the quantities of perceived and of actual safety are similar, as 748 women (plus some in whom false-positive results will be revised) can be assured that there is no evidence of breast cancer.

## Public Enthusiasm for Screening

Americans are enthusiastic about cancer screening. In one recent public opinion poll, Schwartz and colleagues (2004) interviewed a random sample of 500 adults selected from throughout the United States. Eighty-seven percent of the respondents reported that cancer screening is almost always a good idea, and most (74%) endorsed the belief that cancer screening saves lives. Aronowitz (2001) documented the relentless campaign by the American Cancer Society to persuade the public not to delay obtaining cancer tests. In fact, the campaign was prominent throughout the entire 20th century despite continuing questions about the efficacy of early detection. Apparently these messages have been effective. Schwartz and colleagues (2004) noted that only 2% of the population believes that there are too many cancer screening tests. Altogether, 77% of the male respondents said they would continue trying to have the prostate-specific antigen (PSA) test even if their doctor did not recommend it, and 74% said that they would continue to have colonoscopy or sigmoidoscopy although it was not recommended.

Persuasive evidence suggests that Papanicolaou (Pap) smears done every year provide almost no more new information than Pap smears done at 3-year intervals (Eddy, 1987). However, the survey results suggest that 58% of women would try to have Pap smears on their current schedule even if their doctor recommended that there should be more time between tests. Several evidence-based reviews suggest that mammography might provide little or no value for women older than 75 years (Parnes et al., 2001; Harris & Carnes, 2002). The United States is among a small number of countries that have no upper limit on recommended age to stop screening. In Finland screening ends at age 59; and in Australia, Canada, and Iceland it stops at age 69. The United Kingdom stops at age 64, and Sweden screens only until age 69 (Shapiro et al., 1998). Even in the United States, the rate of screening for older women falls off after the age of about 75, suggesting that physicians intuitively know the diminished value of the test and stop ordering it (Kaplan, 2004). Nevertheless, the Schwartz study found that 41% of the population would label an 80-year-old woman who declined a mammogram as "irresponsible."

The public is not deterred by bad experiences with tests. More than one-third of the survey participants had experienced at least one false-positive test. Yet in retrospect, 98% of these individuals were glad they had taken the screening test, and most would do it again. In fact, 100% of those who had experienced a false-positive PSA test were still glad that the tests had been administered (Schwartz et al., 2004).

The public is clearly persuaded that cancer screening is a good idea. At the same time, professional organizations that have systematically reviewed the evidence have raised serious questions about the benefits of common tests, such as mammography (particularly for premenopausal woman) (Arnold, 2002) and the PSA test (U.S. Preventive Services Task Force, 1994; New PSA guidelines for older men, 1998; Farhat et al., 2000; Levenson, 2003; Weston & Parr, 2003).

Over the last decade, the public has become increasingly skeptical about medicine. Why does the public remain enthusiastic about screening while they are becoming critical of other medical services? The Schwartz study offers several hints. Most importantly, screening typically offers a good experience. Most people feel safe and reassured by negative screening results. Those with positive test results perceive benefit because they are guided toward the medical services they need. They are thankful that their disease was discovered. Patients with false-positive results might be frightened, but they gain a great sense of safety once cancer is ruled out.

The perceived benefits of screening often lead to more screening. This is summarized in Figure 21.1, which is based on the work of Welch (2004). The scheme begins with more cancer testing. As a result of increased testing, we might find more cancer (left side of the figure). More cancer detection suggests the development of an "epidemic" of cancer and the need for more aggressive screening. The right side of the figure shows that some early cancer detection is actually

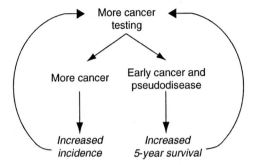

FIGURE 21.1. Screening leads to more screening. (From Welch, 2004.)

pseudodisease, which will never result in early death or reduced quality of life. Although the disease might never have affected a person in his or her lifetime, these persons now become cancer survivors. Because the disease is detected early, the 5-year survival rate increases, which feeds the perception that we are winning the war on cancer. The result is even more aggressive screening for cancer.

## Conclusions

The contribution of clinical economics (CLINECS) can be demonstrated using the example of breast cancer screening. CLINECS provides data to describe the value, not the costs, of health care. It is shown that both benefit and harm—or input/output or profit/effort—are quantified. Benefit includes the proportion of deaths from breast cancer prevented and the proportion of women who experience perceived safety. Harm includes the proportion of false-positive and false-negative results as well as the proportion of pseudodisease.

We do not claim that the lists of benefit and harm are complete. Several additional aspects of breast cancer screening, such as fear of clinical investigation and expected pain induced by mammography, were not discussed. The aim of this chapter was to underline the contribution of the patients' and clinicians' views to an economic evaluation of health care services.

Two other aspects may be discussed as potential benefit from the patient's point of view. Pseudodisease can be seen not only as harm because of unnecessary treatment; the knowledge of pseudodisease may in fact induce hope in the 33 women who received the diagnosis of breast cancer, as these women have a 40% chance (13/33) that the diagnosis of breast cancer and the course of the disease is harmless.

The second benefit of screening is related to certainty. Without mammography, we know that 980 women do not suffer from breast cancer, but we cannot identify which of the 1000 women will not be affected. With mammography, we can tell exactly which women have no sign of breast cancer.

We argue that introducing the concept of perceived safety adds new aspects to the still ongoing discussion about the value of breast cancer screening. If the principle of perceived safety can be accepted in other areas of health care, it may offer new insights and perspectives to many of our patients.

## References

Arnold, K. (2002). Mammography guidelines in the national spotlight again. *Journal of the National Cancer Institute,* 94, 411–413.

Aronowitz, R.A. (2001). Do not delay: breast cancer and time, 1900-1970. *Milbank Quarterly,* 79, 355–386.

Barratt, A., Howard, K. Irwing, L., Alkeld, G., Houssami, N. (2005). Model of outcomes of screening mammography: information to support informed choices. *British Medical Journal (Online First),* DOI:10.1136/bmj.38398.469479.8F.

Eddy, D.M. (1987). The frequency of cervical cancer screening: comparison of a mathematical model with empirical data. *Cancer,* 60, 1117–1122.

Farhat, W.A., Habbal, A.A., Khauli, R.B. (2000). A guideline to clinical utility of prostate specific antigen. *Saudi Medical Journal,* 21, 223–227.

Harris, P., Carnes, M. (2002). Is there an age at which we should stop performing screening Pap smears and mammography? *Cleveland Clinic Journal of Medicine,* 69, 272–273.

Kaplan, R.M. (2004). Shared medical decision making: a new tool for preventive medicine. *American Journal of Preventive Medicine,* 26, 81–83.

Levenson, D. (2003). Routine prostate screening may be unnecessary and harmful. *Report on Medical Guidelines in Outcomes Research* 14, 5–7.

New PSA guidelines for older men (1998). *Johns Hopkins Medical Letter Health After 50,* 10(7), 1–2.

Parnes, B.L., Smith, P.C., Conry, C.M., Domke, H. (2001). When should we stop mammography screening for breast cancer in elderly women? *Journal of Family Practice,* 50, 110–111.

Schwartz, L.M., Woloshin, S., Fowler, F.J., Jr., Welch, H.G. (2004). Enthusiasm for cancer screening in the United States. *Journal of the American Medical Association,* 291, 71–78.

Shapiro, S., Coleman, E.A., Broeders, M., Codd, M., de Koning, H., Fracheboud, J., et al. (1998). Breast cancer screening programmes in 22 countries: current policies, administration and guidelines; International Breast Cancer Screening Network (IBSN) and the European Network of Pilot Projects for Breast Cancer Screening. *International Journal of Epidemiology,* 27, 735–742.

The U.S. Preventive Services Task Force (1994). Screening for prostate cancer: commentary on the recommendations of the Canadian Task Force on the Periodic Health Examination. *American Journal of Preventive Medicine,* 10, 187–193.

Welch, H.G. (2004). *Should I be tested for cancer?* Berkeley, CA: University of California Press.

Weston, R., Parr, N. (2003). New NHS guidelines for PSA testing in primary care. *Lancet,* 361, 89–90.

Zahl, P.H., Strand, B.H., Maehlen, J. (2004). Incidence of breast cancer in Norway and Sweden during introduction of nationwide screening: prospective cohort study. *British Medical Journal,* 328, 921–924.

# 22
# Evidence-Based Health Care Seen from Four Points of View

AMIT K. GHOSH, DIRK STENGEL, NANCY SPECTOR, NARAYANA S. MURALI, AND FRANZ PORZSOLT

Evidence-based health care (EBHC) and its approach to the practice of medicine has gained considerable acceptance among health care professionals. The Association of American Medical Colleges (AAMC) advocates integration of the principles of evidence-based medicine (EBM) into undergraduate training. Promoted as a tool to further learning by inquiry, to steer clear of opinion-based medicine (Sackett et al., 2000), and to help students at all levels of training to assess conscientiously the current best evidence, an increasing number of medical schools in the United States have incorporated it into their curriculum. The 2002–2003 Liaison Committee on Medical Education (LCME) revealed in the Annual Medical School Questionnaire that 122 of 126 LCME-accredited schools included EBM as a required course and devoted a mean of 20 hours to it (Barzansky & Etzel, 2003).

The concept of evidence-based health care ensures that the physician is familiar with the calculated estimate of the patient's probability of having a disease and understands the estimated risks and benefits of tests and treatments. These estimates often derive from the physician's ability to locate critical information from the current medical literature and his or her willingness to incorporate the patient's relevant values into the decision-making process. Hence, the future competence of the physician is not measured by his or her ability to recall facts but by the ability to incorporate the best current evidence into the patient's personal values and come to a shared decision acceptable to both patient and physician.

We here present the views of a surgeon, two internists, a nurse educator, and a health economist on the various aspects of evidence-based practice as perceived in their daily provision of health care services. Although agreement has been reached on the definition of evidence-based health care, there remains considerable debate concerning what constitutes an evidence-based case. Physicians are encountering difficulties in entrenching EBM into mainstream clinical practice owing to conflicting attitudes, different degrees of acceptance, on-site applicability, and (in)ability to appraise articles critically. From a health economist's standpoint, the development of future guidelines requires not only the application of EBM but the ability to distinguish between the effectiveness of treatment and the economic efficiency of the guideline. We discuss new concepts of the steps in EBM, identify the challenges of practicing EBHC, evaluate the current status of evidence-based nursing, and examine the practicality of implementing EBHC in situations of medical uncertainty. We also discuss retrieval and critical appraisal of literature and application of EBHC to patients and enumerate educational interventions to enhance the practice of EBHC.

## Six Steps of Evidence-Based Medicine

The traditional model of EBM as proposed by the Evidence-Based Medicine Working Group involves: (1) transforming the clinical problem into a three- or four-part question; (2) finding external evidence to answer the question; (3) critically appraising the external evidence; (4) applying the evidence to the patient in compliance with the patient's personal values; and (5) evaluating the decision-making process (Sackett et al., 2000).

Recent studies by one of the authors indicate that one encounters numerous difficulties in getting students to accept this strategy of applying the five steps as they advance in their medical training (Porzsolt et. al., 2003). In the presence of well established methods of treatment or diagnosis, there seems to be resistance to accept new information. Recent studies have indicated that students are more likely to accept new information if they are allowed to integrate their *internal evidence* with the existing *external evidence* from the medical literature. Internal evidence is the knowledge that a student has acquired during formal medical education and training and the experience accumulated from daily practice and the clinician–patient relationship. Attempting to answer the patient's questions based on one's own internal evidence, even prior to steps 2 to 5 of the traditional EBM strategy, has not only helped the students critically to appraise and apply the best external evidence but also to assess the accuracy of their internal evidence. The six-step approach, which essentially corresponds to application of the Bayesian model to evidence-based medicine, is outlined in Table 22.1.

As uncertainty often shrouds the medical decision-making process, physicians need to tally the degree of agreement between their internal evidence and the external evidence. When critical appraisal and reflection of internal and external evidence reveal that the result is equivocal, other factors, including the cost of the treatment and the patient's discomfort, become more important. Under conditions of medical uncertainty, one could avoid making an erroneous medical decision based on one's own internal evidence.

## Challenges of Evidence-Based Health Care: Problem of Asymmetry Between Internal and External Evidence

Although much of the progress in medical education and health care has been attributed to the increasing popularity of EBM, there still seems to be considerable resistance in many academic centers. The conventional apprentice approach to imparting medical knowledge revolves around the authoritative decision-making process of a well meaning senior physician. A diagnostician's brilliance

TABLE 22.1. Six Steps of Evidence-Based Medicine

| Step | Action | Explanation |
|---|---|---|
| 1 | Transform the clinical problem into a 3- or 4-part question. | (1) relevant patient characteristics and problem(s); (2) leading intervention; (3) alternative intervention; (4) clinical outcomes or goals. |
| 2 | Additional step: answer the question based on "internal evidence" only. | Internal evidence: acquired knowledge through professional training and experience (in general and applied to the patient). Should be documented before proceeding to step 3. |
| 3 | Find "external evidence" to answer the question. | External evidence obtained from textbooks, journals, databases, experts, etc. The value of the external evidence is highly variable (see step 4). |
| 4 | Critically appraise the external evidence. | Should answer three questions: (1) Are the results valid? (2) Are the results clinically important? (3) Do the results apply to my patient (or is my patient so different from those in the study that the results do not apply)? |
| 5 | Integrate external and internal evidence. | The two sources of information (external and internal) may be supportive, nonsupportive, or conflicting. How the decision is made when the evidence is nonsupportive or conflicting depends on many factors. |
| 6 | Evaluate the decision-making process. | Once the decision has been made, the process and the outcome are considered and opportunities for improvement are identified. |

is measured by the speed at which she or he can make a diagnosis rather than by a careful, reflective, open, shared process of decision making as stressed in EBM. Medical students and residents may face many hurdles when trying to learn the principles of EBM.

The students are exposed to numerous medical educators in the inpatient and outpatient settings who vary considerably in their attitudes toward and expertise in EBM. Application of the tenets of EBM could be perceived as a challenge to authority. A survey of surgical residents from McMaster University in Canada indicates several barriers that limit the application of EBM during daily rounds. Residents perceived a lack of training in EBM, time constraints, lack of priority, and staff disapproval of EBM as major challenges to applying EBM. They also thought that there was a lack of readily available surgical EBM resources in their hospitals (Bhandari et al., 2003). In a study performed in the United States, 33% of community physicians, compared to 5% of full-time academic faculty, did not apply EBM principles when teaching students in outpatient settings (Beasley & Woolley, 2002). Community faculty considered EBM skills to be less important in daily practice than did the full-time academic faculty and were less confident about their knowledge of EBM.

Sackett and colleagues (2000) identified numerous misconceptions of the term evidence-based medicine among many physicians: (1) *It's what we've always done*. Although much of medicine is based on traditional medical education and subjective judgment, this view is no longer totally correct owing to the widespread access to electronic databases. (2) *It will replace clinical judgment*. This is also not true, as we found that agreement of internal and external evidence taken together and external evidence alone affect practice. (3) *I don't have time for it.* Lack of time is a major barrier. However, recent cost-free availability, easy access, and familiarity prompt most clinicians to access MEDLINE/PubMed (a premier bibliographic database of the U.S. National Library of Medicine) for their scientific literature. MEDLINE/PubMed is the world's first and probably largest biomedical literature database, containing citations from more than 4600 journals dating back to 1966. Additionally, secondary analysis of evidence-based guidelines and articles, which can be assessed at a fraction of the time required to read the primary literature, are easily available. (4) *It will lead to "cookbook medicine."* The process of EBM requires the incorporation of patients' values prior to making any medical decision.

The asymmetry of internal and external evidence (int-ext asymmetry) in daily medical decisions occurs because evidence on medical effectiveness is decisive in only 20% of cases. The internal evidence and the external evidence are equivocal in about 80% of the cases in the medical literature (Porzsolt, 2004). In other words, in 80% of cases factors other than medical effectiveness influence doctors' decisions.

This complexity of medical decisions makes it difficult to produce guidelines that can be applied in day-to-day practice. Whether a guideline is applied or simply occupies the bookshelf may depend on the degree of freedom the guideline leaves the decision maker. Guidelines that are highly directive—that is, which indicate that there is only one way to solve the patient's problem—are less likely to be incorporated into the clinical routine than guidelines that explicitly state what and why something should not be done (instead of saying what should be done) and leaving open several alternatives. The frequently observed problem that medical guidelines are carefully produced but subsequently almost completely neglected may depend on the degree to which the health care professional is challenged to contribute her or his knowledge to find the optimal solution of the individual patient's problem. The decision maker is challenged to accept responsibility for his or her part in making the decision. By accepting this responsibility, he or she acquires the right to make this decision (combining action with professional liability). This means the decision maker gets back part of her or his "freedom of medical decision making" by strictly applying the principles of evidence-based health care.

To translate this strong connection between action and professional liability, we have to modify the structure of our medical guidelines. It will no longer be sufficient to write recommendations based on the scientific literature. It will increasingly become necessary to demonstrate either the (medical) effectiveness or the (economic) efficiency of our guidelines. To demonstrate effectiveness and/or efficiency of an action, which are usually not mentioned in a particular guideline, the clinical problem (for example, leg ulcers in diabetic patients) must be addressed explicitly. Second, the problem has to be quantified; that is, its prevalence in the local community must be recorded. Third, the strategies that are expected to be effective and/or efficient must be named and implemented. Finally, effectiveness and/or efficiency of the guideline must be demonstrated by showing a reduction in the prevalence of the clinical problem when using the guideline. Hence, the internal and external asymmetry between medical evidence and freedom of medical decision making needs to be incorporated into future guidelines (Porzsolt, 2004).

## Evidence-Based Health Care in Nursing

Evidence-based nursing (EBN) is integrated into most nursing curriculums today. In the United States, the Institute of Medicine (IOM) report (2003) cited "evidence-based practice" as one of five core competencies that should be taught and practiced across all health professions. The National Council of State Boards of Nursing (NCSBN) surveyed 633 nurses and found that when nurses reported not having been taught to use research findings appropriately for providing care, they had significantly more difficulty with their current workplace assignments (Smith & Crawford, 2002).

In 1966, McKay asked two major questions that are relevant today in EBN: What is valued as an endpoint in nursing, and what can most effectively achieve that end? Romyn and colleagues (2003) raised the question: "Are only some kinds of knowledge termed evidence?" This is a pertinent question to nurses because much of nursing research is qualitative, although the evidence-based databases overwhelmingly review quantitative research. In 1998, the Canadian Nurses Association issued a policy statement defining *evidence* as information that is based on historical or scientific practice evaluations. Types of evidence include experimental and nonexperimental findings, expert opinion, and historical or experiential evidence. This definition considers all forms of knowledge, provided it is subjected to historic or scientific evaluation (Canadian Nurses Association, 1998; Romyn et al., 2003).

Although the definition of evidence-based practice varies among nurses in practice and academic centers, a generally accepted definition is "the integration of the best research evidence with clinical expertise and patient values" (Sackett et al., 2000). Nurses use evidence-based data to deliver effective health care that even exceeds quality assurance standards and introduces innovation (Grinspun et al., 2001). EBN also reduces the variations in nursing care and assists with efficient, effective decision making.

Nursing has always used research findings to support data collection, interventions, and evaluation of patient care. Although there is clearly a difference between EBN and research utilization, it has been difficult for nurses to realize that difference. Therefore, Dr. Kathleen Stevens (Stevens & Cassidy, 1999) of the University of Texas in San Antonio, who has done much work in EBN, calls for jettisoning the term "research utilization" in favor of "evidence-based nursing."

## Implementation of Evidence-Based Nursing

Because one of the most important aspects of evidence-based practice is critical appraisal of the evidence, information literacy is an important element in nursing curriculums. According to Jacobs and colleagues (2003), information literacy goes beyond computer literacy or Internet skills. It focuses on the need for critical appraisal and presumes the capacity to choose appropriate technological tools to obtain information. Thus, faculty members need to teach appropriate search strategies and selection of the best databases, as well as methods to analyze research studies critically. The selection of the best search strategies and databases is increasing in the nursing literature (McGibbon & Marks, 1998a,b; Evans, 2002; Grandage et al., 2002), but this is an area where significant work needs to be done, particularly related to finding databases with qualitative critical appraisals.

Stevens (2002) recommends using the ACE Star Model (Academic Center for Evidence-Based Nursing) as a simple way to organize the five major phases of transforming knowledge from discovery to impact on patient outcomes. The five phases of the star are (1) discovery, (2) summary, (3) translation, (4) implementation, and (5) evaluation. In Steven's ACE Star Model, *discovery* is the original research. When *summarizing* the evidence, all of the research is incorporated into a single meaningful whole. This step is what differentiates research utilization from EBN. Summary is sometimes termed evidence synthesis, systematic review, integrative review, or meta-analysis. A good summary increases the power and effect of the data, reduces bias, and reveals consistencies across a variety of studies. Generalizability is established when the evidence is synthesized, and the information is reduced into a manageable form during this step. *Translation* is where the scientific evidence is considered in the context of clinical expertise, resulting in clinical practice guidelines, best practices, protocols, standards, or clinical pathways. Implementation means translating research into practice. Here is where changes take place, either at the individual or organizational level. The last step in the ACE Star Model is *evaluation*, where the impact of the change (for example, health outcomes, efficiency, cost, or satisfaction) is measured.

## Uncertainty in Clinical Practice and the Application of EBHC

Medical uncertainty is inherent in clinical practice and contributes variability in medical practice. Physicians have differing levels of tolerance to uncertainty. Using a validated Physician Response to Uncertainty Scale, Gerrity and colleagues (1992) demonstrated that primary care physicians (psychiatry, general medicine, family medicine, pediatrics, obstetrics/gynecology) are more tolerant to uncertainty than anesthetists, orthopedists, and urologists.

Despite the availability of well defined, evidence-based guidelines, physicians often fail to implement them in their clinical practice. In a qualitative study conducted in the United Kingdom, six themes were identified that seem to affect the implementation of evidence-based guidelines: (1) the personal and professional experience of the physician; (2) the patient–physician relationship; (3) perceived tensions between primary care physicians and specialists; (4) physicians' attitudes toward their patients and the evidence; (5) the language used by the physicians, and (6) the logistics of general practice (Freeman & Sweeney, 2001). There is a tendency to continue current therapy to which patient is accustomed rather than prescribe a new drug based on the best available evidence. Physicians reported perceived patient stress associated with the initiation of new therapy, as it leads to frequent home visits for dose titration and patient reassurance. In consideration of the patient's domestic situation, physicians were hesitant to begin anticoagulation therapy in their elderly patients.

The complexity of medical problems along with variability in individual physician reaction to uncertainty might alter the perception of a problem. Application of the principles of EBM, although not completely eliminating uncertainty, can provide a common language for discussing causes for disagreement. Shared decision making, meticulous evaluation, exclusion of severe differential diagnoses, and establishing patient trust are all techniques of managing uncertainty (Ghosh, 2004).

## Challenges with Retrieval of Medical Literature

Reading is determined, among other things, by the ease in attaining literature. Scientific articles on MEDLINE/Pub Med are available either as FUTON (Full Text on the Net) or NAA (No Abstracts Available) articles (Wentz, 2002). The innate tendency to pick the low hanging fruit greatly enhances the odds that a FUTON article will be read or cited. This can create a bias, the FUTON or NAA bias, which may influence the visibility of research.

In its effort to keep abreast with rapidly evolving scientific findings, EBM relies on seeking the current best evidence from virtual libraries or online sources and integrating it into patient values after ascertaining the validity of the evidence by critical appraisal. This process helps avoid relying on obsolete and archaic information from traditional textbooks (Sackett et al., 2000). Nevertheless, visibility and easy user availability may determine whether "available evidence" is adopted as "current best evidence" in health care. "Invisible" research may be ignored or overlooked. Ignoring relevant NAA articles may limit the use of medical literature, just as publication bias or citation and language bias do (Murali et al., 2004).

More than 50% of Internet sessions end with the downloading of a full-text article (Delamothe, 2002). Articles available as either full text or an abstract only on the Internet have been found to have a higher impact factor than articles available without an abstract (Murali et al., 2004). As more research is being communicated electronically, health science libraries have increasingly adopted the policy of online subscriptions. This trend, in conjunction with the FUTON bias, may have broad implications on future medical education. Residents and medical students tend to rely heavily on articles that are available online for selective reading on a subject (Wentz, 2002).

## Critically Appraising Medical Literature

Critical appraisal of articles is an essential part of the EBM curriculum. The appraisal of articles in medical schools is taught in small focus groups as team learning and in journal clubs. Several institutions use standard worksheets for critical appraisal, summarize them as CATs (critical appraisal of topics), and post them on their departmental websites. Acquiring skill in critical appraisal is an essential part of EBM workshops worldwide. Having finally identified a suitable article, the physician ought to be able to appraise it critically. The common questions one needs to ask while interpreting an article on primary studies (those that provide original data on a topic) are summarized in Table 22.2.

Articles are appraised for their internal validity (closeness to truth). One can read the abstract and often decide whether the question has been well structured and if the results were collected appropriately and are summarized well. EBM is not restricted to randomized trials and meta-analyses. To be able to answer a question, one needs to identify the best article, check the validity, and see if a more detailed review is indicated to answer the two important questions: What were the results? Can they benefit my patients? Interpretation of the results often requires knowledge of basic statistics and familiarity with EBM terminology. Some commonly used terms when describing the results of a new diagnostic test are sensitivity, specificity, positive predictive value, and likelihood ratio.

In therapy questions, randomized control trials (RCTs) and systemic review of several randomized trials provide the best information to aid in the management of a patient. The number needed to treat (NNT) describes the number of patients who need to be treated to avoid one adverse effect (Cook et al., 1995). This useful parameter considers the patient's baseline risk, in contrast to risk reduction (RR) or relative risk reduction (RRR), which do not tell us the magnitude of the absolute risk. The main problems are lack of physician time to conduct primary appraisal of each article and information overload. A survey of physicians conducted in the United Kingdom revealed that only 5% believed that identifying and appraising the primary literature or systemic reviews was the most important step in moving from opinion-based medicine to EBM (McColl et al., 1998). Most physicians (57%) thought that the most appropriate method for adopting an evidence-based practice was to apply evidence-based guidelines and protocols developed by colleagues. Several secondary sources are available that conveniently provide summaries of critically appraised topics. These sources include the *ACP Journal Club* (USA), *Best Evidence* (USA), InfoPOEMS (http://www.infopoems.com), Bandolier (UK), and the Cochrane Library. InfoPOEMs is also

TABLE 22.2. Checklist for critical appraisal of articles with valid results

| | |
|---|---|
| Diagnosis: | Was there an independent, blinded comparison with a gold standard? |
| | Did the patient sample include an appropriate spectrum of patients similar to those found in general practice? |
| Therapy: | Was the study randomized and double-blinded? |
| | Were all enrolled patients included in the conclusion of the study? |
| Harm: | Were the exposures and outcomes measured similarly in both groups? |
| | Was the comparison group similar to the outcome group in all respects except for the variable in question? |
| Prognosis: | Was the patient sample selected from a well defined point during the course of the disease? |
| | Was the follow-up adequate and complete? |

available for palmtop computers (PDAs), which are frequently used by residents and physicians and provide updated information on medication and medical texts. It is unclear at present how helpful these secondary sources of information are in clinical decision making. In one study, physicians reported that they were helpful in 15% to 17% of cases (McColl et al., 1998).

## Applying Evidence to Patients

Having carefully evaluated the patient's condition and the best available evidence, clinicians need to understand the patient's preferences to identify the best available treatment for that particular patient. Table 22.3 provides some common rules to aid the clinician in assessing the external validity of an article. It is becoming increasingly clear that evidence alone is not enough to make a good clinical decision. Patients may vary quite widely in their tolerance of side effects, thus nullifying anticipated therapeutic benefit. Communicating risks and benefits in language understood by patients could greatly influence their decision in making a well informed choice (Borgardus et al., 1999; Paling, 2003). A combination of quantitative (ARR – absolute risk reduction, NNT – number needed to treat, RRR – relative risk reduction) and qualitative (unlikely, very likely) terms can be applied to explain the results of a study to a patient (Borgardus et al., 1999).

While explaining the risk to patients, clinicians often provide the details of the risk and the probability that it may occur (objective information), whereas the patient is also interested in knowing how important a bad outcome would be for him or her (subjective information). It is important to identify the risk (death, disability, pain), its inception (early versus late), and the nature of the bad event (temporary, permanent).

The mnemonic CARE is often used to improve risk communication: Cite basic risk in general terms; add estimated probabilities for positive and negative outcomes to descriptive terms (such as low risk); reinforce effectiveness by using visual aids for risk communication; express encouragement and hope to the patient (Paling, 2003).

TABLE 22.3. Application of the result(s) of a study

| | |
|---|---|
| Diagnosis: | Is the test affordable, accurate, and available in my hospital? |
| | Can I estimate the pretest probability of the disease in question? |
| | Will the posttest probability affect my management? |
| Therapy: | Is the patient so different from the study group that the results cannot be applied? |
| | According to the study results, how much would my patient truly benefit from the treatment? |
| | Are the treatment and consequences consistent with my patient's values and beliefs? |
| Harm: | Can the study results be extrapolated to my patient? |
| | What is the patient's risk of adverse events? |
| | Can the patient's preferences and expectations be met by an alternative therapy? |
| Prognosis: | Is my patient similar to the patients in the study group? |
| | Will the evidence alter the choice of treatment? |

## *Educational Interventions to Enhance Evidence-Based Practice*

Numerous workshops and training sessions on how to teach and learn EBM have been developed at various local, national, and international levels. These sessions are mainly directed toward improving technical EBM and cognitive skills. The main focus of these sessions has been to enhance specific aspects of EBM skills, especially asking a clinical question, conducting literature searches, and critically appraising topics. Although most of these sessions test the EBM knowledge and skills of learners, there is good evidence that other factors inhibit practitioners' ability to practice EBM, such as time pressures, lack of peer support, and limited accessibility to quality sources (articles and secondary critically appraised topics). Hence, recent efforts have been dedicated not only to the EBM curriculum but also to the learning environment. Although there are several validated tools to assess EBM knowledge and skills of learners, the attitude of learners toward EBM (knowledge, attitude, behavior—KAB) must also be understood (Johnston et al., 2003).

Despite a few enthusiastic reports about using EBM in inpatient medical wards, pediatrics, and general practice (Ellis et al, 1995; Gill et al., 1996; Kenny et al., 1997), numerous personal, interpersonal, and institutional barriers still impair the uniform application of EBM in many institutions. Strategies to overcome this inertia could include hiring preceptors and role models who are experts in EBM, improving EBM training, reducing innumeracy among physicians and patients, implementing strategies for improving patient–physician communication, and improving attitudes toward EBM. Shaughnessy and colleagues (1994) described the usefulness of medical information in an equation.

$$\text{Usefulness of information} = \frac{\text{relevance} \times \text{validity}}{\text{work}}$$

The most relevant information should be relevant to the practice, highly valid, and should take little work to acquire.

Numerous developments have made the practice of evidence-based health care more practical. Ebell and colleagues (1997) found that 85% of family physicians were willing to carry a hand-held computer. Among the most desired software were drug information, current treatment recommendations, ability to update information, and ability to print patient educational material. Many hospitals currently provide computers at or near care units. The development of organizations such as the Cochrane Collaboration, evidence-based journals of secondary publications (*ACP Journal Club, Best Evidence, Evidence Based Nursing*), availability of information systems that bring relevant evidence in seconds (InfoPOEMs), and learning the strategies of EBM for lifelong learning have created an invigorating environment to bring EBM into the mainstream of medical education.

Self-reflection and evaluation of ones' attitude toward critical inquiry of medical problems, as well as periodically checking one's skills in practicing and communicating about evidence-based health cases, could greatly enhance the practitioner's ability to keep up with ever-changing medical information and to answer questions posed by the patient.

## References

Barzansky, B., Etzel, S.I. (2003). Educational programs in US medical school, 2002-2003. *Journal of the American Medical Association*, 290, 1190–1196.

Beasley, B.W., Woolley, D.C. (2002). Evidence-based medicine knowledge, attitudes and skills of community faculty. *Journal of General Internal Medicine*, 17, 632–640.

Bhandari, M., Montori, V., Devereaux, P.J., Dosanjh, S., Sprague, S., Guyatt, G.H. (2003). Challenges to the practice of evidence-based medicine during residents' surgical training: a qualitative study using grounded theory. *Academic Medicine*, 78, 1183–1190.

Borgardus, S.T., Holmboe, E., Jekel, J.F. (1999). Perils, pitfalls and possibilities in talking about medical risks. *Journal of the American Medical Association*, 281, 1037–1041.

Canadian Nurses Association (1998). *Policy statement: evidence-based decision-making and nursing practice*. Ottawa: Canadian Nurses Association.

Cook, R.J., Sackett, D.L., Roberts, R.S. (1995). An assessment of clinically useful measures of treatment effect. *British Medical Journal*, 310, 452–454.

Delamothe, T. (2002). Is that it? How online articles have changed over the past five years. *British Medical Journal*, 290, 1475–1478.

Ebell, M.H., Gaspar, D.A., Khurana, S. (1997). Family physicians' preference for computerized decision-support hardware and software. *Journal of Family Practice*, 45, 137–141.

Ellis, J., Mulligan, I., Rowe, J., Sackett, D.L. (1995). Inpatient general medicine is evidence based. *Lancet*, 346, 407–410.

Evans, D. (2002). Database searches for qualitative research. *Journal of the Medical Library Association,* 90(3), 298–293.

Freeman, A.C., & Sweeney, K. (2001). Why general practitioners do not implement evidence: quantitative study. *British Medical Journal*, 323, 1–5.

Gerrity, M. S., Earp, J.A.L., DeVilles, R.F. (1992). Uncertainty and professional work: Perceptions of physicians in clinical practice. *American Journal of Sociology*, 97, 1022–1051.

Ghosh, A.K. (2004). Dealing with medical uncertainty: a physicians' perspective. *Minnesota Medicine*, 87, 48–51.

Gill, P., Dowell, A.C., Neal, R.D., Smith, N., Heywood, P., Wilson, A.E. (1996). Evidence based general practice: a retrospective study of interventions in one training practice. *British Medical Journal*, 312, 819–821.

Grandage, K.K., Slawson, D.C., Shaughnessy, A.F. (2002). When less is more: a practical approach to searching for evidence-based answers. *Journal of the Medical Library Association,* 90(3), 298–304.

Grinspun, D., Virani, T., Bajnok, I., (2001–2002). Nursing best practice guidelines: The RNAO project. *Hospital Quarterly*, 5(2), 56–60.

Institute of Medicine (2003). *Health professions education: a bridge to quality*. Washington, DC: National Academy Press.

Jacobs, S.K., Rosenfeld, P., Haber, J. (2003). Information literacy as the foundation for evidence-based practice in graduate nursing education: a curriculum-integrated approach. *Journal of Professional Nursing*, 19(5), 320–328.

Johnston, J.M., Leung, G.M., Fielding, R., Tin, K.Y., Ho, L.M. (2003). The development and validation of a knowledge, attitude and behaviour questionnaire to assess undergraduate evidence-based practice teaching and learning. *Medical Education*, 37, 992–1000.

Kenny, S.E., Shankar, K.R., Rintala, R., Lamont, G.L., Lloyd, D.A. (1997). Evidence-based surgery: intervention in a regional surgical unit. *Archives of Diseases in Childhood*, 76, 50–53.

McColl, A., Smith, H., White, P., Field, J. (1998). General practitioners' perceptions of the route of evidence based medicine: a questionnaire survey. *British Medical Journal*, 316, 361–365.

McKay, R. (1966). *The process of theory development in nursing*. Unpublished doctoral dissertation, Columbia University, New York.

McKibbon, K.A., Marks, S. (1998a). Searching for the best evidence. Part 1. Where to look. *Evidence-Based Nursing*, 1, 68–70.

McKibbon, K.A., Marks, S. (1998b). Searching for the best evidence. Part 2: searching CINAHL and Medline. *Evidence-Based Nursing*, 1, 105–107.

Murali, N.S., Murali, H.R., Auethavekiat, P., Erwin, P.J., Mandrekar, J.N., Manek, et al. (2004). Impact of FUTON and NAA bias on visibility of research. *Mayo Clinic Proceedings*, 79, 1001–6.

Paling, J. (2003). Strategies to help patients understand risk. *British Medical Journal*, 327, 745–748.

Porzsolt, F. (2004). Synopse der Nutzenbewertung medizinischer Gesundheitsleistungen aus der Sicht unterschiedlicher Autoren: Erstellung einer Matrix. [Synopsis of the evaluation of the benefit of medical health care services from the viewpoint of different authors: creation of a matrix] [editorial]. *Der Chirurg BDC*, 11, M302–M304.

Porzsolt, F., Ohletz, A., Thim, A., Gardner, D., Ruatti, H., Meier, H., et al. (2003). Evidence-based decision making: the 6-step method [editorial]. *American College of Physicians Journal Club*, 139, A11–A12.

Romyn, D., Allen, M., Boschma, G., Duncan, S.M., Edgecombe, N., Jensen, L.A., et al. (2003). The notion of evidence in evidence-based practice by the nursing philosophy working group. *Journal of Professional Nursing*, 19(4), 184–188.

Sackett, D.L., Straus, S.E., Richardson, W.S., Rosenberg, W., Haynes, R.B. (2000). Introduction. In: D.L. Sackett, S.E. Straus, W.S. Richardson, W. Rosenberg, R.B. Haynes (Eds.) *Evidence-based medicine: how to practice and teach* EBM (2nd ed.). Edinburgh: Churchill Livingstone; p. 1–261.

Shaughnessy, A.F., Slawson, D.C., Bennett, J.H. (1994). Becoming an information master: a guidebook to the medical information jungle. *Journal of Family Practice*, 39, 489–499.

Smith, J., Crawford, L. (2002, spring). *Practice and professional issues survey*. Chicago: National Council of State Boards of Nursing.

Stevens, K.R., Cassidy, V. (Eds.) (1999). *Evidence based teaching: current research in nursing education*. Sudbury, MA: Jones & Bartlett.

Stevens, K.R. (2002). ACE star model of EBP: the cycle of knowledge transformation. San Antonio, Texas: Academic Center for Evidence-Base Practice (http://www.acestar. uthscsa.edu).

Wentz, R. (2002). Visibility of research: FUTON bias. *Lancet*, 360, 1256.

# 23
# Efficacy, Effectiveness, and Efficiency of Diagnostic Technology

DIRK STENGEL AND FRANZ PORZSOLT

"Everything should be made as simple as possible, but not simpler."

—Albert Einstein

No goal-oriented action in health care would be possible without a reliable diagnosis. There are distinct demands on the test procedures leading to a diagnosis and the diagnosis itself.

- Results must be precise and reproducible (efficacy).
- Test findings must prompt medical actions that are different from those considered without knowledge of test results (effectiveness).
- Actions based on the results must lead to improved quality of life, a prolonged lifetime, or both (efficiency).

A potential value can be assigned only if a test clears all these hurdles. Efficacy is a mandatory, minimal qualification of a test to allow its further assessment. Figure 23.1 summarizes the hierarchy of appraising the value of a test (described in the next sections).

## Diagnostic Test Performance

### *What a Diagnostic Test Does*

We claim that a diagnostic test discriminates between two imaginable states: health and disease. In real life, there is a smooth transition between those two expressions. For practical reasons, we must admit the arbitrary thresholds that shift us from health to disease because the biological or anatomical truth is rarely available to us. A common surrogate for this truth is the result of a diagnostic reference test, the so-called gold standard (that is, a test that has proved to explain reality as precisely as possible).

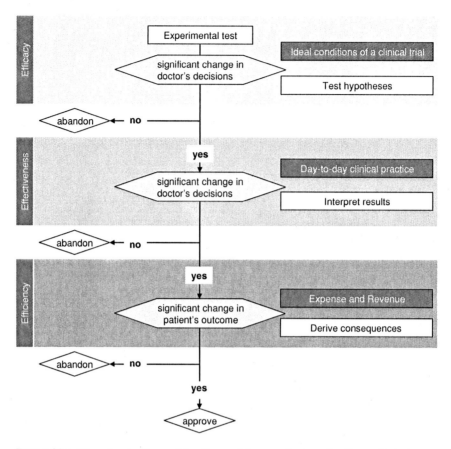

FIGURE 23.1. Three levels of appraising the usefulness and value of a diagnostic test.

## Quantitative Expressions of Diagnostic Test Accuracy

How to Investigate a Group of Patients in a Clinical Study

We stress that findings from a diagnostic test depend on the scientifically accepted threshold in the continuity between health and disease, the choice of the proper gold standard, and the individual test characteristics.

Figure 23.1 shows the three levels of appraising the usefulness and value of a diagnostic test. At the first level (efficacy), epidemiologists are responsible for defining the degree of correlation between test findings and biological truth (that is, the findings from the diagnostic gold standard). Given the controlled conditions of a clinical study, the null hypothesis claims the test cannot discriminate between health and disease.

However, if the collected data support rejection of this hypothesis (in other words, the test is likely to distinguish a diseased patient from a healthy subject), the clinician must decide at the second level (effectiveness) whether test results contribute exciting, novel, or unexpected information to his or her initial impression. If the test findings considerably change the doctor's therapeutic behavior, it is time to ask the patient whether she or he will accept the test because of its consequences or invasiveness. This is also an economic decision. Patients must decide whether the possible benefit from a test finding justifies the expenses (efficiency).

Figure 23.1 also stresses an important conflict between science and practice. Epidemiologists are extremely careful people and difficult to nail down to provide a definite answer. They come up with a certain probability of the observed findings (that is, the most likely range of data). Unfortunately, clinicians must unequivocally opt for or against a particular treatment choice. This requires translating the continuous probability scale used by epidemiologists into a binary (yes or no) management decision. Excellent doctors are artists; they switch quickly between facts and expertise and can often decide reliably and correctly even in a state of uncertainty. Other doctors prefer to wait until they have collected compelling facts to reach safe decisions, which may be too late for the patient. Some doctors even trust in inspirations rather than facts and act rapidly, which is dangerous for the patient.

A vital precondition to appraising the discriminatory features of a test is the occurrence of the target disease in the investigated population, the so-called *prevalence*, or *prior probability* of disease.

The term prevalence describes the number of persons suffering from a particular disease in a *defined population* (for example, the number of breast cancer patients in the United States). The prior or pretest probability has a similar meaning but refers to the probability of disease in an *individual subject* before test results are available.

The pretest probability may be known (because somebody else investigated this problem earlier in a similar group of individuals), or it may be just an estimate. In any case, it describes the expected number of persons suffering from a particular disease in a *defined sample*. For example, you are planning a study to determine the frequency of breast cancer in a group of 200 young women at the university college. Is it likely that the pretest probability of breast cancer in this group of college students will be higher or lower than the prevalence in the United States, which includes all American women? You are right to assume the pretest probability of breast cancer in college students will be much lower than the prevalence in the U.S. population.

Let us consider someone who consults his or her doctor because of pain on the right side of the wrist. If she or he cannot remember a recent injury, the chance that the pain is caused by a distal radius fracture is close to null (there is, of course, still a small chance of a pathological fracture caused by osteoporosis or a tumor). However, if she or he sustained high velocity trauma from a fall during inline skating, the probability of a fracture would be very high. In the first case, we would doubt a radiograph showing a fracture line; in other words, we would consider this a false-positive test result. In the second case, we would question a negative radiograph; that is, we would consider this a false-negative test result.

It is clear in these extreme clinical scenarios, in which common sense generates so much prior information, that a diagnostic test has only a minor impact on clinical reasoning. Consequently, any diagnostic test performs best when there is diagnostic uncertainty, or a fifty-fifty chance of health or disease.

In the above-mentioned situation, a fall at home may lead to a painful contusion or a fracture of the distal radius with a similar probability, and the radiographic findings considerably influence the clinically estimated likelihood of a fracture. The prior probability of a disease may also influence the purpose of testing. Whereas in the first scenario a radiograph is not necessary to rule the condition out, it may reassure both the doctor and the patient and avoid further consultations. In the second scenario, a radiograph is not needed to confirm the fracture but to decide about casting or surgical fixation.

These brief reflections clarify the two opposite directions of diagnostic test performance. A test can either detect or exclude the condition of interest, but few tests are jacks-of-all-trades. These opposite directions are classified by the terms *sensitivity* and *specificity*. A highly sensitive test correctly detects most individuals affected by the disorder being investigated and produces few false-negative results. This test, if negative, confidently excludes the disorder of interest. A highly specific test correctly detects most nonaffected individuals and produces very few false-positive results. This test, if positive, confidently rules in the disorder of interest.

We already mentioned the necessity of agreement on a threshold between health and disease. A radiograph of the wrist shows a fracture line or not; its result is binary (yes or no). Because a binary result creates a well defined number of true-positive, false-negative, false-positive, and true-negative results, it is easy to communicate in terms of sensitivity and specificity.

In contrast, a laboratory test (for example, to determine the blood glucose level) provides a result on a continuous scale and, thus, an infinite number of sensitivity-specificity pairs. This needs a cutoff value with optimal sensitivity and specificity. A popular method for deriving an appropriate threshold value is the receiver operating characteristics (ROC) curve, which demonstrates the trade-off between sensitivity and 1 − specificity.

Sensitivity explains the proportion of individuals affected by the disorder who turn out to be test-positive; 1 − specificity describes the proportion of healthy patients with a positive test finding. In other words, the ROC curve quantifies the ratio between the number of false-positive findings that must be accepted to obtain a certain number of true-positive findings. A classic example is the derivation of threshold blood levels for the tumor marker carcinoembryonic antigen (CEA) in patients with colorectal cancer.

The diagnostic accuracy of CEA for identifying tumor load was proven during the early 1980s (Fletcher, 1986). Figure 23.2 depicts the ROC curves for varyious disease stages (Dukes, 1951). The bisecting line (dotted line) indicates a worthless test with an accuracy close to chance. The area under the curve (AUC), a convenient global measure of test accuracy, would be 50% in this case. The curve of a perfect test rises perpendicularly along the $y$ axis (for a specificity of 100% for any given sensitivity) and, after reaching the upper left-hand corner of the ROC space, runs horizontally along the top to the upper right-hand corner (for a

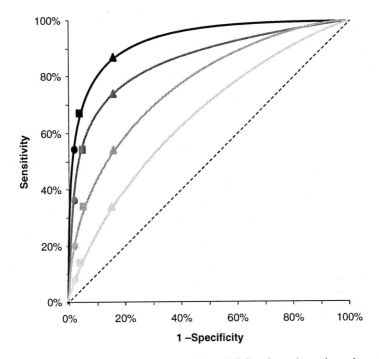

FIGURE 23.2. Receiver operating characteristics (ROC) of carcinoembryonic antigen (CEA) in varying clinical stages of colorectal carcinoma. Triangles indicate a cutoff point of 2.5 ng/ml, squares 5.0 ng/ml, and circles 10 ng/ml. Dukes A: cancer limited to the inner layers of the bowel or rectum. Dukes B: cancer grown into the muscle layer of the bowel or rectum. Dukes C: cancer has spread into locoregional lymph nodes. Dukes D: metastatic disease.

sensitivity of 100% for any given specificity). Obviously, the AUC would be 100% in this case.

Consider a patient with locally advanced disease (Dukes B). If the cutoff point is set at 5 ng/ml, the sensitivity and the specificity are about 35% and 95%, respectively. In other words, a patient who had undergone, for example, left-sided hemicolectomy (removal of part of the large intestine) for a Dukes B tumor and has a CEA level above 5 ng/ml on follow-up has a 95% chance of a residual tumor, a local recurrence, or a distant metastasis because the false-positive rate is less than 5%. On the other hand, a CEA level below 5 ng/ml does not exclude the presence of tumor cells. The false-negative rate would still be 65% at this cutoff level. The lower the cutoff level (for example, 2.5 ng/ml), the higher the sensitivity (55%) and the confidence in a negative result. Vice versa, the higher the cutoff level (for example, 10 ng/ml), the higher the specificity (99%) and the confidence in a positive result.

The shape of the curves indicates how difficult it is to exclude reliably the presence of a tumor on the basis of the CEA value. In Dukes B tumors, a sensitivity higher than 80% could only be achieved with an unacceptably high 50% false-positive rate.

We are now able to determine the accuracy or efficacy of a test by appraising its sensitivity, specificity, and the trade-off between the two measures in an ROC curve.

## Diagnostic Meta-analysis

As in therapy, systematic reviews and meta-analyses provide the best available evidence for scrutinizing the efficacy of a diagnostic test. During the last decade, scientific progress was made in developing advanced search strategies for diagnostic studies in electronic databases (Haynes & Wilczynski, 2004), assessing the methodological quality of individual studies (Whiting et al., 2004), and compiling the data into a summary measure of test accuracy (Rutter & Gatsonis, 2001; Stengel et al., 2003).

The most popular method of meta-analyzing diagnostic test data is the summary receiver operating characteristics (SROC) curve. Readers interested in the mathematical framework of SROC are referred to the original publication (Moses et al., 1993).

Although similar at a glance, the ROC and the SROC have different statistical backgrounds, features, and interpretations. Whereas the ROC is derived from single observations made in one study only, the SROC represents the fitted line amid the results from multiple studies. The ROC uses the entire range of data from a test with measures expressed on a continuous scale (for example, CEA values). In contrast, the SROC employs binary test results (either from tests with a yes-or-no answer or continuous data that had already been dichotomized at a certain cutoff point). Figure 23.3 shows an SROC example for the CEA scenario derived from six published studies ($n = 2249$).

# Influence of Diagnostic Test Results on Management Decisions

Common sense tells us that if additional information does not change our world view, we do not need it, especially not at considerable extra cost. In health care, this principle is not widely accepted. Sparse information is available on the effectiveness or influence of diagnostic test results on management decisions.

# Melsungen Experiment

## Design

The Melsungen experiment was conducted to determine the effectiveness of diagnostic tests using the tumor marker CEA as an example. Physicians were provided with typical clinical scenarios and a choice of appropriate interventions. Each scenario was presented in two alternative forms, whereby the clinical baseline data remained unchanged but the result of the CEA assay was either normal

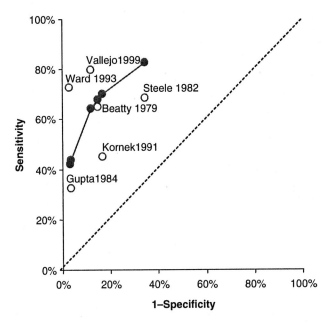

FIGURE 23.3. Summary receiver operating characteristics (SROC) of studies investigating the diagnostic accuracy of carcinoembryonic antigen (CEA) for detecting recurrent or metastatic colorectal cancer. Continuous data were already dichotomized in the original studies, and the distinction between CEA-positive and CEA-negative results was made at a threshold of 5 ng/ml. Generalized linear model (GLM) with maximum-likelihood estimation. The estimated common area under the curve (AUC) is 0.82 [95% confidence interval (CI) 0.69 – 0.95]. The method was described by Walter (2002). Obviously, there is strong diversity between single studies. The lower limit of the 95% CI exceeds the 50% threshold (a worthless test) by 19%. The upper limit of the confidence interval, however, is close to 100% (a perfect test). Circles = original data; solid dots = fitted model.

or elevated (that is, CEA plasma concentrations were either higher or lower than 5 ng/ml). Three paper cases (Tables 23.1–23.3)—medical histories of patients with colorectal cancer—were developed by a surgeon and a medical oncologist. Each scenario depicted a common clinical situation, provided the result of a CEA assay, and offered several possible consequences.

It was hypothesized that different CEA test results in otherwise identical scenarios prompt different patterns of consequences. Second, the pattern of interventions chosen by the study participants depends on the degree of clinical experience, the number of patients treated, and the type of hospital or institutional affiliation.

Questionnaires containing the clinical scenarios were distributed to the 370 participants of a conference on good clinical practice guidelines in surgery. Detailed instructions on how to complete the forms and how to indicate refusal to participate in the experiment were provided. The questionnaires were handed out to the conference participants at the registration desk, and screen messages in the

TABLE 23.1. Scenario 1

Mrs. S. is a 60-year-old woman who was operated on for Dukes' B colon cancer 5 years ago with curative intent and did not receive any adjuvant therapy. She felt well until 4 weeks ago, when she started complaining about abdominal cramps that increased during deep inspiration. Among her laboratory results, aminotransferases are nearly doubled, whereas γ-glutamyl transferase and phosphatase (liver values) are in the upper reference range.

*Questionnaire A*: The CEA assay turned out to be normal (1.9 ng/ml).
*Questionnaire B*: The CEA assay turned out to be pathologically elevated (19.1 ng/ml).

Please select the next step of further diagnostic workup (only one answer possible).

Ultrasonography – Chest radiography – CT scan – MRI – PET – Endoscopy

CEA = carcinoembryonic antigen; CT = computed tomography; MRI = magnetic resonance imaging; PET = positron emission tomography.

TABLE 23.2. Scenario 2

Mr. K. is a 48-year-old healthy male politician who is admitted to your department because of lower gastrointestinal bleeding. Six weeks ago he recognized traces of blood in his stool for the first time. The digital rectal examination reveals a suspicious palpation finding.

*Questionnaire A*: The CEA assay turned out to be pathologically elevated (18.5 ng/ml).
*Questionnaire B*: The CEA assay turned out to be normal (1.8 ng/ml).

Please select all diagnostic modalities considered necessary, in addition to endoscopy and biopsy (multiple answers possible).

Ultrasonography – CT scan – MRI – PET – Repeat CEA assay – Endoscopy only

TABLE 23.3. Scenario 3

Mr. T. is a 51-year-old man who underwent right-sided hemicolectomy (surgical removal of part of the large intestine) for advanced colon cancer, stage: T3 N2 M0. He is receiving his third cycle of adjuvant chemotherapy with 5-FU, which is well tolerated. Following surgery, the CEA assay remained elevated (9.3 ng/ml).

*Questionnaire A*: The CEA assay remains stable during treatment (9.1 ng/ml).
*Questionnaire B*: The CEA assay shows steadily rising values (16.2 ng/ml).

Please mark the interventions required in this setting (multiple answers possible).

Ultrasonography – Chest radiography – CT scan – MRI – PET – Watchful waiting

T3 = tumor size and depth of invasion; N2 = lymph node involvement; M0 = no metastases; 5-FU = fluorouracil.

main auditorium reminded the attendees to fill in the questionnaire before the conference convened.

Neither the participants nor the conference staff was aware that two versions of each of the three scenarios had been prepared. The questionnaires were randomly mixed and put into eight stacks to be supplied by eight conference secretaries. The secretaries distributed the study forms one after another from their individual stacks, which comprised an unknown sequence of both types of questionnaire. One questionnaire provided normal CEA values for scenario 1 (Table 23.1), elevated values for scenario 2 (Table 23.2), and stable values during therapy for scenario 3 (Table 23.3), whereas the alternative questionnaire presented elevated, normal, and increasing values, respectively. To meet the requirements of post-allocation informed consent, one author who was an invited speaker at the conference collected the completed questionnaires at the beginning of his presentation, explained the study design, and requested the participants who did not agree with this type of informed consent to leave a note at the conference registration desk. Participants remained anonymous throughout the study.

## Results

Questionnaires were received, completed, and returned by 143 conference participants. Following the explanation of the study design (postallocation informed consent), none of the participants raised objections against this procedure. Complete demographic data were available from 137 questionnaires. Demographic details are summarized in Table 23.4.

There was no significant difference in the proportions of diagnostic interventions selected in the first two clinical settings, regardless of CEA levels (Figure 23.4). In scenario 3, the physicians selected the watchful waiting policy less often when CEA concentrations were increasing than in the presence of stable CEA concentrations [difference in proportions: 20% and 95%, respectively; confidence interval (CI) 7.6%–32.5%; $p = 0.003$]. Accordingly, abdominal imaging by

TABLE 23.4. Demographic characteristics of the participating surgeons

| Item | Questionnaire A (n = 66) | Questionnaire B (n = 77) | p |
|---|---|---|---|
| Gender | | | 0.55 |
| Male | 57 (86%) | 64 (83%) | |
| Female | 8 (12%) | 12 (16%) | |
| Missing | 1 (2%) | 1 (1%) | |
| Affiliation | | | 0.35 |
| University | 16 (24%) | 28 (36%) | |
| Teaching hospital | 44 (67%) | 45 (58%) | |
| Others | 3 (5%) | 3 (4%) | |
| Missing | 3 (5%) | 1 (1%) | |
| Surgical experience | | | 0.91 |
| < 2 years | 4 (6%) | 2 (3%) | |
| 2–4 years | 3 (5%) | 4 (5%) | |
| 5–8 years | 11 (17%) | 11 (14%) | |
| 9–6 years | 13 (20%) | 13 (17%) | |
| >16 years | 34 (52%) | 45 (58%) | |
| Missing | 1 (2%) | 2 (3%) | |
| Patients treated annually | | | 0.30 |
| <10 | 2 (3%) | 2 (3%) | |
| 10–20 | 6 (9%) | 4 (5%) | |
| 21–40 | 21 (32%) | 11 (14%) | |
| 41–80 | 18 (27%) | 30 (39%) | |
| > 80 | 16 (24%) | 27 (35%) | |
| Missing | 3 (5%) | 3 (4%) | |

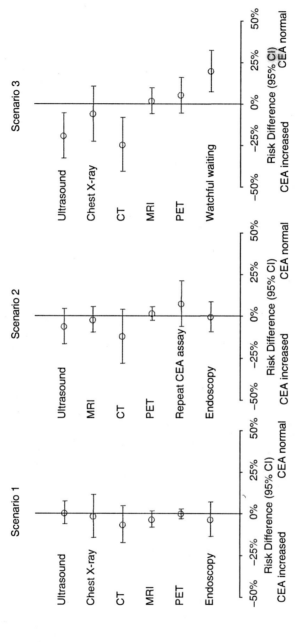

FIGURE 23.4. Results of the Melsungen experiment. There were no differences in treatment decisions made for normal or increased CEA values in the first two scenarios. In scenario 3, surgeons would have scheduled their patients for computed tomography more often when the CEA assay showed abnormal findings.

ultrasonography (US) and computed tomography (CT) was ordered significantly more often (88% vs. 65%, $p = 0.003$ and 61% vs. 32 %, $p = 0.001$) for rising CEA levels compared to stable CEA levels.

The CT scans were selected more frequently for increasing CEA concentrations in scenario 3 by participants affiliated with nonuniversity hospitals (difference in proportions: 47% and 95%, respectively; CI 24.6%–68.7%; $p = 0.001$) but not by university staff (difference in proportions: 17% vs. 95%; CI –3.6% to 46.9%).

Possible Interpretations

Our data indicate that virtually the same decisions are made in two of the clinical scenarios, regardless of whether CEA values are elevated or normal. This was true for CEA in both a follow-up situation (scenario 1) and at the primary diagnosis of colorectal cancer (scenario 2). Thus, CEA has poor effectiveness in changing management decisions in these clinical situations.

In the third scenario, which described surveillance during adjuvant chemotherapy, more subsequent US and CT investigations were requested when CEA was increasing compared to stable CEA values.

In the first two scenarios, CEA was not helpful for clinical decision making, and no further scientific investigations were requested. In contrast, in the third scenario, findings from the CEA assay influenced management decisions. It remains to be demonstrated that a higher rate of CT scanning results in improved patient outcomes.

Ultimate Goal of Improving Outcomes by Diagnostics

After proving efficacy and effectiveness, a diagnostic test may finally attain the top level of usefulness—its benefit for patients and society. The simplest imaginable design to address the efficiency of a test is a pre–post study, in which outcomes are compared for two consecutive populations before and after introducing the test. This design is, however, susceptible to bias. Alternatively, one might consider a parallel-group design, either randomized or nonrandomized. There are various options to estimate efficiency in this setting.

- Patients undergo either the new test or the established reference standard.
- Patients undergo the established and the new test or the established reference standard alone.
- Patients undergo the established and the new test in both groups, but doctors receive either one or the other test result.

Regardless of the chosen format, an efficient test should significantly improve outcomes (in terms of quality or quantity of life), reduce complications, or cut costs. If a test fails to pass even the first level of evaluation, it would be senseless to judge its effectiveness or efficiency. In a Cochrane Review, we found no evidence that emergency US for suspected blunt abdominal trauma reduces morbidity or mortality (Stengel et al., 2005b). This is not surprising because its sensitivity is at the same level as tossing a coin (Stengel et al., 2005a).

However, assume a test is highly accurate but does not improve outcomes. There are two possible reasons for this failure.

- The test result does not affect management decisions (that is, poor effectiveness).
- It affects management decisions, but these decisions do not affect patient's outcomes.

We have already stressed that studies of diagnostic effectiveness are rare. Unless this lack is comprehended and aggressively abolished, efficiency will remain an unsatisfying proxy for both effectiveness and efficiency.

Theoretically, CEA may signal tumor recurrence or systemic spread early. Four randomized trials of intensive follow-up (including abdominal US, CT, endoscopy, and chest radiography) showed a significant advantage in 5-year survival over standard care, as shown in Figure 23.5.

All authors except Ohlsson employed CEA testing in both experimental and control arms of their studies. Thus, the observed survival benefit may have been caused by other components of the follow-up programs but not the CEA assay. One may speculate whether the decision to schedule patients presenting with pathological CEA values for CT (as noted in the previous experiment) increases the resection rate of liver metastases and thereby improves outcomes. However, this hypothesis can neither be confirmed nor rejected on the basis of the available information. In conclusion, in addition to the results from the effectiveness study, there is no compelling evidence that measurement of CEA is efficient in prolonging life after curative resection of colorectal cancer.

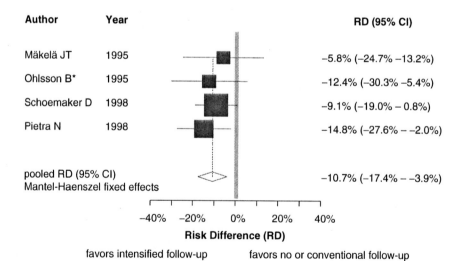

FIGURE 23.5. Summarized data on overall survival from four randomized trials of intensive versus conventional follow-up after surgery for colorectal cancer.
*CEA was determined only in the experimental arm.

# Summary

We have briefly sketched the complexity of diagnostic test research. Evaluating the usefulness of a diagnostic test does not end, but begins, after proving efficacy. We demonstrated how a test with proven efficacy (that is, the CEA assay) can fail on the level of effectiveness and efficiency. Although still underrepresented compared to the therapeutic setting, there is awareness of the need for diagnostic meta-analyses. This has also been recognized by the Cochrane Collaboration, which has welcomed diagnostic reviews before the end of 2005. We must accept that a detailed look at the efficacy of our diagnostic battery can change our attitudes toward therapeutic efficacy.

Imagine what would happen if a thorough diagnostic meta-analysis shows weak accuracy of a test that is commonly used to diagnose a condition. If it creates more false-positive results than expected, patients might have erroneously been recruited into a therapeutic trial. This may dilute absolute measures of efficacy. Differential and nondifferential misclassification may introduce bias toward and away from the null. Although desirable, adding diagnostic meta-analyses to the Cochrane Library may lead to severe conflicts with current knowledge.

Few studies have addressed the efficiency of tests, and very few are available that have investigated the effectiveness of diagnostic methods. Therefore, it is difficult if not impossible to judge whether negative efficiency was caused by the missing impact of test findings on management decisions or lacking effects of the interventions applied because of test results. This is of minor relevance for tests that have already been abandoned because of poor efficiency. However, distinguishing between poor effectiveness and efficiency is mandatory for future research to avoid recruitment of patients into comparative trials aiming at proving beneficial outcomes with new test technology. If a test is ineffective, such trials are useless, potentially harmful, and expensive.

Although defining the value of testing needs some simplification, the hierarchy of scientific appraisal must be maintained.

## References

Dukes, C.E. (1951). The surgical pathology of tumours of the colon. *Medical Press*, 226, 512–515.

Fletcher, R.H. (1986). Carcinoembryonic antigen. *Annals of Internal Medicine*, 104, 66–73.

Haynes, R.B., Wilczynski, N.L. (2004). Optimal search strategies for retrieving scientifically strong studies of diagnosis from MEDLINE: analytical survey. *British Medical Journal*, 328, 1040.

Moses, L.E., Shapiro, D., Littenberg, B. (1993). Combining independent studies of a diagnostic test into a summary ROC curve: data-analytic approaches and some additional considerations. *Statistics in Medicine*, 12, 1293–1316.

Rutter, C.M., Gatsonis, C.A. (2001). A hierarchical regression approach to meta-analysis of diagnostic test accuracy evaluations. *Statistics in Medicine*, 20, 2865–2884.

Stengel, D., Bauwens, K., Sehouli, J., Ekkernkamp, A., Porzsolt, F. (2003). A likelihood ratio approach to meta-analysis of diagnostic studies. *Journal of Medical Screening*, 10, 47–51.

Stengel, D., Bauwens, K., Rademacher, G., Mutze, S., Ekkernkamp, A. (2005a). Association between compliance with methodological standards of diagnostic research and reported test accuracy: meta-analysis of focused assessment of sonography for trauma (FAST). *Radiology*, 236, 102–111.

Stengel, D., Bauwens, K., Sehouli, J., Rademacher, G., Mutze, S., Ekkernkamp, A., et al. (2005b). Emergency ultrasound-based algorithms for diagnosing blunt abdominal trauma. *Cochrane Database of Systematic Reviews*, 2:CD004446.

Walter, S.D. (2002). Properties of the summary receiver operating characteristic (SROC) curve for diagnostic test data. *Statistics in Medicine*, 21, 1237–1256.

Whiting, P, Rutjes, A. W., Dinnes, J., Reitsma, J., Bossuyt, P.M., Kleijnen, J. (2004). Development and validation of methods for assessing the quality of diagnostic accuracy studies. *Health Technology Assessment*, 8(25), 1–234.

# Additional References

### Randomized Trials Assessing the Efficiency of Intensive Follow-up with CEA After Curative Resection for Colorectal Cancer

Mäkelä, J.T., Laitinen, S.O., Kairaluoma, M.I. (1995). Five-year follow-up after radical surgery for colorectal cancer: results of a prospective randomized trial. *Archives of Surgery*, 130, 1062–1067.

Ohlsson, B., Breland, U., Ekberg, H., Graffner, H., Tranberg, K.G. (1995). Follow-up after curative surgery for colorectal carcinoma: randomized comparison with no follow-up. *Diseases of the Colon and Rectum*, 38, 619–626.

Pietra, N., Sarli, L., Costi, R., Ouchemi, C., Grattarola, M., Peracchia, A. (1998). Role of follow-up in management of local recurrences of colorectal cancer: a prospective, randomized study. *Diseases of the Colon and Rectum*, 41, 1127–1133.

Schoemaker, D., Black, R., Giles, L., Toouli, J. (1998). Yearly colonoscopy, liver CT, and chest radiography do not influence 5-year survival of colorectal cancer patients. *Gastroenterology*, 114, 7–14.

### Studies of CEA Accuracy

Beatty, J.D., Romero, C., Brown, P.W., Lawrence, W., Terz, J.J. (1979). Clinical value of carcinoembryonic antigen: diagnosis, prognosis, and follow-up of patients with cancer. *Archives of Surgery*, 114, 563–567.

Steele, G., Ellenberg, S., Ramming, K., O'Connell, M., Moertel, C., Lessner, H., et al. (1982). CEA monitoring among patients in multi-institutional adjuvant G.I. therapy protocols. *Annals of Surgery*, 196, 162–169.

Gupta, M.K., Arciaga, R., Bocci, L., Tubbs, R., Bukowski, R., Deodhar, S.D. (1985). Measurement of a monoclonal-antibody-defined antigen (CA19-9) in the sera of patients with malignant and nonmalignant diseases: comparison with carcinoembryonic antigen. *Cancer*, 56, 277–283.

Kornek, G.V., Depisch, D., Rosen, H.R., Temsch, E.M., Scheithauer, W. (1992). Comparative analysis of CA72-4, CA195 and carcinoembryonic antigen in patients with gastrointestinal malignancies. *Journal of Cancer Research and Clinical Oncology*, 118, 318–320.

Ward, U., Primrose, J.N., Finan, P.J., Perren, T.J., Selby, P., Purves, D.A., et al. (1993). The use of tumour markers CEA, CA-195 and CA-242 in evaluating the response to chemotherapy in patients with advanced colorectal cancer. *British Journal of Cancer*, 67, 1132–1135.

Vallejo, J., Torres-Avisbal, M., Contreras, P., Rodriguez-Liñán, M., Rebollo, A., González, F., et al. (1999). CEA, CA 19.9 y CA 195 en pacientes con carcinoma colorrectal: análisis ROC. (CEA, CA 19.9, and CA 195 in patients with colorectal carcinoma: ROC analysis.( *Revista Espanola de Medicina Nuclear*, 18, 281–286.

# 24
# Reduced Mammographic Screening May Explain Declines in Breast Carcinoma Among Older Women

ROBERT M. KAPLAN AND SIDNEY L. SALTZSTEIN

Life expectancy in the United States continues to lengthen (Buttler, 2003; Lubitz et al., 2003). There are many explanations for the increasing life expectancy; evidence suggests that an increasing portion of the population lives to be older than 85 years (Tuljapurkar et al., 2000; Centers for Disease Control, 2003). Some estimates suggest that by 2050 about 1 of every 43 persons will be 90 years of age or older (Day, 1996).

One consequence of increasing age is the increasing incidence of chronic diseases. We have been developing a disease reservoir hypothesis. The hypothesis suggests that disease is common, particularly among older adults; but much of the disease is not clinically significant (Kaplan, 2003). Black and Welch (1997) drew the distinction between true disease and pseudodisease. Pseudodisease is disease that, although detectable, has no clinical significance because it neither affects life expectancy nor causes symptoms or dysfunction (Kaplan, 2003). True disease either shortens life expectancy or causes symptoms. The disease reservoir hypothesis argues that the incidence of disease systematically increases with age but that most of the disease in older adults is pseudodisease. Efforts to screen for disease yield many cases in older adults because disease is there to be found (Welch & Black, 1997). Yet discovery of this disease may be of no practical importance because the disease is not clinically meaningful.

Considerable evidence suggests that the incidence of cancer systematically increases with age (American Cancer Society, 2003) up to a point. However, most analyses lump together all age groups older than 65, 75, or 85 years. It has been rare to include separate categories for those 85 to 89, 90 to 94, or 95 to 99 years of age. Saltzstein and Behling (2003) described cancer incidence in California and U.S. populations and included separate categories for the oldest age groups. They found that the incidence of many cancers declines for adults beyond 80 years of age. It is unclear whether the incidence of cancer actually has declined

Major portions of this chapter were previously published as Kaplan, R.M. & Saltzstein, S.L. (2005). Reduced mammographic screening may explain declines in breast carcinoma among older women. *Journal of the American Geriatrics Society*, 53, 862–866.

with increasing age or if cases are missed because there is less surveillance in the oldest age groups. The purpose of this study is to examine whether declines in cancer among the oldest old correspond with declines in the use of cancer testing. We use invasive carcinoma in situ (CIS) of the breast as an example.

## Methods

Data for this study came from three sources: the California Cancer Registry (CCR); the Surveillance, Epidemiology, and End Results (SEER) Program; and the Behavioral Risk Factor Surveillance System (BRFSS).

### *California Cancer Registry and SEER*

Cancer became a reportable disease in California in 1988. Since that time, all cases of cancer have been reported to the California Cancer Registry. This analysis uses data reported between 1988 and 1997. The file contains 1,346,859 cancer cases. Among them, 1,204,960 are invasive, and 141,888 are cancer in situ. The system contains demographic information including age, race/ethnicity, sex, marital status, place of birth, county of residence, and date of diagnosis. It also includes stage of disease and pathological data specifying cell differentiation and in situ versus invasive status. In addition to the California data, national U.S. data (California excluded) were added from Surveillance, Epidemiology, and End Results (SEER) Program sites of the National Cancer Institute (NCI) for the same 10 parallel years used for comparison (National Cancer Institute, Cancer Statistics Branch, 2000). The data have been described in detail elsewhere (Saltzstein & Behling, 2003). In the group 90 years of age and older, 94% of breast CIS is ductal CIS (DCIS) (in women under 70, only 70% is DCIS), the remainder being mostly lobular CIS (LCIS), mixed DCIS, and LCIS, with a small percentage of unspecified types (Saltzstein, 2004).

### *BRFSS*

The Behavioral Risk Factor Surveillance System (BRFSS) is a collaborative project between the Centers for Disease Control and Prevention (CDC) and the various U.S. territories and states. The BRFSS samples the adult population 18 years and older through telephone surveys. The study uses a random sample in each state of all households with a telephone. Approximately 95% of all households have telephone service. Interviews are conducted through Computer-Assisted Telephone Interviewing (CATI). A set of core questions that are given to all states is included in the BRFSS. These questions consider health status, health insurance, diabetes, tobacco use, and selected cancer screening including mammography. The core questions also include demographic characteristics of the sample. We employed the 2002 BRFFS, which included 99,262 male and 148,708 female respondents.

Our analysis considered whether a woman had undergone mammography within the past 2 years. In the 2002 BRFFS, women were selected if they were aged 40 or above. There were 98,809 female respondents aged 40 or older. Two questions were used to determine if mammography had been completed during the previous 2 years. The first question asked if the woman had ever had mammography, and the second asked how long ago the test had been given. Altogether, 2464 of the responses were missing, leaving 96,345 cases for analysis.

## Results

Between 1988 and 1997 there were 181,313 cases of invasive breast cancer among California women, with 2967 cases observed in women 90 years of age or older. Breast cancer in situ accounted for about 20% of all female cancers for women 69 years or younger (19,747 cases). The breast was the most common site of in situ cancer for women ages 70 to 89, accounting for 41.5% of all in situ female cancers (6775 case). However, among women 90 years or older, mammary CIS was the third most common cause of in situ cancer, with only 108 cases.

Figure 24.1 shows the rate of in situ breast cancer per 100,000 women broken down by age. The figure shows that cases peak at the 70- to 74-year age category and then systematically decline with advancing age.

Table 24.1 shows the number of women responding to BRFFS in each age category and the number in each category undergoing mammography during the last 2 years. The percentage undergoing mammography in the last 2 years is also shown in Figure 24.1. The decline after age 70–74 paralles the decline in incident cases.

Figure 24.2 shows the percentage of women who reported undergoing mammography during the past 2 years in the BRFSS. The Figure compares states with SEER registries with all other states Rates of mammography in SEER and non-SEER states appear to be equivalent.

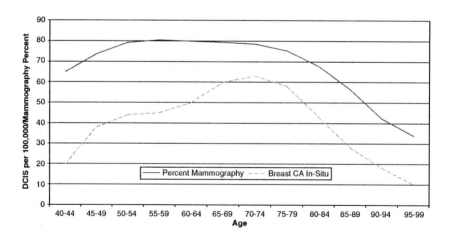

FIGURE 24.1. Mammography and in situ breast cancer by age. DCIS = ductal carcinoma in situ. (Based on data reported by Saltzstein and Behling, 2003.)

TABLE 24.1. Participation in the Behavioral Risk Factor Surveillance System and mammography during the past 2 years, by age

| Age (years) | No. | % | Mammogram during past 2 years | Percent in age group undergoing mammography |
|---|---|---|---|---|
| 40–44 | 15,276 | 15.68 | 9,928 | 65.0 |
| 45–49 | 14,607 | 14.99 | 10,780 | 73.8 |
| 50–54 | 13,731 | 14.10 | 10,878 | 79.2 |
| 55–59 | 11,517 | 11.83 | 9,273 | 80.5 |
| 60–64 | 9,505 | 9.76 | 7,596 | 79.9 |
| 65–69 | 8,945 | 9.18 | 7,105 | 79.4 |
| 70–74 | 8,478 | 8.70 | 6,663 | 78.6 |
| 75–79 | 7,349 | 7.55 | 5,532 | 75.3 |
| 80–84 | 5,077 | 5.21 | 3,442 | 67.8 |
| 85–89 | 2,112 | 2.17 | 1,191 | 56.4 |
| 90–94 | 669 | 0.69 | 282 | 42.2 |
| 95–94 | 127 | 0.13 | 43 | 33.9 |
| Total | 97,393 | 100 | 72,713 | |

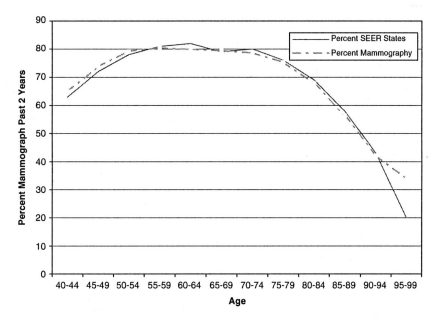

FIGURE 24.2. Percentage of women reporting having undergone mammography in the United States and Surveillance and Epidemiology End Results (SEER) states during the last 2 years from the Behavioral Risk Factor Surveillance System (BFFRS).

## Discussion

Evidence from the California Cancer Registry, SEER, and the BRFSS demonstrate that the incidence of in situ breast cancer increases with age until about age 75. After age 75, both mammary CIS and breast cancer testing decline with age.

These results are important for two reasons. First, they illustrate the importance of using separate age categories for individuals older than 75. Previous analyses that lumped together all participants in the old age categories missed these trends toward declining breast cancer in older women (Saltzstein & Behling, 2003).

The second reason these results are important is that they provide evidence relevant to the disease reservoir hypothesis. This hypothesis suggests that disease is common, particularly among the oldest members of society. If disease is present, the more we look for it, the more likely it is to be found. Yet much of detected disease may be pseudodisease, which is of little or no clinical importance. The observation by Saltzstein and Behling ( 2003) appears to be inconsistent with the disease reservoir hypothesis. According to this hypothesis, the incidence should increase with age. Saltzstein and Behling demonstrated that the incidence of mammary CIS peaks at age 75 and then declines. However, a corollary of the disease reservoir hypothesis is that pseudodisease goes undetected unless there is surveillance. Evidence from this study suggests that testing for mammary CIS increases and then decreases with advancing age. Thus, one explanation for the decline in mammary CIS with advancing age is that physicians simply are not ordering the tests that would detect it.

Welch and Black (1997) used autopsy data to estimate the reservoir of DCIS. Using hospital-based and forensic autopsy data, they estimated the prevalence of occult invasive breast cancer or DCIS over a series of autopsy evaluations. Among seven autopsy series of women who were not known to have breast cancer during their lifetimes, they found a median DCIS prevalence of 8.5%. All of the series had potential selection biases. Furthermore, the autopsy studies differed in the number of slides per breast that were examined. There was a relation between the number of slides examined and the probability of detecting mammary DCIS. Overall, these results indicated that there is a substantial reservoir of undetected mammary DCIS; and that the closer the scrutiny, the higher the probability that CIS will be detected. Much of the detected DCIS, however, may be pseudodisease, which is of little or no clinical significance. Our analysis did not separate carcinoma in situ into subcategories of ductal, lobular, and mixed; but 94% of the observed cases in women 90 years of age and older were ductal CIS.

Our study has significant limitations. We are not able to explain why the rate of ordering mammography declines with age. It is possible that physicians intuitively know that breast cancer declines with age and therefore do not order the tests. There are at least two reasons for ordering mammography: screening and clinical evaluation. Because mammography is often ordered in response to lump identification, it may be that declining breast cancer may explain the decline in mammography. This would serve as an alternative explanation for our suggestion that the declining identification of breast cancer results from failure to order mammography for older women. We cannot rule out the possibility that the true incidence of CIS declines with age. However, the report by Welch and Black suggests that there is, indeed, a substantial reservoir of undiagnosed CIS that would be identified through greater surveillance. The reduced incidence in the oldest age groups is not unique to mammary CIS. Saltzstein and Behling (2003) found that many cancers, including those of the female reproductive system and the prostate, become less common after age 85. We focused on CIS because we were able to find data on the rates of testing and because we believe identification of new cases may not lead to better health outcomes among the oldest members of the population.

Another limitation of our study is that we used cancer cases from California but estimates of mammography from the entire U.S. population. However, the Saltzstein and Behling analysis demonstrated that the California pattern of declining CIS in the older adult population mirrors that observed at other SEER registries (see also Figure 24.2). Thus, our conclusions would not change if we used national data.

## Summary

To understand the incidence of breast cancer in older women, it is important to include separate categories of women for age groups 85 to 89, 90 to 94, 95 to 99, and 100+ years. Studies using these older age categories show a decline in CIS and invasive breast cancer with advancing age. These declines may be explained by decreased surveillance in older women. To rule out alternative explanations, we believe that systematic autopsy studies including older people and examining breast tissue as thoroughly as with surgical specimens and including mammography must be conducted.

## *References*

American Cancer Society (2003). *Cancer facts and figures—2003*. Atlanta, GA: American Cancer Society.

Black, W.C., Welch, H.G. (1997). Screening for disease. *American Journal of Roentgenology, 168*, 3–11.

Buttler, G. (2003). [Increasing life expectancy: what are the promises of demography?] *Zeitschrift für Gerontologie und Geriatrie, 36*(2), 90–94.

Centers for Disease Control (2003). *Health, United States, 2003 with chartbook on trends in the health of Americans*. Atlanta, GA: Centers for Disease Control.

Day, J. (1996). *Populations projections of the United States by age, sex, race and Hispanic origin: 1995–2050*. Washington, DC: US Government Printing Office.

Kaplan, R.M. (2003). The significance of quality of life in health care. *Quality of Life Research, 12(Suppl), 1*, 3–16.

Lubitz, J., Cai, L., Kramarow, E., Lentzner, H. (2003). Health, life expectancy, and health care spending among the elderly. *New England Journal of Medicine, 349*, 1048–1055.

National Cancer Institute, Cancer Statistics Branch (2000). *Surveillance, epidemiology, and end results (SEER) program public-use CD-ROM (1973–1997)*. Rockville, MD: National Cancer Institute, Cancer Statistics Branch.

Saltzstein, S.L. (2004). Unpublished data. California Cancer Registry.

Saltzstein, S.L., Behling, C.A. (2003). *Cancer in the chronologically gifted: a study of 45,000 cases of cancer in people 90 years of age and older*. San Diego, CA: San Diego and Imperial Organization for Cancer Control.

Tuljapurkar, S., Li, N., Boe, C. (2000). A universal pattern of mortality decline in the G7 countries. *Nature, 405*, 789–792.

Welch, H.G., Black, W.C. (1997). Using autopsy series to estimate the disease "reservoir" for ductal carcinoma in situ of the breast: how much more breast cancer can we find? *Annals of Internal Medicine, 127*, 1023–1028.

# 25
# "Fading of Reported Effectiveness" Bias: Longitudinal Meta-Analysis of Randomized Controlled Trials

BERNHARD T. GEHR, CHRISTEL WEISS, AND FRANZ PORZSOLT

Meta-analyses have become an instrument that is fundamental to the idea of best medical care. Meta-analyses combine the results of a large number of randomized controlled trials (RCTs) on a certain topic to gain more significant results. Should the reported effect size of RCTs change with time, the result of a meta-analysis would depend on when it was performed. Thus, the validity of a meta-analysis could be impaired.

Although an extensive literature search on this topic yielded no results in the medical field, we identified one relevant study in the field of biology. Jennions and Moeller (2002) recently examined 44 meta-analyses covering topics such as animal behavior, parasitism, and plant growth. They found a small but highly significant decline in the strength of reported correlations with the publication date (best model: $p < 0.0001$; R = −0.133) and the sample size (best model: $p < 0.002$; R = −0.188). In other words, the investigated meta-analyses estimated higher intervention effects if they were performed earlier. The authors attributed the decrease to *publication bias* (underreporting of studies with small sample sizes and little effect) and *time of publication bias* (studies that report large effect sizes are published sooner than other studies). Unfortunately, they did not investigate whether sample size increased with the publication year, and they failed to describe the time lag between study completion and publication date for the individual studies, which would have been necessary to verify their hypotheses. Moreover, as it remains unclear whether results from the field of biology also apply to medical research. This chapter describes a meta-analysis of clinical drug trials to examine the reported effectiveness of a specific medical treatment over time.

The objective of our longitudinal meta-analysis was to determine if the effect size of medical therapies reported in RCTs changes with time. We also intended to identify reasons for any possible change. The unit of analysis was the individual study, not the individual trial participant.

Why should the effect size of a medical intervention change with time? Our hypothesis is based on the assumption that we have to distinguish between the "real" effectiveness of a medical therapy and the effectiveness reported in RCTs and that the latter may change with time.

- The "real" size of the biological effect of a medical therapy is constant over time, which means it should be possible to obtain similar results when a trial is repeated at a later date. If a study investigating, for example, the effectiveness of beta-blocker therapy in patients with arterial hypertension is conducted today, 10 or 20 years does not alter the effect size of the pharmaceutical. We know that in some cases this does not apply. For example, bacteria can become resistant to antibiotics, so the effectiveness of these pharmaceuticals may decline with time. However, these examples are rare, and the real effect size should be constant in most cases.
- The sum of all kinds of bias influencing the reported effect size of a medical therapy is not necessarily constant over time. During the course of time, social, political, and economic circumstances surrounding medical research and its publication change. Therefore, it can be assumed that the impact of the various potential sources of bias also changes dynamically with time. In consequence, the effect size of a medical therapy reported in RCTs may change over time.

Because we presumed that if there were any change at all the reported effectiveness of medical therapies was more likely to decrease than to increase, we tested three hypotheses that might explain a decrease in the reported effect size.

- *Decreasing publication bias.* The problem of publication bias is well known in the medical literature (Dickersin et al., 1987; Easterbrook et al., 1991; Callaham et al., 1998; Egger & Smith, 1998). Studies with positive outcomes and significant results are more likely to get published, leading to underrepresentation of studies with negative or nonsignificant results in meta-analyses. Because the level of significance rises with increasing study size, the problem of publication bias more likely applies to studies with smaller sample sizes. New medical therapies are first tried in small selected populations, followed by larger trials to validate the benefits in larger populations. Increasing study size should lead to a decrease in publication bias and to lower reported effect sizes over time.
- *Selection bias.* New medical interventions tend to be studied in severely ill patients in whom significant benefits can be expected. After a therapy has been established, physicians tend to broaden its use and prescribe it to a wide range of patients, including a large number of less sick patients. In addition, specific treatment goals have been developed in recent years for several diseases, such as hypertension, diabetes mellitus, and glaucoma. Patients who might not have been treated a decade ago receive therapy today. In less sick patients, less improvement of the study parameter can be expected. Over time, the effectiveness of the therapy seems to diminish.
- *"Shift of treatment group" bias.* Although the studies were conducted as RCTs, expectations of patients, physicians, and study authors may play a role by favoring the therapy used in the experimental treatment group. Over time, medical therapies become established and are used as control new therapies in later studies. This may lead to a decrease in the reported effect size over time.

To answer our questions, we examined data from a large number of RCTs dealing with the effectiveness of four pharmaceuticals. The primary outcome measure was the reported effect size. Secondary outcome measures were the publication year, study size, mean preintervention level of the investigated parameter, and treatment assignment to experimental or control group.

## Methods

### Selection of Pharmaceuticals

The pharmaceuticals to be investigated in this experiment had to meet the following requirements: (1) their effectiveness was measurable in terms of commonly accepted, quantitative parameters that are reported in most studies; (2) the pharmaceuticals were administered as a monotherapy and in a fixed dosage to obtain a large number of studies with comparable results; (3) the therapies were of clinical importance and of general interest. For our investigation, we arbitrarily chose the lipid-lowering drugs pravastatin and atorvastatin [route of administration: oral; outcome measure: change in serum low-density lipoprotein (LDL) cholesterol] and the antiglaucoma drugs timolol and latanoprost (eye drops; change in intraocular pressure).

### Date Sources

A standardized literature search was performed with emphasis on transparency and repeatability rather than on completeness. Our MEDLINE search strategy included the following text strings (PubMed, 2003): "pravastatin LDL," "atorvastatin LDL," "timolol glaucoma," and "latanoprost glaucoma." The literature search was performed for the time up to and including December 2001. The MEDLINE search was limited to studies on human subjects and to items with abstracts only. A filter for randomized controlled trials was used. Non-English studies were included.

### Study Selection

A study was included if it met the following criteria: (1) baseline value and postintervention value of the parameter of interest were reported, that is, LDL cholesterol for pravastatin and atorvastatin and intraocular pressure for timolol and latanoprost; (2) the pharmaceutical was administered as monotherapy and after a washout period; (3) the pharmaceutical was administered in the most commonly used dosage, that is, pravastatin 40 mg once daily, atorvastatin 10 mg once daily, timolol 0.5% twice daily, and latanoprost 0.005% once daily; and (4) the study was conducted as an RCT. One investigator (B.T.G.) reviewed 625 citations and selected appropriate studies. A total of 274 studies were considered for more detailed evaluation. Figure 25.1 shows the selection process for the 206 studies finally deemed appropriate for inclusion.

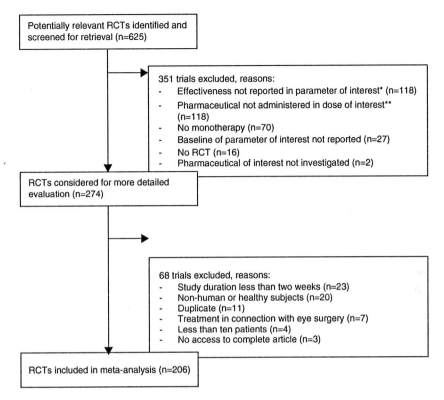

FIGURE 25.1. Flow diagram. RCT, randomized controlled trial; *n*, number of trials. Reported effectiveness of the pharmaceutical is measured as the change in intraocular pressure (timolol, latanoprost) or in low-density lipoprotein cholesterol (pravastatin, atorvastatin). The dose of interest were measured in comparability studies. Studies that did not use the pharmaceutical in the most common dosage were excluded, as were studies that increased the individual dosage until a certain outcome was reached.

## Data Extraction

One of the authors (B.T.G.) extracted the following data for each study: publication year, study size (number of evaluated patients), pre- and postintervention mean values of LDL cholesterol/intraocular pressure, and assignment to experimental or control group. Whenever necessary, means were approximated from figures in the manuscripts or calculated from individual patient data. In each study, the effect size for the intervention was calculated by the difference between the means of the group before and after intervention. In some studies, more than one postintervention mean was reported, for example, for different follow-up visits or for different hours of the day. In these cases, the arithmetic mean of the given means was calculated instead of choosing one of the given means arbitrarily.

A study was designated a "control group" if the pharmaceutical of interest was compared with at least one newer pharmaceutical. The designation "experimental group" was chosen if the pharmaceutical of interest was compared with older pharmaceuticals or if no other pharmaceuticals were involved in the study (for instance, placebo-controlled studies or studies comparing the effectiveness of different dosages of the same pharmaceutical).

## Statistical Analysis

Statistical analysis was performed with SAS software (SAS release 8.02; SAS Institute, Cary, NC, USA). Arithmetic means and standard deviations were calculated for each of the variables (publication year, reported effect size, baseline, study size). The reported effect size was measured in the most commonly reported dimension: pravastatin and atorvastatin, change in LDL cholesterol (%); timolol and latanoprost, change in intraocular pressure (mmHg). As the variable treatment group is dichotomous, with the two possibilities "experimental group" and "control group," exact frequencies are reported.

The primary outcome parameter (reported effect size) and the secondary outcome parameters (baseline, study size, treatment group) were regressed against the publication year. For the variable treatment group, point biserial correlation was used (control group = 0, experimental group = 1). For every correlation, the equation of the regression line and the limits of its 95% confidence interval (CI) were calculated. This enabled the mean change of every parameter during an interval of 5 years (± 95% CI) to be calculated.

Bivariate qualitative analyses of the investigated parameters in all possible combinations were performed (analysis of covariance). Pearson's correlation coefficients and p values were calculated. We used a standard approach for statistical significance (α = 0.05). The funnel plot technique was used to detect publication bias (Egger et al., 1997; Macaskill et al., 2001; Sterne & Egger, 2001). Diagrams of the relation between study size and reported effect size were drawn and visually checked for asymmetry.

We performed a multiple regression analysis, with reported effect size as the outcome variable and publication year, baseline, study size, and treatment group as possible predictors. Up to two predictors were entered into the model to quantify the impact of the various predictors on the outcome variable.

We investigated whether measuring the primary outcome parameter in absolute or relative dimensions changes the significance levels of the results. Bivariate qualitative analysis and multiple regression analysis were performed, with reported effect size measured in absolute terms (pravastatin and atorvastatin: LDL cholesterol change in mg/dl, timolol and latanoprost: intraocular pressure change in mmHg) and in relative terms (change in outcome parameter in percentages).

We could not investigate the change of reported effectiveness in the control therapies of the pharmaceutical of interest because the control therapies were different in almost all of the studies. The chance to find a study comparing exactly the same control and experimental group several years later is small.

# Results

## Included Trials and Their Characteristics

A total of 206 studies were included in the final analysis, as shown in Figure 25.1. (A list of the individual trials and the extracted raw data are available from the corresponding author.) A total of 64 of the included studies investigate pravastatin, 35 atorvastatin, 75 timolol, and 32 latanoprost.

Table 25.1 shows the mean ± SD year of publication, reported effect size, baseline value, and study size for each of the four investigated medical therapies. Exact effect sizes are given for the dichotomous variable treatment group (experimental/control group). Pravastatin lowered the LDL cholesterol (LDL-C) on average by 29.50% ± 4.16% and atorvastatin by 36.07% ± 3.70%; timolol lowered the intraocular pressure (IOP) on average by 6.55 ± 1.56 mmHg and latanoprost by 6.83 ± 1.53 mmHg.

## Effect of Time on the Investigated Parameters

Over time, the reported effect size decreased significantly for three of the four investigated pharmaceuticals, as shown in Figure 25.2 and Tables 25.2 and 25.3. Pravastatin on average was reported to lower the patient's LDL-C by 3.22% less every 5 years [95% confidence interval (CI): ± 1.28] ($p < 0.0001$), in other words, by 29.74% in 1995 and by 26.52% in 2000. Timolol was reported to reduce the intraocular pressure by 0.56 ± 0.22 mmHg less every 5 years ($p < 0.0001$) and latanoprost by 1.78 ± 1.26 mmHg less every 5 years ($p = 0.0074$). The reported effect size of atorvastatin did not change significantly over time ($p = 0.8618$).

Most of the other investigated parameters changed over time as well, as shown in Tables 25.2 and 25.3. The baseline values of the parameter of interest decreased over time for all investigated pharmaceuticals. This relation was significant for pravastatin (–41.80 mg/dl LDL-C every 5 years) ($p < 0.0001$) and timolol (–0.70 mmHg IOP every 5 years) ($p = 0.0004$). The study size increased over time for three of the four pharmaceuticals; this relation was significant only for timolol (+80.55 patients every 5 years) ($p < 0.0001$). The variable treatment group changed over time from the experimental group toward the control group for all investigated pharmaceuticals. This relation was significant for pravastatin (–0.20 every 5 years), meaning that in all pravastatin studies 20% less used pravastatin in the experimental treatment arm every 5 years and 20% more in the control arm ($p = 0.0008$). For timolol the figure was –0.12 every 5 years ($p < 0.0001$).

## Other Bivariate Analyses

For pravastatin, timolol, and latanoprost, the reported effect sizes correlated significantly with the baseline values of the parameter of interest, as shown in Table 25.3. The reported effect size was related to the treatment group for atorvastatin ($p = 0.0092$). There was no significant correlation between study size and

TABLE 25.1. Trial characteristics

| Parameter | Pravastatin (n = 64) | | | | Atorvastatin (n = 35) | | | | Timolol (n = 75) | | | | Latanoprost (n = 32) | | | |
|---|---|---|---|---|---|---|---|---|---|---|---|---|---|---|---|---|
| | Mean | ± SD | Min. | Max. | Mean | ± SD | Min. | Max. | Mean | ± SD | Min. | Max. | Mean | ± SD | Min. | Max. |
| Year of publication | 1995.28 | ± 3.46 | 1990 | 2001 | 1999.40 | ± 1.82 | 1996 | 2001 | 1992.68 | ± 6.99 | 1978 | 2001 | 1999.06 | ± 2.00 | 1995 | 2001 |
| Reported effect size[a] | −29.50 | ± 4.16 | −19.0 | −39.0 | −36.07 | ± 3.70 | −28.4 | −44.2 | −6.55 | ± 1.56 | −3.65 | −11.3 | −6.83 | ± 1.53 | −3.5 | −9.8 |
| Baseline[b] | 205.62 | ± 47.78 | 134.4 | 344.0 | 198.05 | ± 35.05 | 143.0 | 340.3 | 25.94 | ± 2.49 | 20.8 | 38.7 | 24.07 | ± 2.13 | 19.3 | 28.2 |
| Study size[c] | 595.77 | ± 1511.59 | 10 | 9014 | 328.71 | ± 686.64 | 22 | 3916 | 197.96 | ± 249.59 | 12 | 1198 | 152.81 | ± 195.57 | 20 | 829 |
| Treatment group[d] | EG: 56 (87%); CG: 8 (13%) | | | | EG: 31 (89%); CG: 4 (11%) | | | | EG: 12 (16%); CG: 63 (84%) | | | | EG: 29 (91%); CG: 3 (9%) | | | |

n = number of trials that met selection criteria; EG = experimental group; CG = control group.

[a] Unit of measurement for reported effect size: change of intraocular pressure (IOP) measured in millimeters of mercury (timolol, latanoprost), change in low-density lipoprotein cholesterol (LDL-C) measured in percent (pravastatin, atorvastatin).

[b] Unit of measurement for baseline: IOP measured in millimeters of mercury (timolol, latanoprost), LDL-C measured in milligrams per deciliter (pravastatin, atorvastatin). To convert LDL-C from milligrams per deciliter to millimoles per liter, multiply the milligrams per deciliter by 0.0259.

[c] Unit of measurement for study size: number of patients included in final analysis.

[d] As the variable "treatment group" is either the "experimental group" or the "control group," exact frequencies and percentages are given.

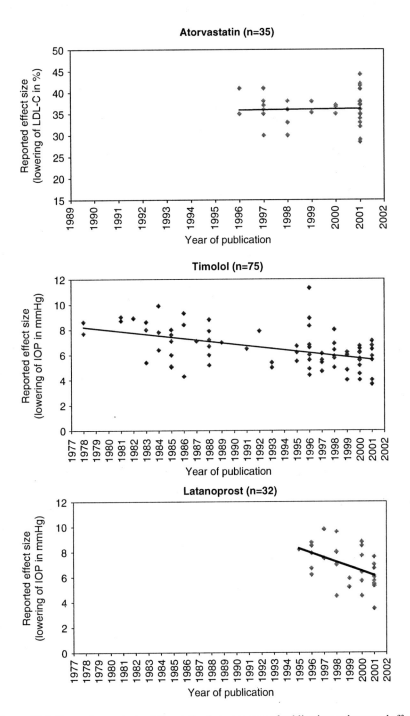

FIGURE 25.2. Regression analysis of the relation between year of publication and reported effectiveness of pravastatin ($y = 90.818 - 0.643x$; $p < 0.0001$), atorvastatin ($y = 29.900 + 0.062x$; $p = 0.8618$, not significant), timolol ($y = 16.983 - 0.113x$; $p < 0.0001$), and latanoprost ($y = 42.069 - 0.356x$; $p = 0.0074$). IOP = intraocular pressure; LDL-C = low-density lipoprotein cholesterol; x = reported effectiveness—for timolol and latanoprost change of IOP (mmHg), for pravastatin and atorvastatin change of LDL-C (%); y = year of publication minus 1900.

TABLE 25.2. Bivariate quantitative analyses of all investigated parameters in dependence of year of publication

| Parameter | Pravastatin | Atorvastatin | Timolol | Latanoprost |
|---|---|---|---|---|
| Reported effect size[a] | | | | |
| Change in | | | | |
| 5 years | −3.22 | +0.31 | −0.56 | −1.78 |
| 95% CI limits | −4.50/−1.93 | −3.29/+3.91 | −0.79/−0.34 | −3.04/−0.51 |
| Baseline[b] | | | | |
| Change in | | | | |
| 5 years | −41.80 | −14.63 | −0.70 | −1.82 |
| 95% CI limits | −55.74/−27.86 | −48.38/+19.11 | −1.08/−0.32 | −3.69 / +0.05 |
| Study size[c] | | | | |
| Change in | | | | |
| 5 years | +533.54 | +233.63 | +80.55 | −16.94 |
| 95% CI limits | −3.94/+1071.01 | −429.97/+897.23 | +43.38/+117.71 | −199.23/+165.35 |
| Treatment group[d] | | | | |
| Change in | | | | |
| 5 years | −0.20 | −0.28 | −0.12 | −0.23 |
| 95% CI limits | −0.31/−0.08 | −0.58/+0.01 | −0.17/−0.06 | −0.50/+0.03 |

All given data are calculated from the equations of the regression lines. For statistical significance ($p$), see Table 25.3.

CI = confidence interval; LDL-C = low-density lipoprotein cholesterol.

[a]Unit of measurement for reported effect size: change of intraocular pressure (IOP) measured in millimeters of mercury (timolol, latanoprost); change in LDL-C measured in percent (pravastatin, atorvastatin).

[b]Unit of measurement for baseline: IOP measured in millimeters of mercury (timolol, latanoprost); LDL-C measured in milligrams per deciliter (pravastatin, atorvastatin). To convert LDL-C from milligrams per deciliter to millimoles per liter, multiply milligrams per deciliter by 0.0259.

[c]Unit of measurement for study size: number of patients included in final analysis.

[d]The parameter treatment group has two possibilities: control group = 0, experimental group = 1. Point biserial correlation was used to obtain the equation of the regression line and to calculate the given data.

reported effect size (in the most commonly reported dimension) for any of the investigated pharmaceuticals.

## Measuring Effect Size in Relative or Absolute Dimensions

Some results of the lipid-lowering drugs were altered when the reported effect size was measured in absolute, not relative, terms. When measuring the change of LDL-C in milligrams per deciliter and not in percentages, (1) the relation between reported effect size and baseline value *was significant* for atorvastatin ($p < 0.0001$ vs. $p = 0.4045$); (2) the relation between the reported effect size and the treatment group *was no longer significant* for atorvastatin ($p = 0.3731$ vs. $p = 0.0092$); and (3) the relation between reported effect size and study size *was significant* for pravastatin ($p = 0.0139$ vs. $p = .1327$). For timolol and latanoprost, the results were not altered if the reported effect size was measured in relative terms and not in absolute terms.

TABLE 25.3. Bivariate qualitative analyses of all investigated parameters

| Parameter | Reported effect size[a] | | | Baseline | | | Study size | | | Treatment group[b] | | |
|---|---|---|---|---|---|---|---|---|---|---|---|---|
| | Ph | R | p | Ph | R | p | Ph | R | p | Ph | R | p |
| Year of publication | P: | −0.5360 | <.0001 | P: | −0.6056 | <.0001 | P: | 0.2444 | 0.0517 | P: | −0.4092 | 0.0008 |
| | A: | 0.0305 | 0.8618 | A: | −0.1518 | 0.3840 | A: | 0.1237 | 0.4789 | A: | −0.3207 | 0.0603 |
| | T: | −0.5043 | <.0001 | T: | −0.3955 | 0.0004 | T: | 0.4512 | <.0001 | T: | −0.4513 | <.0001 |
| | L: | −0.4642 | 0.0074 | L: | −0.3413 | 0.0559 | L: | −0.0346 | 0.8508 | L: | −0.3167 | 0.0774 |
| Reported effect size | 1.00 | | | P: | 0.2591 | 0.0387 | P: | −0.1899 | 0.1327 | P: | 0.1598 | 0.2073 |
| | | | | A: | −0.1454 | 0.4045 | A: | 0.0381 | 0.8281 | A: | −0.4339 | 0.0092 |
| | | | | T: | 0.6949 | <.0001 | T: | −0.1364 | 0.2432 | T: | 0.1565 | 0.1801 |
| | | | | L: | 0.8745 | <.0001 | L: | 0.2206 | 0.2251 | L: | 0.0289 | 0.8753 |
| Baseline | | | | 1.00 | | | P: | −0.2897 | 0.0202 | P: | 0.0872 | 0.4933 |
| | | | | | | | A: | −0.0868 | 0.6201 | A: | 0.0848 | 0.6282 |
| | | | | | | | T: | −0.1923 | 0.0983 | T: | 0.0686 | 0.5587 |
| | | | | | | | L: | 0.2673 | 0.1392 | L: | −0.1069 | 0.5604 |
| Study size | | | | | | | 1.00 | | | P: | 0.0566 | 0.6568 |
| | | | | | | | | | | A: | 0.1106 | 0.5269 |
| | | | | | | | | | | T: | −0.2723 | 0.0181 |
| | | | | | | | | | | L: | −0.3557 | 0.0457 |

Ph = pharmaceutical; T = timolol; L = latanoprost; P = pravastatin; A = atorvastatin ; R = Pearson's correlation coefficient.

[a] Reported effect size for pravastatin and atorvastatin is measured in relative terms (%), for timolol and latanoprost in absolute terms (mmHg).

[b] As the parameter treatment group only has the possibilities control group (= 0) or experimental group (= 1), point biserial correlation was used.

Significant correlations ($p < 0.05$) are highlighted with gray background.

## Multiple Regression Analysis

The results of the multiple regression analysis differed depending on whether the effect size was measured in absolute or relative terms. If measured in absolute terms, the parameter *baseline* was the most reliable predictor and explained 80.37% of the variability of the reported effect size of pravastatin ($R^2$) (Table 25.4), 69.59% of atorvastatin, 48.29% of timolol, and 76.47% of latanoprost. If the parameters *publication year* or *treatment group* were entered, an additional 3.11% to 6.24% of the variability was explained by the model. The variable *study size* accounted for not more than 0.23%.

If the effect size was measured in relative terms, the results of the multiple regression analysis were less homogenous; but overall the *year of publication* was the most important predictor for the reported effect size. For pravastatin and timolol the parameter publication year alone explained 28.73% and 19.58%, respectively, of the variability in effect size ($R^2$) (Table 25.4). For pravastatin other parameters did not add more than 0.68% when entered in the model. For timolol, the *baseline value* added 3.93% and the *study size* 2.48%. For the

TABLE 25.4. Multiple regression analysis to explain the variability of the parameter "reported effect size"

| Ranking of model | Effect size measured in absolute terms | | Effect size measured in relative terms | |
| --- | --- | --- | --- | --- |
| | Variables in model | $R^2$ | Variables in model | $R^2$ |
| Pravastatin | | | | |
| 1 | B, Y | 0.8477 | Y, B | 0.2941 |
| 2 | B, T | 0.8077 | Y, T | 0.2916 |
| 3 | B, n | 0.8060 | Y, n | 0.2910 |
| 4 | B | 0.8037 | Y | 0.2873 |
| Atorvastatin | | | | |
| 1 | B, T | 0.7473 | T, Y | 0.2014 |
| 2 | B, Y | 0.6961 | T, B | 0.2001 |
| 3 | B, n | 0.6960 | T, n | 0.1957 |
| 4 | B | 0.6959 | T | 0.1882 |
| Timolol | | | | |
| 1 | B, Y | 0.5453 | Y, B | 0.2351 |
| 2 | B, T | 0.4948 | Y, n | 0.2206 |
| 3 | B, n | 0.4829 | Y, T | 0.1979 |
| 4 | B | 0.4829 | Y | 0.1958 |
| Latanoprost | | | | |
| 1 | B, Y | 0.7958 | B, Y | 0.5636 |
| 2 | B, T | 0.7798 | B, T | 0.5306 |
| 3 | B, n | 0.7649 | B, n | 0.5030 |
| 4 | B | 0.7647 | B | 0.5030 |

Shown are the top four models taking into account one or two variables with the effect size measured in absolute or in relative dimensions.
Y = year of publication; B = baseline of parameter of interest; T = treatment group; n = study size; $R^2$ = determination coefficient.

reported effect size of atorvastatin, *treatment group* was the most important predictor ($R^2 = 0.1882$) and of latanoprost the parameter *baseline value* ($R^2 = 0.5030$).

## Evaluation of Potential Bias

The funnel plot technique was used to evaluate publication bias. The study size was plotted against the reported effect size of the study, as shown in Figure 25.3. The plots of atorvastatin and latanoprost did not show relevant asymmetry, indicating that significant publication bias was unlikely. The plots of pravastatin and

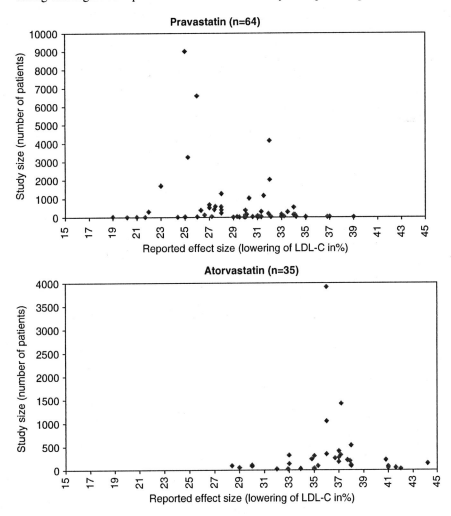

FIGURE 25.3. Funnel plots showing the relation between study size and reported effectiveness. None of the relations are statistically significant (pravastatin $p = 0.1327$; atorvastatin $p = 0.8281$; timolol $p = 0.2432$; latanoprost: $p = 0.2251$). n, number of trials; IOP, intraocular pressure; LDL-C, low-density lipoprotein cholesterol.

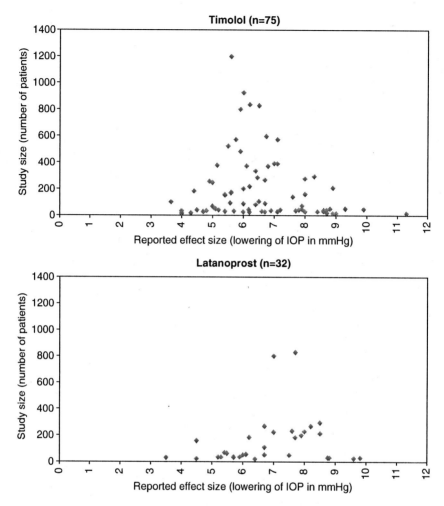

FIGURE 25.3. (*Continued*)

timolol showed slight asymmetry. For example, the timolol studies, including more than 500 patients, reported effect sizes of about 6 mmHg. More of the smaller studies than represented on the funnel plot should report effect sizes of less than 6 mmHg.

## Discussion

It must be stressed that the investigated medical interventions were chosen arbitrarily based on the criteria stated in the methods section. We chose to conduct our investigation using pharmaceutical interventions for methodological reasons, but our theory is not limited to drug therapies.

## Reported Effect Size Decreases Over Time

Our empirical evaluation of 206 RCTs shows that the reported effect size of three of the four investigated pharmaceuticals decreased significantly over time. When pravastatin, timolol and latanoprost were new, studies reported them to be more effective than studies that were conducted in later years. We call this a "FORE[1] bias" (fading of reported effectiveness bias).

The FORE bias may contribute to many clinicians' impression that the "real" clinical improvement is not as impressive as publications in medical journals suggest. For example, in 1978, when the antiglaucoma beta-blocker timolol was new, it was reported to lower the IOP by an average of 8.17 mmHg (calculated from Figure 25.2). By 1995, this had decreased to an average of 6.25 mmHg. More recently, the prostaglandin analogon latanoprost was introduced for glaucoma therapy. In 1995, latanoprost was reported to lower the IOP by an average of 8.25 mmHg. Compared to timolol during the same year, latanoprost was 2.00 mmHg more effective; compared to timolol in 1978, latanoprost was equally effective. Improvement may have been more a matter of perception than reality. Being aware of the risk of FORE bias can contribute to improving our understanding of medical progress.

For one of the investigated pharmaceuticals, there was no significant change in the reported effectiveness over time. For atorvastatin, analyses in relation to time may not yet be feasible, as this pharmaceutical is relatively new, and there is little variability of the publication dates ($1999.40 \pm 1.82$) (Table 25.1).

When conducting different trials about the same topic, perfect consistency of the results certainly cannot be expected. Even the best designed studies may differ in several parameters, leading to a broad continuum of reported effect sizes, as shown in Figure 25.2. This finding is expected, but a temporal trend in the development of the continuum, as described above, must be the result of other factors.

## Reasons for the Decline in Reported Effectiveness

We investigated whether the decrease in reported effectiveness was influenced by the patients' baseline levels of disease, by the treatment assignment to the experimental or the control group, or by the study size.

### Selection Bias

For all of the investigated medical therapies we studied, the baseline values of the parameter of interest decreased over time; that is, patients who had been included in the earlier trials were sicker than patients in later trials. This was highly significant for pravastatin and timolol and just short of the chosen level of significance for latanoprost (Tables 25.2 and 25.3). The baseline values were, again, the most important predictors of the reported effect size. Our multiple regression analysis

---

[1]"Fore!" is a shout given to warn people that a golf ball is about to hit another player and is therefore a matter of transparency. The adjective "fore" means "situated in the front part of a vehicle." Because the FORE bias is situated mainly in the front part of a series of publications and because we strive for maximum transparency in meta-analyses, we chose this acronym.

showed that up to 80.37% of the effect size variability was explained by the baseline value differences (Table 25.4). We conclude that most of the decline in reported effectiveness over time was explained by the baseline value differences.

Decreasing Publication Bias

We found only weak evidence for the hypothesis that the decline in reported effectiveness could be mediated by study size. In theory, the combination of publication bias and increased study size could contribute to the gradual decrease in reported effect size. We found an increase in study size over time for timolol ($p < 0.0001$) (Table 25.3) and pravastatin ($p = 0.0517$, not significant). The relation between study size and reported effect size was weak. It was significant only for pravastatin and then only when the outcome parameter was measured in absolute terms ($p = 0.0139$). We conclude that very little of the loss of reported effectiveness was influenced by the study size.

"Shift of Treatment Group" Bias

We did not find evidence for the hypothesis that the treatment assignment to experimental or control group influenced its reported effect size, although there was a strong correlation between publication year and treatment group (Table 25.3). The latter correlation was to be expected because a medical therapy would be typically studied as the experimental therapy when new and as the control therapy when established. The relation between treatment group and effect size was very weak. The correlation was significant only for atorvastatin and only if the treatment effect was measured in relative terms, surprisingly favoring the *control group*. Nevertheless, the treatment group parameter is involved in several of the best multiple regression analysis models (Table 25.4). These results must be interpreted with care because of the problem of multicolinearity, especially between publication year and treatment group.

Other Potential Influencing Factors

Our study was limited in that we did not explore whether parameters other than baseline value, treatment group, and study size contribute to the decrease of the reported effect size over time. From the statistical viewpoint, there must be other factors that play a role in the temporal development of the reported effect size.

The influence of the time of publication bias, study quality, and financial conflicts of interest on study outcome are known; but to the best of our knowledge, it has not yet been studied how temporal trends in these factors influence the reported effectiveness of medical therapies over time.

The "time of publication bias," which has been described in recent years, leads to an apparently decreasing effect size. Several reports indicate that studies with positive or significant results are published an average of 2 to 3 years more rapidly than studies with negative or nonsignificant results (Stern & Simes, 1997; Ioannidis, 1998; Misakian & Bero, 1998). Although the publication of studies with negative results is delayed during the first years after a new pharmaceutical has become available, studies with positive outcomes dominate in meta-analyses. The size of the treatment effect may thus be overestimated. Little by little, the average reported effect size decreases to a lower level when studies with negative results are also published. In future meta-analyses, this bias could be addressed by taking into account the date of study completion and not the date of publication.

Changes in study quality may be related to the decrease in reported effect size. During the last decades, methodological trial quality has improved significantly in many areas of medicine (Kidwell et al., 2001; Kjaergard et al., 2002). There are a substantial number of reports that higher study quality is associated with lower estimates of treatment effects (Schulz et al., 1995; Moher et al., 1998; Goetsche & Olsen, 2000; Ioannidis et al., 2001; Nieuwenhoven et al., 2001). This may contribute to our observation that the reported effectiveness of medical therapies fades over time. In our meta-analysis we did not assess study quality because of the well known lack of established quality scores (Jüni et al., 1999; Balk et al., 2002) and because it is often impossible to distinguish study quality from reporting quality. Nevertheless, future meta-analyses should take into consideration the effect of trial quality development.

Unlike the other described factors, the problem of financial conflicts of interest on the part of scientists is likely to lead to an *increase* in reported effectiveness over time. In our meta-analysis, this effect may have mitigated the size of the observed decrease in reported effect size. In the United States, industry's share of total investment in biomedical research and development grew from approximately 32% in 1980 to 62% in 2000 (Bekelman et al., 2003); and more and more industry sponsorship is being reported in many areas of medicine (Dorman et al., 1999; Hussain & Smith, 2001; Kidwell et al., 2001). It is well known in the literature that studies funded by for-profit organizations are more likely to recommend the experimental therapy as the treatment of choice and less likely to report unfavorable conclusions (Friedberg et al., 1999; Kjaergard & Als-Nielsen, 2002; Als-Nielsen et al., 2003; Bekelman, 2003). Therefore, the reported effectiveness could improve with time. We did not investigate the role of competing financial interests in our meta-analysis because we could not determine which authors had adhered to the disclosure guidelines (Hussain & Smith, 2001; Gross et al., 2003), but further studies should address this issue.

## Consequences for the Validity of Meta-Analyses

This study suggests that the effectiveness of medical therapies reported in RCTs is not necessarily constant, and that it may decline with time (FORE bias). A meta-analysis sums up evidence from a large number of RCTs that have usually been conducted over an extensive period of time. If a FORE bias is present, the result of a meta-analysis depends on when it was performed.

- A meta-analysis investigating the effectiveness of a single medical therapy that was conducted when the therapy was relatively new may estimate higher treatment effects than a meta-analysis that was conducted later.

- A meta-analysis comparing the effectiveness of two or more medical therapies produce distorted results favoring the newer therapies or therapies that are less subjected to the FORE bias.

We conclude that the validity of a meta-analysis may be impaired when a FORE bias is present. To establish maximal transparency, we propose to include a test for FORE bias in future meta-analyses. In our view, it would be sufficient to plot effect size against publication year, as shown in Figure 25.2, and to calculate the significance level and the equation of the regression line of this correlation. Given this information, the reader could make up his or her own mind if the validity of the meta-analysis is undermined.

## Summary

The current meta-analysis suggests that the effectiveness of medical therapies, as reported in RCTs, may decrease over time. We call this phenomenon the "fading of reported effectiveness" (FORE) bias. Baseline differences could be identified as the main factor contributing to this effect; changes in study size or treatment group did not play a significant role. As the validity of a meta-analysis where a FORE bias is present may be undermined, we propose to include a test for FORE bias in future meta-analyses. Furthermore, we encourage others to replicate this study with a focus on other clinical areas and interventions. Future research should include the analysis of additional factors, such as time of publication bias, trial quality, and financial conflicts of interest. We need to learn more about the implication of the FORE bias for the interpretation of meta-analyses.

*Acknowledgements.* The authors thank Ernst Pöppel for his general support and Stefan Stein and Kathleen M. Schoennagel for reviewing the manuscript.

## *References*

Als-Nielsen, B., Chen, W., Gluud, C., Kjaergard, L.L. (2003). Association of funding and conclusions in randomized drug trials. *Journal of the American Medical Association,* 290, 921–928.

Balk, E.M., Bonis, P.A.L., Moskowitz, H., Schmid, C.H., Ioannidis, J.P., Wang, C., et al. (2002). Correlation of quality measures with estimates of treatment effect in meta-analyses of randomized controlled trials. *Journal of the American Medical Association,* 287, 2973–2982.

Bekelman, J.E., Li, Y., Gross, C.P. (2003). Scope and impact of financial conflicts of interest in biomedical research. *Journal of the American Medical Association,* 289, 454–465.

Callaham, M.L., Wears, R.L., Weber, E.J., Barton, C., Young, G. (1998). Positive-outcome bias and other limitations in the outcome of research abstracts submitted to a scientific meeting. *Journal of the American Medical Association,* 280, 254–257.

Dickersin, K., Chan, S., Chalmers, T.C., Sacks, H.S., Smith, H., Jr. (1987). Publication bias and clinical trials. *Controlled Clinical Trials,* 8, 343–353.

Dorman, P.J., Counsell, C., Sandercock, P. (1999). Reports of randomized trials in acute stroke, 1955 to 1995: what proportions were commercially sponsored? *Stroke*, 30, 1995–1998.

Easterbrook, P.J., Berlin, J.A., Gopalan, R., Metthews, D.R. (1991). Publication bias in clinical research. *Lancet*, 337, 867–872.

Egger, M., Smith, G.D. (1998). Bias in location and selection of studies. *British Medical Journal*, 316, 61–66.

Egger, M., Smith, D.S., Schneider, M., Minder, C. (1997). Bias in meta-analysis detected by a simple, graphical test. *British Medical Journal*, 315, 629–634.

Friedberg, M., Saffran, B., Stinsons, T.J., Nelson, W., Bennett, C.L. (1999). Evaluation of conflict of interest in economic analyses of new drugs used in oncology. *Journal of the American Medical Association*, 282, 1453–1457.

Goetsche, P.C., Olsen, O. (2000). Is screening for breast cancer with mammography justifiable? *Lancet*, 355, 129–134.

Gross, C.P., Gupta, A., Krumholz, H.M. (2003). Disclosure of financial competing interests in randomised controlled trials: cross sectional review. *British Medical Journal*, 326, 526–527.

Hussain, A., Smith, R.( 2001). Declaring financial competing interests: survey of five general medical journals. *British Medical Journal,* 323, 263–264.

Ioannidis, J.P.A. (1998). Effect of the statistical significance of results on the time to completion and publication of randomized efficacy trials. *Journal of the American Medical Association*, 279, 281–286.

Ioannidis, J.P.A., Haidich, A.B., Pappa, M., Pantazis, N., Kokori, S.I., Tektonidou, M., et al. (2001). Comparison of evidence of treatment effects in randomized and nonrandomized studies. *Journal of the American Medical Association,* 286, 821–830.

Jennions, M.D., Moeller, A.P. (2002). Relationships fade with time: a meta-analysis of temporal trends in publication in ecology and evolution. *Proceedings of the Royal Society of London Series B: Biological Sciences*, 269, 43–48

Jüni, P., Witschi, A., Bloch, R., Egger, M. (1999). The hazards of scoring the quality of clinical trials for meta-analysis. *Journal of the American Medical Association,* 282, 1054–1060.

Kidwell, C.S., Liebeskind, D.S., Starkman, S., Saver, J.L. (2001). Trends in acute ischemic stroke trials through the 20th century. *Stroke*, 32, 1349–1359.

Kjaergard, L.L., Als-Nielsen, B. (2002). Association between competing interests and authors' conclusions: epidemiological study of randomised clinical trials published in the BMJ. *British Medical Journal*, 325, 249–252.

Kjaergard, L.L., Frederiksen, S.L., Gluud, C. (2002). Validity of randomized clinical trials in gastroenterology from 1964–2000. *Gastroenterology*, 122, 1157–1160.

Macaskill, P., Walter, S.D., Irwig, L. (2001). A comparison of methods to detect publication bias in meta-analysis. *Statistics in Medicine*, 20, 641–654.

Misakian, A.L., Bero, L.A. (1998). Publication bias and research on passive smoking. *Journal of the American Medical Association*, 280, 250–253.

Moher, D., Pham, B., Jones, A., Cook, D.J., Jadad, A.R., Moher, M., et al. (1998). Does quality of reports of randomised trials affect estimates of intervention efficacy reported in meta-analyses? *Lancet*, 352, 609–613.

Nieuwenhoven, C.A., Buskens, E., van Tiel, F.H., Bonten, M.J.M. (2001). Relationship between methodological trial quality and the effects of selective digestive decontamination on pneumonia and mortality in critically ill patients. *Journal of the American Medical Association*, 286, 335–340.

PubMed (2003). National Library of Medicine and National Center for Biotechnology Information, USA (http://www.ncbi.nlm.nih.gov/entrez/query.fcgi).

Schulz, K.F., Chalmers, I., Hayes, R.J., Altman, D.G. (1995). Empirical evidence of bias: dimensions of methodological quality associated with estimates of treatment effects in controlled trials. *Journal of the American Medical Association*, 273, 408–412.

Sterne, J.A.C., Egger, M. (2001). Funnel plots for detecting bias in meta-analysis: guideline for choice of axis. *Journal of Clinical Epidemiology*, 54, 1046–1055.

Stern, J.M., Simes, R.J. (1997). Publication bias: evidence of delayed publication in a cohort study of clinical research projects. *British Medical Journal*, 315, 640–645.

# 26
## Clinical Research and Outcomes Research: Common Criteria and Differences

Franz Porzsolt, Dirk Stengel, Amit K. Ghosh, and Robert M. Kaplan

With rapid changes and new challenges in global health care, there is increasing awareness of the limits with current measures of effectiveness. Promoting the use and reimbursement of a certain health technology requires evidence of its value for patients by means of improved quality or extended quantity of life. The term "outcomes research" has been introduced as a catch-all phrase for scientific approaches of determining the impact of health care interventions on the population level. However, because there is still debate as to the definition of outcome, the goals of outcomes research remain to be defined. We herein propose concepts and criteria that may suit the principle of outcomes research, and we sketch the major differences to clinical research.

Continuing biomedical progress remains the expectation of progressive societies and is almost taken for granted. Knowledge gain, refinement of previous ideas, and invention of new technologies, however, does not always change clinical practice or enhance benefit for patients (Bast et al., 2001). Contopoulos-Ioannidis and colleagues (2003) noted that of 101 scientific advancements published in recognized periodicals (for example, *Science*, *Nature*, *Cell*), only 5 subsequently achieved consensus approval, and only 1 of 101 innovations resulted in significant changes in medical practice two decades after first publication. There is also a serious discrepancy between inputs of resources and patient outcomes that is prevalent in several health care systems in the world. Although the United States spends the most on health care among 29 industrialized countries, it remains in the lowest quartile when judged by outcomes indicators, such as quality of life and infant mortality (Anderson, 1997).

Outcomes research was proposed as a theoretical construct to address this problem. Unfortunately, there is still no generally accepted definition of outcomes research, and there remains a lack of consensus on the methods to study and document health outcomes (Rothwell, 2005a,b,c). A comprehensive treatise on the history of outcomes research by Lee and colleagues (Lee et al., 2000) defined what does not constitute outcomes research rather than enumerating what characteristics could define an ideal approach to outcomes research. A series of articles by Rothwell (2005a,b,c) outlined the message of randomized trials and its application to individual patients. In this chapter we propose differences between clinical and outcomes research at three levels: goals, applied methods, and results.

## Current Conflicts Between Research and Practice

Strong therapeutic effects noted in clinical studies are not regularly observed in clinical practice. The American Society of Clinical Oncology (ASCO) distinguished the activity and the effectiveness of a treatment based on the description of cancer outcomes (response rate) from patient outcomes (quantity and quality of life) (American Society of Clinical Oncology, 1996). Patient outcomes were assigned a higher priority than cancer outcomes.

These recommendations have neither been systematically applied in clinical practice nor by international regulatory authorities, such as the Food and Drug Administration (FDA) or the European Agency for the Evaluation of Medicinal Products (EMEA). In the clinical setting, response rates are often used as decision nodes in treatment algorithms. Although experts recommend the evaluation of quality of life, these data are usually not assigned much importance when approving new treatments (Schilsky, 2002; Apolone, 2003; Johnson et al., 2003).

Survival rates associated with new interventions are often poor indicators of treatment success. Changes in life expectancy are generally small, and their value remains controversial. Moreover, although quality-of-life data are increasingly published, they are difficult to interpret. Members of the jury of a quality-of-life prize awarded in Germany to support outcomes research analyzed 146 submitted papers. In these papers, about 200 instruments, including several newly developed ones, were used to measure quality of life. Authors of articles in which several instruments were compared lamented *in unison* the lack of comparability of data.

We deliberately introduce bias when assessing *all* dimensions of the quality of life of our patients. Determining the underlying cause for a critical symptom requires broad knowledge of the most likely pattern of health impairments accompanying various conditions. Moreover, there is a need for instruments that identify specific indicators of well-being or disease in distinct populations (Porzsolt et al., 2003).

Further difficulties arise from extrapolating the results of clinical studies to clinical practice. Stringent inclusion and exclusion criteria generate patient groups who represent only a small portion of the population normally referred to the clinical practitioner. This bears the risk of uselessly applying treatments to patients who would probably have been excluded from clinical trials.

## Objectives of Clinical and Outcomes Research

The National Institutes of Health (NIH) roadmap (Zerhouni, 2003) claims to have sensitive and validated instruments to measure the outcomes of patient care. When following the development of an innovation in health care, we can distinguish several phases of research. In vitro experiments (basic research) are followed by in vivo (animal) experiments (preclinical research) and research in humans under experimental conditions (clinical research).

In each of these research phases we try to get closer to the final goal, that is, to offer effective, efficient health services. We may consider outcomes research the last link in the research chain in which the proof of efficacy must be supplemented by the proof of effectiveness. Effectiveness of a therapy must be assessed under everyday conditions (Last, 1998).

Clinical research is usually performed to demonstrate the efficacy of a new treatment in comparison to a conventional approach. In a clinical trial, the efficacy of specific treatments are compared under ideal (and artificial) experimental conditions in a selected population generated by predetermined exclusion and inclusion criteria. This maintains the internal validity of the findings. External validity and effectiveness are often neglected in these studies. In clinical trials, nonrepresentativeness of the study population is the rule rather than the exception (Schmoor et al., 1996).

Outcomes research is carried out in an environment in which perceived effectiveness, knowledge framing (Porzsolt et al., 2004a,b), and other psychological variables are deliberately applied and desired as integral elements of overall effect estimates. It is difficult to assume efficacy of a distinct intervention (as observed under experimental conditions) if the noted effects are too small to be detected under the influence of confounders arising in daily clinical practice.

## Methods

Posing a precise hypothesis is mandatory for both clinical and outcomes research. Both are conducted in a deductive manner: Data are gathered to support or reject the hypothesis. Outcomes research must not be confused with clinical practice, in which inductive processes are common ways of gaining knowledge. Observations made while treating more and more patients strengthen the belief in pathophysiological relationships and the effectiveness of a certain intervention.

Both clinical and outcomes research demand methods to control for confounding. The most critical confounder is a mismatch in biological baseline risks of patients included in any trial. Most scientists tend to interpret differences in outcomes as a result of different interventions rather than differences in baseline risks or confounders. The double-blind, randomized, controlled trial is widely considered the gold standard to address the clinical objective in therapeutic studies and to distribute known and unknown confounders equally between the treatment arms.

Outcomes research describes effects achieved under usual clinical situations, when eligible patients undergo treatments according to the doctors' and patients' choice or preference, not by chance. Consequently, randomized controlled trials (RCTs) are probably inappropriate tools for determining outcomes in clinical practice. One of the important challenges for evidence-based medicine is that clinical patients are heterogeneous. Evidence-based reviews usually consider average treatment effects. This can mask the complex mixture of benefits and harms for a particular population. On the basis of evidence-based reviews, some patients are denied treatments that may help them, and other patients receive treatments that can cause harm (Kravitz et al., 2004).

Patients differ in their baseline risks of adverse events, their responsiveness to treatment, their vulnerability to side effects, and their propensity for various outcomes. For example, evidence-based reviews suggest that low-dose aspirin reduces the risk of myocardial infarction (MI). However, some patients are at very low risk for MI and may be at high risk for gastrointestinal bleeding (Lip & Lowe, 1996), and they may be better off without aspirin. Other patients, such as those with atrial fibrillation or abnormal heart valves, may gain much greater benefit from aspirin use. Warfrin (an anticoagulant) greatly reduces the risk of atrial fibrillation for most patients. However, patients with atrial fibrillation who are under 65 years of age with no history of hypertension, diabetes, or previous stoke have less than a 1% chance of stroke per year. Warfarin may increase their chances of bleeding and could cause harm (Anonymous, 1994). Many interventions that show benefit for certain diagnoses may have little benefit for the very old because they will not live long enough for the positive outcomes to be realized.

Baseline profiles of subgroups generated by choice may not be comparable, and modeling the distinct benefits and harms of a certain treatment in a certain risk group represents both an opportunity and a challenge. Basically, outcomes research in clinical practice must employ the principle of subgroup analysis on a larger scale. It investigates which of the benefits derived from small, highly selected patient samples in a randomized trial can be detected in particular subgroups of subjects counseled in daily practice.

The description of the target groups of an outcomes research study needs two sets of data. First, we must sketch characteristics that all of the study subjects have in common. We call these items common clinical characteristics (CCC). Second, characteristics are needed that distinguish individuals among subgroups. We call these items diverse demographics and diseases (DDD).

Both CCC and DDD must be defined before the outcomes in individual patients can be described. The definitions of CCC and of DDD determine both the eligible patients who should be included in the analysis and the allocation of each individual patient to one of the risk groups. In outcomes research, identical risk groups may receive different treatments (as in clinical research studies). In addition, outcomes research includes different risk groups that receive the same treatments. An example is shown in Figure 26.1. The example of applied interventions makes it possible to compare interventions 1 and 3 in low risk patients (DDD 1) and interventions 1 and 2 in intermediate risk patients (DDD 2).

Individual risk groups as defined by DDD and matching interventions are distributed differently among the cells of a cross table. Some interventions are preferably applied to patients with a certain DDD profile (because of findings from clinical research, practice guidelines, or preference), whereas others are rarely or never used (Figure 26.1). To describe this complex pattern reliably, large cohort studies are needed.

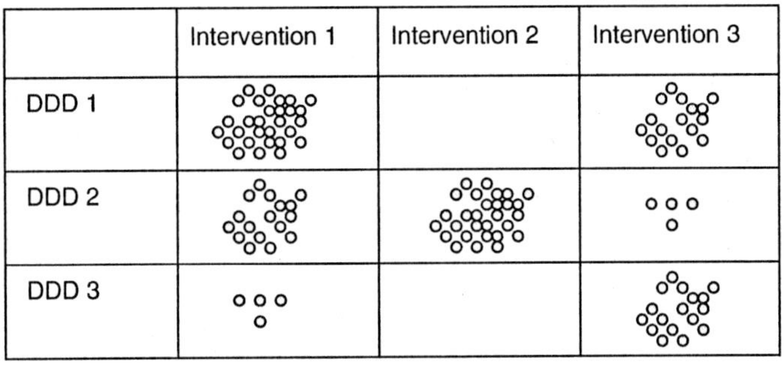

| | Intervention 1 | Intervention 2 | Intervention 3 |
|---|---|---|---|
| DDD 1 | | | |
| DDD 2 | | | ○ ○ ○ ○ |
| DDD 3 | ○ ○ ○ ○ | | |

FIGURE 26.1. Cross-table of a hypothetical frequency of various interventions applied to certain risk groups as defined by diverse demographics and diseases (DDD). All DDD subgroups have specific common clinical characteristics (CCC) criteria. In this example, intervention 2 is used in neither subgroup DDD 1 nor DDD 3. Intervention 1 is more frequently applied to subgroup DDD 1 than DDD 3. DDD 1 = low risk group; DDD 2 = intermediate risk group; DDD 3 = high risk group.

Outcomes research is not exclusively conducted at academic institutions but at primary care facilities as well, where several treatment options might be considered to target disorders and disabilities of subjects with similar CCC.

The essential differences between clinical research and outcomes research are summarized in Table 26.1. The discussed example is confined to treatment interventions. In clinical research, entry criteria must be defined before individual patients can be randomly allocated to treatment groups. In outcomes research, data are generated in daily clinical practice; in other words, it is not possible to exclude patients. Physicians select a certain treatment according to individual preferences and skills, availability, and cost considerations. Applying CCC and DDD criteria generate subgroups with comparable baseline risks. To avoid selection bias, all patients have to be included in the final analysis.

## Summary and Prospects

The results obtained from clinical trials are needed to plan and conduct outcomes studies. Outcomes research provides additional data on effectiveness, external validity, and outcomes. Outcomes supply vital information for providers, consumers, and payers of health care services.

Clinical and outcomes research are not competitive, but complementary, methods. Unfortunately, data about the efficacy of certain medical and surgical interventions are, at best, sparse. Nowadays, many new treatments are rapidly adopted by doctors and requested by patients before data from randomized trials become available. For example, laparoscopic cholecystectomy, navigated surgery, and percutaneous vertebroplasty, among many other interventions, have established themselves in clinical practice even without formal proof of efficacy under the rigor of a clinical trial.

TABLE 26.1. Differences between clinical and outcomes research in treatment studies

| Parameter | Clinical research | Outcomes research |
|---|---|---|
| Objectives | Comparison of new and established treatments under the conditions of a clinical trial (confirming efficacy and internal validity) using the perspective of clinical epidemiology | Comparison of new and established treatments under everyday conditions (confirming effectiveness and external validity) using various perspectives, such as the patient's perspective |
| Methods | Step 1: definition of characteristics of study groups (inclusion and exclusion criteria) and of treatment options<br>Step 2: random allocation of individual patients to the treatment options<br><br>Step 3: evaluation of patients in the groups to which they were allocated by randomization (intent to treat principle) | Step 1: preference-based allocation of patients to various treatments (all patients are included)<br>Step 2: definition of characteristics of study groups (DDD, CCC, and included treatment options)<br>Step 3: allocation of all individual patients for evaluation to subgroups defined by DDD, CCC, and treatment |
| Results | Provision of information that is necessary to plan and conduct outcomes research | Description of the effectiveness and external validity from the perspectives of various partners of the system based on the results of clinical research |

CCC = common clinical characteristics; DDD = diverse demographics and diseases.

Outcomes research offers the possibility of comparing health interventions by assessing patient-related outcomes of established interventions even if their efficacy is still unknown. This poses some danger of having a fine excuse for not conducting clinical research; and clinicians, scientists, and authorities must counter this trend early.

Clinical research investigates the activity of individual interventions but cannot be used to evaluate system performance. To achieve this, one must compare the frequency of use of a certain service with the frequency of attaining the achieved goals. Thus, outcomes research may also apply to the investigation of effects of newly established structural facilities, such as cancer centers, trauma centers, or stroke units, as well as various types of integrated health care.

It is likely that outcome studies require larger groups of patients than clinical studies. In fact, the size of outcome studies mainly depends on the definition of investigated subgroups. Outcomes studies can be kept at a reasonable size if study groups (CCC) are compared that are represented in similar proportions in the overall group (DDD), that is, only frequently occurring patterns or only rarely occurring patterns are compared within one study. Large numbers of patients do not necessarily increase the quality of a study, but they definitely increase the cost.

As randomization cannot be applied in outcomes research, other methods, such as multiple regression analysis or propensity scores (Rubin, 1997), have to be included to control for differences among the CCC groups that receive different treatments.

Evaluating efficiency in outcomes research from the economic perspective (in analogy to classic cost-effectiveness analysis) must consider the available, not theoretical, resources. The public has a right to participate in the decision about funding of health care services. Outcomes research needs data that are collected and analyzed by independent scientists, and, finally, evaluated by all stakeholders.

So long as we apply identical methods to conduct clinical and outcomes research, we cannot expect different results. Outcomes research is necessary to confirm the assumed quality, to pose new scientific perspectives, and to increase the efficiency and affordability of health care provision. Above all, we must not forget the essential goal of health care service—the value for patients.

## References

American Society of Clinical Oncology (1996). Outcomes of cancer treatment for technology assessment and cancer treatment guidelines. *Journal of Clinical Oncology*, 14, 671–679.

Anderson, G.F. (1997). In search of value: an international comparison of cost, access, and outcomes. *Health Affairs*, 16, 163–171.

Anonymous. (1994). Risk factors for stroke and efficacy of antithrombotic therapy in atrial fibrillation: analysis of pooled data from five randomized controlled trials. *Archives of Internal Medicine*, 154, 1449–1457.

Apolone, G. (2003). Clinical and outcome research in oncology: the need for integration. *Health Quality of Life Outcomes*, 1, 3.

Bast, R.C., Mills, G.B., Young, R.C. (2001). Translational research: traffic on the bridge. *Biomedicine and Pharmacotherapy*, 55, 565–571.

Contopoulos-Ioannidis, D.G., Ntzani, E., Ioannidis, J.P. (2003). Translation of highly promising basic science research into clinical applications. *American Journal of Medicine*, 114, 477–484.

Johnson, J.R., Williams, G., Pazdur, R. (2003). Endpoints and United States Food and Drug Administration approval of oncology drugs. *Journal of Clinical Oncology*, 21, 1404–1411.

Kravitz, R.L., Duan, N., Braslow, J. (2004). Evidence-based medicine, heterogeneity of treatment effects, and the trouble with averages. *Milbank Quarterly*, 82, 661–687.

Last, J. M. (1988). *A dictionary of epidemiology*. Oxford: Oxford University Press.

Lee, S.J., Craig, C.E., Weeks, J.C. (2000). Outcomes research in oncology: history, conceptual framework, and trends in the literature. *Journal of National Cancer Institute*, 92, 195–204.

Lip, G.Y., Lowe, G.D. (1996). ABC of atrial fibrillation: antithrombotic treatment for atrial fibrillation. *British Medical Journal*, 312, 45–49.

Porzsolt, F., Kumpf, J., Coppin, C., Pöppel, E. (2003). Stringent application of epidemiological criteria changes the interpretation of the effects of immunotherapy in advanced renal cell cancer. In: C. Williams, V. Bramwell, X. Bonfill, J. Cuzick, J. Forbes (Eds.), *Evidence-based oncology*. Oxford: BMJ Books. pp. 34–38.

Porzsolt, F., Kojer, M., Schmidl, M., Greimel, E.R., Siegle, J., Richter, J., et al. (2004a). A new instrument to describe indicators of well-being in old-old patients with severe dementia: the Vienna List. *Health Quality of Life Outcomes*, 2, 10.

Porzsolt, F., Schlotz-Gorton, N., Biller-Andorno, N., Thim, A., Meissner, K., Roeckl-Wiedmann, I., et al. (2004b). Applying evidence to support ethical decisions: is the placebo really powerless? *Science in Engineering and Ethics*, 10, 119–132.

Rothwell, P.M. (2005a). External validity of randomised controlled trials: "to whom do the results of this trial apply?" *Lancet*, 365, 13–14.

Rothwell, P.M. (2005b). Treating individuals, 2. Subgroup analysis in randomised controlled trials: importance, indications, and interpretation. *Lancet*, 365, 176–186.

Rothwell, P.M. (2005c). Treating individuals. 3. From subgroups to individuals: general principles and the example of carotid endarterectomy. *Lancet*, 365, 256–265.

Rubin, D.B. (1997). Estimating causal effects from large data sets using propensity scores. *Annals of Internal Medicine*, 127, 757–763.

Schilsky, R.L. (2002). Endpoints in cancer clinical trials and the drugs approval process. *Clinical Cancer Research*, 8, 935–938.

Schmoor, C., Olschewski, M., Schumacher, M. (1996). Randomized and non-randomized patients in clinical trials: experiences with comprehensive cohort studies. *Statistics in Medicine*, 15, 263–271.

Zerhouni, E. (2003). The NIH roadmap. *Science*, 302, 63–72.

# 27
# Are the Results of Randomized Trials Influenced by Preference Effects? Part I. Findings from a Systematic Review

DIRK STENGEL, JALID SEHOULI, AND FRANZ PORZSOLT

The randomized controlled trial (RCT), presently accepted as the undisputed gold standard of study formats to prove the effectiveness of a treatment over its control, has experienced criticism during the last decade (Kramer & Shapiro, 1984; Jack et al., 1990; Kotwall et al., 1992; Plaisier et al., 1994; Andrews, 1999; Prescott et al., 1999; Ross et al., 1999; McCormack & Greenhalgh, 2000; Kaptchuk, 2001; McCulloch et al., 2002). Some arguments raised against RCTs are scientifically founded, whereas others emanate from reasons such as lack of understanding the theoretical background or emotional conflicts. Clinicians who believe in the need of controlled trials for scientific progress but are uncomfortable with prescribing their patients a treatment by chance have earned support from statisticians and epidemiologists. Several authors found no evidence of a difference in outcomes between randomized and observational studies (Benson & Hartz, 2000; Concato et al., 2000; MacLehose et al., 2000; Peppercorn et al., 2004). Interpretation of these findings is still pending.

Patients' preferences gained much attention when dealing with the ethics of randomization and maintenance of the equipoise principle[1] (Kassirer, 1994; Silverman & Altman, 1996; Chard & Lilford, 1998; Jansen et al., 2000; Lambert & Wood, 2000; Stiggelbout & de Haes, 2001; Lilford, 2003). Also, a mathematical construct was developed for additive and two-way interactions between preference, guessed and actual treatments, and treatment outcomes (McPherson, 1994; McPherson et al., 1997; Halpern, 2003).

In a recent systematic review of 32 studies, King and colleagues (2005) failed to demonstrate differences in baseline and outcome effect sizes between randomized and preference cohorts. The authors confined their conclusion to the statement that "intervention preferences appear to have limited impact on the external or internal validity of randomized trials."

---

[1]Equipoise means therapeutic uncertainty: neither doctors nor patients must know which of two or more possible treatments for a certain disease or condition leads to better/best outcomes. In this and only this setting, it is justified to allocate subjects randomly to one or the other intervention.

In a short communication published in the *British Medical Journal* in 1989, Brewin and Bradley introduced the partially randomized patient preference trial (PRPPT) as a new design to address preference effects. Both authors must be rewarded for recognizing the importance of the *proper decisional sequence* in obtaining informed consent. In the PRPPT, potentially eligible subjects are asked *first* whether they have a clear preference for one or the other treatment under investigation and, *if undecided*, are offered randomization. This schedule is essentially different from the order of information adopted by other study formats, such as the comprehensive cohort design (CCD), in which patients are primarily asked if they are willing to participate in a randomized trial (Olschewski and Scheurlen, 1985). Those who refuse randomization for any reason are invited to take part in an observational study (Moher et al., 2001). Thus, different approaches have been proposed to test the hypothesis that results of randomized trials are influenced by patient preferences.

In the first part of this chapter, we describe the results of a systematic review addressing the same problem as King et al. (2005). We extracted additional data that allow an alternative interpretation of the findings from preference trials. In the second part of the chapter, we draw special attention to how established methods can solve the preference problem, potential sources of bias, and consequences for research and clinical practice.

# Methods

## Eligibility Criteria

We included clinical trials that comprised (1) observational treatment arms comprised of subjects who clearly preferred the experimental or the control intervention, and (2) an additional RCT, enrolling patients without a preference who were willing to be randomized. We also included studies in which patients declining random allocation were given the opportunity to participate in an observational study or consented to providing health-related data to set up a registry.

We excluded studies that did not allow the possibility of assigning subjects to parallel randomized or observational arms (for example, studies in which patients were exclusively treated according to their preferences). We also excluded studies that used the patient's preference solely as an outcome measure or randomly allocated patients to treatment groups, regardless of their preference stated at the beginning of a trial.

## Search Strategy

We scanned MEDLINE, Embase, Cancerlit, Scisearch, Cinahl, the Cochrane Central database, and Google for potentially eligible studies published between 1966 and August 2004. We made no restrictions for language. Search terms meeting the MeSH, Emtree, or other database-specific indices are listed in Table 27.1.

TABLE 27.1. Search strategy

| No. | MeSH | Retrievals |
|---|---|---|
| 1 | Patient preference *or* patient choice *or* patient convenience *or* prefer* *or* choice *or* convenience | 286253 |
| 2 | Clinical study *or* clinical trial *or* clinical investigation *or* survey *or* study *or* trial *or* investigation | 3833880 |
| 3 | Random* | 345710 |
| 4 | Nonrandom* *or* nonrandom* *or* observ* | 1324187 |
| 5 | Nos. 1 *and* 2 *and* 3 *and* 4 | 2690 |
| 6 | Arm *or* group *or* subgroup *or* set | 1213255 |
| 7 | Nos. 5 *and* 6 | 1163 |
| 8 | Nos. 5 *and* 6. Limits: human | 1061 |
| 9 | Nos. 5 *and* 6 *not* (blind* OR review). Limits: human | 687 |
| 10 | Nos. 5 *and* 6 *not* (blind* *or* review *or* cross-sectional) Limits: human | 670 |
| 11 | Prefer* *or* choice *or* convenience *or* discretion *or* wish *or* want | 280817 |
| 12 | Investigation *or* study *or* trial | 3239157 |
| 13 | Arm *or* group *or* subgroup *or* set *or* sample | 1369010 |
| 14 | Nos. 11 *and* 12 *and* 3 *and* 4 *and* 13 | 1053 |
| 15 | No. 14 *not* (blind*) | 839 |
| 16 | No. 14 *not* (blind*), Field: all fields. Limits: human | 731 |

Additional search terms for Embase, Cancerlit, Scisearch, and Cinahl using the XMEDALL superbase provided by the German Institute of Medical Documentation and Information (DIMDI).

All authors jointly made a first selection of studies according to titles and abstracts. If both were inconclusive, we retrieved the full text article. All bibliographies of identified papers were surveyed for potentially relevant work missed by the electronic search. We also collected articles containing subset analyses of the core studies or related methodological work.

## Quality Assessment

Two of the authors (D.S. and F.P.) independently evaluated the methodological quality of eligible studies according to an a priori defined checklist containing 14 standards. Discrepant views were solved by discussion with a third reviewer (J.S.).

We specifically counted the number of inclusion and exclusion criteria; counted the number of patients screened, included, and evaluated; and recorded institutional review board approval, risk stratification, concealment of random codes, blinding of outcome assessors, presentation of a study flowchart according to the Consolidated Standards of Reporting Trials (CONSORT) (Moher et al., 2001), and maintenance of the intent-to-treat principle (all patients are statistically evaluated according to the group in which they actually participated, regardless of the group to which they were originally assigned). We also graded the reliability of outcome measures as weak (for example, pain measurement), intermediate (for example, validated quality of life assessment tools), and high (for example, mortality). Finally, we checked whether the authors had presented measures of variability of their outcome estimates.

Data were extracted independently by both reviewers and entered into a Microsoft Access Database.

## Statistical Analysis

Quantitative analysis was conducted in an exploratory fashion. We counted imbalances in patients' baseline characteristics as a possible source of bias. An imbalance was assumed if the upper or lower 95% confidence limit of a difference in proportion (for example, the percentage of male patients) was beyond 0%. Likewise, a 95% confidence limit beyond 0 pointed to an imbalance in baseline values expressed on a continuous scale (for example, a difference in mean age). The numbers of items describing baseline profiles and those showing an imbalance were graphically compared by box-and-whiskers plots.[2]

To gain an impression of the direction and magnitude of preferences, we divided the number of subjects choosing the control treatment by the number of subjects choosing the experimental treatment. The odds of preferring the control over the experimental intervention was illustrated on a dot plot.

Addressing primary outcomes, we calculated risk differences (RD) or standardized mean differences (SMD) with 95% confidence intervals (CI) between the experimental and the control arms in the randomized and preference groups. If multiple scales were tested as the primary endpoint and no emphasis was placed on a certain dimension, we calculated weighted mean differences (WMD) in a random-effects model. The STATA 8.0 software package was employed for all analyses.

## Results

## Systematic Review

We identified 781 citations, of which 229 papers were retrieved in full text. A list of these papers is available from the authors on request. A total of 57 articles reporting the findings from 33 core studies were eligible for this review. Information was available for 20,025 patients. The study profile is sketched in Figure 27.1.

Trials were published between 1984 and 2004 and covered a broad range of conditions and interventions (Table 27.2). Of note, the term "randomizable" patients (that is, subjects fulfilling entry criteria for an RCT but either refusing random allocation or not being randomized by their physicians) first appeared in the Coronary Artery Surgery Study (CASS) (CASS principal investigators and

---

[2]In box-and-whiskers plots, the box represents the interquartile range (that is, observations between the 25th and the 75th percentile, or 50% of all observations). The box normally includes a transverse bar representing the median, or the 50th percentile. Whiskers extend to a length 1.5 times the box size. Outliers are indicated by dots.

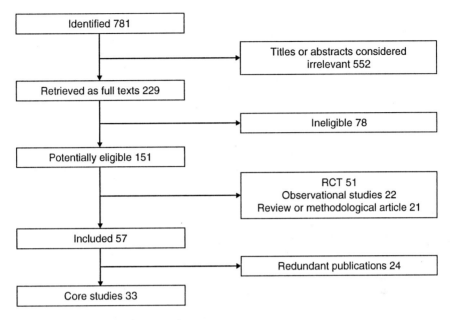

FIGURE 27.1. Trial selection procedure.

their associates, 1984). Despite CASS, two other major cardiology trials enrolled subjects on both a random and a nonrandom basis (BARI Investigators, 1996; Chaitman et al., 1997; Detre et al., 1999; Morrison et al., 1999, 2001, 2002a,b; Brooks et al., 2000; Feit et al., 2000; Sedlis et al., 2002, 2004).

Thirteen studies focused on women's health issues, such as breast cancer (Schmoor et al., 1996, 2000, 2002; Rauschecker et al., 1998; Julien et al., 2000; Sauerbrei et al., 2000; Bijker et al., 2002; Coward, 2002, 2003), endometrial ablation for dysfunctional menstrual bleeding (Cooper et al., 1997a,b; Bain et al., 2001; Wallage et al., 2003), medical and surgical abortion (Henshaw et al., 1993; Howie et al., 1997; Ashok et al., 2002), hormone replacement therapy for preventing osteoporotic fractures (Mosekilde et al., 2000, 2001), the acceptability of land birth and water birth (Woodward & Kelly, 2004), surveillance for pathological cervical smears (Kitchener et al., 2004), and fetal karyotyping (Nicolaides et al., 1994).

Treatment of psychiatric disorders (Bakker et al., 1999, 2000; Bedi et al., 2000; Bower et al., 2000; King et al., 2000; Ward et al., 2000; Chilvers et al., 2001; Renjilian et al., 2001; Miller et al., 2003), drug withdrawal (Gossop et al., 1986; McKay et al., 1995, 1998), pain management (de C Williams et al., 1999; Kerry et al., 2000; Kendrick et al., 2001; Melchart et al., 2002; Kennedy et al., 2003), and education of diabetic patients (Noel et al., 1998) were other typical scenarios covered by hybrid designs. Two studies investigated chemotherapy versus best supportive care for sarcomas (Antman et al., 1984, 1985) and non-small-cell lung cancer (NSCLC) (Helsing et al., 1998) in a composite format.

TABLE 27.2. Publication dates, recruitment periods, conditions, and interventions

| Study | Year | Papers | Recruited | Design | Target condition | Experimental treatment | Control treatment |
|---|---|---|---|---|---|---|---|
| Antman | 1985 | 2 | 1978–1982 | CCS | Surgery for sarcoma | Adj. radiotherapy + doxorubicin | Adj. radiotherapy |
| Ashok | 2002 | 1 | – | PRPPT? | Abortion | Medical | Vacuum |
| AWESOME | 1999 | 6 | 1995–1999 | CCS | Unstable angina | Bypass surgery | Percutan. coronary intervention |
| Bain | 2001 | 1 | 1998–1999 | PRPPT | Microwave endometrial ablation for dysfunctional uterine bleeding | Local anesthesia and intravenous sedation | General anesthesia |
| Bakker | 2000 | 2 | – | CCS | Panic disorder | Random: cognitive therapy, paroxetine, clomipramine, placebo | Choice: cognitive therapy |
| BARI | 2000 | 5 | 1988–1991 | CCS | Coronary artery disease | Percut. Coronary intervention | Bypass surgery |
| Bedi | 2000 | 3 | – | PRPPT? | Major depression | Antidepressants | Counseling |
| CASS | 1984 | 1 | 1974–1979 | CCS | Stable angina pectoris | Coronary artery bypass surgery | Medical therapy |
| Cooper | 1997 | 2 | 1994–1995 | TSTD | Heavy menstrual bleeding | Medical | Transcervical endometr. resection |
| Coward | 2002 | 2 | 1996–1997 | PRPPT? | Self-transcendence in breast cancer | Eight-week, closed support group | Not specified |
| de C Williams | 1999 | 1 | – | CCS | Chronic pain | Inpatient treatment | Outpatient treatment |
| DOPS | 2000 | 2 | 1990–1993 | CCS | Osteoporotic fracture prevention | Hormone replacement therapy | No hormone replacement therapy |
| EORTC | 2002 | 2 | 1986–1996 | CCS | DCIS | Local resection + radiotherapy | Local resection |
| GBSG 2 | 1996 | 2 | 1983–1983 | CCS | Node-pos. breast cancer | Mastectomy + CMF + tamoxifen | Mastectomy + CMF |
| GBSG 3 | 1996 | 3 | 1983–1986 | CCS | Node-pos. breast cancer | Mastectomy + CMF + radiother. | Mastectomy + CMF |
| Gossop | 1986 | 1 | 1984–1985 | CCS | Opiate addiction | Inpatient withdrawal program | Outpatient withdrawal program |
| Helsing | 1998 | 1 | 1990–1995 | CCS | NSCLC | Carboplatin + etoposide | Best supportive care |
| Henshaw | 1993 | 2 | 1990–1991 | PRPPT | Abortion | Medical | Vacuum |
| Kendrick | 2001 | 1 | 1995–1999 | PRPPT | Low back pain for > 6 weeks | Usual care + spine radiography | Usual care |
| Kerry | 2000 | 1 | 1996–1999 | CCS | Low back pain | Usual care + spine radiography | Usual care |
| King | 2000 | 3 | 1996–1997 | PRPPT | Depression and anxiety | Nondirective counseling | Cognitive-behavior therapy |
| Kitchener | 2004 | 1 | 1998–1999 | Zelen I | Mildly abnormal cervical smears | Choice: surveillance or colposcopy | Surveillance |
| Mattila | 2003 | 1 | 1996–1999 | Zelen I | Prevention of otitis media | Tympanostomy + adenoidectomy | Tympanostomy |
| McKay | 1995 | 1 | – | PRPPT? | Alcoholism | Day hospital | Inpatient |

| McKay | 1998 | 1 | – | CCS | Cocaine abuse | Day hospital | Inpatient |
| Melchart | 2002 | 1 | 1996–1998 | PRPPT? | Pre-treatment for gastroscopy | Acupuncture | Midazolam |
| Nicolaides | 1994 | 1 | 1990–1993 | CCS | Fetal karyotyping at 10–13 weeks | Early amniocentesis | Chorionic villous sampling |
| Noel | 1998 | 1 | – | TSTD | Diabetes mellitus | Nutrition curriculum | Standard curriculum |
| Paradise | 1984 | 2 | 1971–1982 | CCS | Recurrent throat infection | Tonsillectomy w/o adenoidectomy | Observation |
| Reddihough | 1998 | 1 | – | CCS | Cerebral palsy | Conductive education | Traditional neurodevelopment |
| Renjilian | 2001 | 1 | – | 2 × 2 factorial | Obesity | Group therapy | Individual therapy |
| Wallage | 2003 | 1 | 1999–2000 | PRPPT? | Microwave endometrial ablation for dysfunctional uterine bleeding | Local anesthesia and intravenous sedation | General anesthesia |
| Woodward | 2004 | 1 | – | PRPPT? | Delivery | Water birth | Land birth |

CCS = comprehensive cohort design; PRPPT = partially randomized patient preference trial; TSTD = two stage trial design; NSCLC = non-small-cell lung cancer; CMF = cyclophosphamide/methotrexate/fluorouracil; Adj. = adjuvant; Percut. = percutaneous.

Three studies were conducted in pediatric populations (Paradise et al., 1984, 1990; Reddihough et al., 1998; Mattila et al., 2003). Here, given preference for a certain treatment, if any, was issued by parents, not by the patients themselves.

Only four trials unequivocally met the original PRPPT design (Henshaw et al., 1993; Howie et al., 1997; Bower et al., 2000; King et al., 2000; Ward et al., 2000; Bain et al., 2001; Kendrick et al., 2001). It was not clear whether another five studies indexed as preference trials merely represented comprehensive cohort studies (McKay et al., 1995; Bedi et al., 2000; Chilvers et al., 2001; Ashok et al., 2002; Melchart et al., 2002; Miller et al., 2003; Wallage et al., 2004). For example, although the trial published by Bedi and others was named a preference trial, the authors noted that "the patient was first offered randomization and, if willing, was randomized. . . . Patients who refused randomization but nevertheless agreed to participate, provided they were given the treatment of their choice, were then entered into a patient preference trial." (Bedi et al., 2000; Chilvers et al., 2001; Miller et al., 2003).

Another typical statement was that "patients refused randomization because of a strong preference" (Wallage et al., 2003). Explanations of allocation procedures are listed in Table 27.3. We noted some discrepant definitions in multiple publications of the same study. For example, King asked patients whether they "wished to choose their treatment" (King et al., 2000). In the accompanying paper, Ward stressed that "participants were encouraged to accept randomization" (Ward et al., 2000).

Our impression that the unique sequence of information mandated by the PRPPT was rarely maintained was strengthened by a phone call with one of the principle investigators. He admitted that "the conceptual difference between asking patients first for their preference or their willingness to be randomized was not fully comprehended."

Twenty-two investigations represented comprehensive cohort studies in which subjects who refused random allocation, but agreed in trial participation, were scheduled for similar follow-up examinations. Two studies used a two-stage trial design as proposed by Rücker (1989) in which eligible subjects were prerandomized first to a choice cohort, a PRPPT, or an RCT (Cooper et al., 1997a,b; Noel et al., 1998). In another trial, children with otitis media (infection of the middle ear) were prerandomized to tympanostomy (incision of the eardrum) with adenoidectomy (removal of the adenoids) or tympanostomy alone (Mattila et al., 2003). Children whose parents refused the random assignment were treated according to the parent's choice, thus combining Zelen's design (Zelen, 1979) with a comprehensive cohort study.

Renjilian stratified obese patients according to their preference for group or individual therapy in a $2 \times 2$ factorial randomized trial yielding subjects whose treatment did and did not meet their preferred choice (Renjilian et al., 2001).

Studies enrolled a median of 137 patients in the randomized cohort (range 6–1796) and a median of 102 patients in the observational or preference cohort (range 20–1814). Study details are summarized in Tables 27.4 and 27.5.

TABLE 27.3. Sequence of allocation procedures

| Study | Statement on allocation sequence |
|---|---|
| Antman | "Those who were offered participation in the study **but refused randomization** were considered nonparticipants by virtue of patient choice." |
| Ashok | "Women **who agreed to be randomized** were assigned to a method by opening consecutive sealed envelopes. . . . The women willing to participate if they received their preferred treatment option constituted a non-randomized prospective cohort." |
| AWESOME | "The 327 patients who **refused random allocation** elected either CABG or PCI for themselves and are referred to as the patient-choice registry." |
| Bain | "Each individual was informed about both methods and was randomly allocated to one or, **if a preference was expressed, that method was offered.**" |
| Bakker | "Thirty-one patients who had **refused randomized treatment** . . . received cognitive therapy by preference. . . . There were no patients who refused randomization because they only wanted to accept treatment with medication." |
| BARI | "Clinically eligible patients who **consented to random assignment** entered the randomized trial. An additional 2010 clinically eligible patients who did not consent to randomization but consented to provide follow-up data were entered into the registry." |
| Bedi | "The **patient was first offered randomization** and, if willing, was randomized. . . . Patients who refused randomization but nevertheless agreed to participate, provided that they were given the treatment of their choice, were then entered into a patient preference trial." |
| CASS | "Randomized patients met the criteria for randomization and **gave informed consent for randomization.** . . . The randomizable patients were those patients at the 11 randomizing institutions who . . . met criteria for randomization but who were not randomized." |
| Cooper | "Those in the PRPP arm were counseled in a similar way, but it was pointed out that if they had a **strong preference for one of the treatments they should have it.**" |
| Coward | "Twenty-three women . . . **indicated a strong preference for being in a support group.** . . . Only 6 women were willing to be randomized." |
| de C Williams | "Patients who accepted the offer of treatment **were asked if they were willing to be randomized.** . . ." |
| DOPS | "DOPS is an ongoing long-term **comprehensive cohort multicenter study.** . . ." |
| EORTC | "Apart from reasons for ineligibility, also **doctors' and patients' preferences for trial participation or a particular treatment were searched for.**" |
| GBSG 2 | "The **majority of patients had a treatment preference** mainly due to treatment options being qualitatively quite different." |
| GBSG 3 | "**All subjects were asked if they were prepared to accept either inpatient or outpatient withdrawal.** Those subjects who were willing to accept either were then assigned randomly to one of the two randomized groups. The 40 subjects who expressed a strong preference. . . . were assigned to the appropriate group." |
| Gossop | "One year after commencement of the trial, it became obvious that **some of the participating centers were unable to obtain patients' consent for the randomization.** It was then decided that those centers would have the option to continue enrolling patients on a treatment preference basis." |

*(Continued)*

TABLE 27.3. (*Continued*)

| Study | Statement on allocation sequence |
| --- | --- |
| Helsing | Henshaw: "... eligible women ... **were asked if they were willing to be allocated to a method of abortion at random. Women who declined randomization invariably did so because one of the alternatives seemed much more attractive. ...**" |
| Kendrick | Howie: "**Women were allocated to an abortion method using a patient-centered, partially randomized study design.**" |
|  | "The study included **a preference arm, in which participants who did not consent to randomization** could choose whether to have an X-ray or not." |
| Kerry | "Patients who **refused to be take part in the RCT** or patients whom the GP did not wish to randomize were invited to take part in the observational study." |
|  | King King: "**Patients were asked whether they wished to choose their treatment or were willing to be randomized.**" Ward: "After the assessment, the researcher took each patient through a series of explanations about the treatments and the allocation procedure. **We encouraged participants to accept randomization.** Those who continued to express a strong preference were allowed to choose their treatment." |
| Kitchener | "**Prerandomized women who refused the experimental option** were offered standard treatment." |
| Mattila | "However, **if the parents expressed willingness to participate, the randomly allocated treatment was revealed to them.** At this point, the parents were given the chance not to participate. After the allocation was revealed, those children whose parents gave written consent were enrolled in the randomized trial and operated on according to the allocation of the randomization." |
| McKay | "... alcohol patients were **invited to participate in a random assignment study.** ... Patients who accepted randomization were assigned ..." |
| McKay | "Patients who **accepted randomization** were assigned to their treatment by a research technician. ... The final study sample consisted of randomized and nonrandomized patients. ..." |
| Melchart | "**They were then asked whether they agreed to being randomly assigned to receive sedation or acupuncture.** If they did not agree they received the treatment of their preference." |
| Nicolaides | "**Women were counseled as to the available options** of noninvasive screening or invasive testing by mid-trimester amniocentesis, early amniocentesis (EA), or chorionic villus sampling (CVS), or randomization to EA or CVS at 10–13 weeks." |
| Noel | "**Eligible patients were randomly assigned to either a choice or no choice condition** using a computer-generated randomization scheme carried out by a secretary who was unaware of baseline patient characteristics. Patients in the choice condition were then provided with written neutral descriptions of the two curricula and then were assigned to the curriculum of their choice." |
| Paradise | "**The 114 children whose parents withheld consent were ... assigned according to parental preference.**" |
| Reddihough | "Early in the study, it became clear that some families were **unwilling to accept the randomization process.** These children were still studied but their outcomes were treated separately." |
| Renjilian | "The remaining 75 individuals **who expressed a clear preference** ... were stratified on the basis of treatment preference and then randomly assigned to receive treatment in either their preferred or nonpreferred modality." |
| Wallage | "Women who **declined randomization because of a strong preference** for one type of anesthetic were treated under the anesthetic of their choice ..." |
| Woodward | "The trial design incorporated a nonrandomized 'preference arm'. Consent was obtained from 20 women—10 who definitely wanted a water birth and 10 who definitely wanted a land birth." |

TABLE 27.4. Primary and secondary endpoints

| Study | Primary endpoint | Secondary endpoint |
|---|---|---|
| Antman | 4-year disease-free survival | ? |
| Ashok | Level of acceptability | Complete uterine evacuation, medical sequelae at 2 and 8 weeks of F/U |
| AWESOME | 5-year survival | Survival free of unstable angina, survival free of unstable angina + repeat revascularization |
| Bain | McGill semantic differential scale | Postoperative analgesia, postoperative discharge time |
| Bakker | Panic frequency | CGI-S, PGE, HAMA, MSPS, SDS, ACQ, BSQ, MADRS |
| BARI | Mortality from all causes | Cardiac death |
| Bedi | change in Beck depression scale | Good outcome, good or moderate outcome, remission, relapse |
| CASS | 5-year survival | ? |
| Cooper | Satisfaction with treatment | Acceptability, bleeding score, pain score, hemoglobin increase, SF-36 at 4 months F/U |
| Coward | Change in Self-Transcendence Scale | ? |
| de C Williams | ≥50% Improvement in walk distance | ≥25% Improvement in function (SIP), ≥1 SD reduction in BDI, no further pain medication |
| DOPS | Fracture incidence | Incidence of forearm, vertebral, and femoral neck fractures, BMD, adverse events |
| EORTC | Local recurrence at 4 years F/U | DCIS recurrence, invasive recurrence, distant metastasis, death, contralateral cancer |
| GBSG 2 | 5-year disease-free survival | 5-year survival |
| GBSG 3 | 5-year disease-free survival | 5-year survival |
| Gossop | Abstinence at end of withdrawal regimen | ? |
| Helsing | Quality of life (EORTC QLQ-C30) | 1-year survival |
| Henshaw | Acceptability of treatment | Semantic differential rating scores |
| Kendrick | Still low back pain at 6 months F/U | Roland and Morris disability score, VAS for pain, EuroQol-5, satisfaction and expectations, reassurance and belief in the value of radiography, duration of low back pain, sick leave, use of health and other services, pain dairy, cost-effectiveness |
| Kerry | Roland and Morris disability at 1 year F/U | SF-36, HADS, EuroQol, cost-effectiveness |
| King | Beck depression scale at 12 months F/U | BSI, SAS, EuroQol, patient satisfaction, experience of treatment, cost effectiveness |
| Kitchener | General Health Questionnaire (GHQ-28) | Negative repeat smear, CIN |
| Mattila | Episodes of otitis media | Episodes of otitis media by S. pneumoniae, H. influenzae, M. catarrhalis |
| McKay | Number of drinking days at 12 months F/U | Days of alcohol intoxication/cocaine use, return to rehabilitation, entering of detoxification program, no. of days paid for working, welfare, conflicts with family or others, illegal income, incarceration |
| McKay | days of cocaine use at 12 months F/U | Drug composites, days of alcohol use, positive urine tests, family-social and psychiatric composites |

*(Continued)*

TABLE 27.4. (*Continued*)

| Study | Primary endpoint | Secondary endpoint |
|---|---|---|
| Melchart | perceived trouble on 100-mm VAS | Opt for same treatment in future, physician assessment, physiological variables |
| Nicolaides | total fetal loss | Spontaneous death, termination, chromosomal defect, congenital defects |
| Noel | knowledge | Self-care behaviors, HbA1c, BMI, SF-36 |
| Paradise | episodes of throat infections at F/U | Moderate or severe throat infections, group A streptococcal infections, cervical lymphadenopathy, sore-throat days, school absence |
| Reddihough | Vulpe Assessment Battery (VAB) videotapes | Gross Motor Function Measure (GMFM), Reynell Developmental Language Scale (RDLS), QRS-F, Parenting Stress Index (PSI) |
| Renjilian | net change in BMI | Net change in body weight |
| Wallace | acceptability of treatment after two weeks | Hospital Anxiety and Depression Scale, analgesia, total opiates, sickness, time to discharge |
| Woodward | length of first stage of labor | Length of second stage of labor, delivery method, analgesia, maternal temp., babies' outcomes |

TABLE 27.5. Patient flow (published data)

| Study | Screened | Included | Randomized | Observed |
|---|---|---|---|---|
| Antman | ? | 90 | 42 | 48 |
| Ashok | 486 | 445 | 368 | 77 |
| AWESOME | 22662 | 2431 | 454 | 1650 physician-directed, 327 patient-choice |
| Bain | 114 | 98 | 36 | 62 |
| Bakker | 154 | 66 | 35 | 31 |
| BARI | 4107 | 3839 | 1829 | 2010 |
| Bedi | ? | 323 | 103 | 220 |
| CASS | 24959 | 2099 | 780 | 1315 |
| Cooper | 273 | 135 randomized to PRPPT, 138 randomized to RCT | 90 randomized in PRPPT | 40 observed in PRPPT |
| Coward | 54 | 39 | 6 | 33 |
| de C Williams | 412 | 249 | 121 (33 to waiting list group) | 128 |
| DOPS | 47720 | 2016 | 1006 | 1010 |
| EORTC | ? | 1010 | 1010 | Five hospitals, 27% of subjects (LE+RT: 29 excluded, 133 random- ized, LE: 93 excluded, 135 randomized |
| GBSG 2 | ? | 720 | 247 | 473 |
| GBSG 3 | ? | 328 | 129 | 199 |
| Gossop | ? | 60 | 20 | 40 |
| Helsing | 151 | 151 | 49 | 102 |
| Henshaw | 373 | 363 | 195 | 168 |
| Kendrick | 9453 | 476 | 421 | 55 |
| Kerry | 659 | 659 | 153 | 506 |
| King | 627 | 464 | 327 (130 2-way, 197 3-way) | 137 |
| Kitchener | 739 | 712 prerandomized, 476 included | 243 no choice (surveillance), 103 surveillance and 130 colposcopy by choice | |
| Mattila | 2497 | 306 prerandomized | 137 accepted allocation | 169 declined random allocation |
| McKay | 125 | 108 | 28 | 80 |
| McKay | 663 | 144 | 48 | 96 |
| Melchart | 308 | 171 | 115 | 56 |
| Nicolaides | 2094 | 534 selected noninvasive screening, 35 amniocentesis, 1301 randomized or observed | 488 | 813 |
| Noel | ? | 305 assigned to choice, 291 assigned to RCT | 291 | 305 |
| Paradise | 2043 | 187 | 91 | 96 |
| Reddihough | 69 | 60 | 34 | 26 |
| Renjilian | 135 | 75 (39 matching, 36 nonmatching preference) | 75 | |
| Wallage | 359 | 322 | 191 | 131 |
| Woodward | 148 | 80 | 60 | 20 |

TABLE 27.6. Methodological standards

| Study | No. of exclusion criteria | No. of inclusion criteria | Risk stratification? | Concealment? | Outcome assessors blinded? | Flowchart of study profile? | Intent-to-treat analysis? | No. baseline criteria provided | Reliability of outcome criteria? | Measures of variance provided? | IRB approval? |
|---|---|---|---|---|---|---|---|---|---|---|---|
| Antman | 0 | 5 | Yes | Unclear | Unclear | No | Yes | 17 | High | No | Unclear |
| Ashok | 6 | 6 | Unclear | Yes | Unclear | Yes | Unclear | 6 | Intermediate | Yes | Yes |
| AWESOME | 0 | 3 | Unclear | Yes | Unclear | No | Unclear | 23 | High | No | Yes |
| Bain | 0 | 3 | Unclear | Yes | Unclear | No | Unclear | 9 | Low | Yes | Yes |
| Bakker | 2 | 3 | Unclear | Unclear | Yes | No | Yes | 4 | Intermediate | Yes | Yes |
| BARI | 0 | 3 | Unclear | Yes | Unclear | Yes | Yes | 35 | High | Yes | Yes |
| Bedi | 5 | 2 | Unclear | Unclear | Unclear | No | Unclear | 20 | Intermediate | Yes | Unclear |
| CASS | 12 | 4 | Yes | Yes | Unclear | Yes | Unclear | 65 | High | Yes | Unclear |
| Cooper | 5 | 2 | Unclear | Yes | Unclear | Yes | Unclear | 8 | Intermediate | Yes | Yes |
| Coward | 0 | 0 | Unclear | Unclear | Unclear | No | Unclear | 31 | Intermediate | Yes | Yes |
| de C Williams | 7 | 7 | Unclear | Unclear | Yes | Yes | Yes | 18 | Intermediate | Yes | Unclear |
| DOPS | 6 | 2 | Unclear | Yes | Unclear | Yes | Yes | 14 | High | Yes | Yes |
| EORTC | 5 | 2 | Unclear | Yes | Unclear | No | Yes | 7 | High | No | Yes |
| GBSG 2 | 0 | 4 | Yes | Yes | Unclear | No | Unclear | 13 | High | Yes | Yes |
| GBSG 3 | 0 | 4 | Yes | Yes | Unclear | No | Unclear | 13 | High | Yes | Yes |
| Gossop | 0 | 2 | Unclear | Unclear | Unclear | No | Unclear | 0 | Intermediate | No | Unclear |
| Helsing | 0 | 12 | Unclear | Unclear | Unclear | Yes | Unclear | 15 | Intermediate | Yes | Yes |
| Henshaw | 0 | 1 | Yes | Yes | Yes | No | Yes | 10 | Low | Yes | Unclear |
| Kendrick | 10 | 2 | Unclear | Yes | Unclear | Yes | Yes | 32 | High | Yes | Yes |
| Kerry | 3 | 1 | Unclear | Yes | Unclear | Yes | Yes | 32 | Intermediate | Yes | Yes |
| King | 6 | 2 | Yes | Yes | Unclear | Yes | Yes | 4 | High | Yes | Yes |
| Kitchener | 1 | 2 | Unclear | Unclear | Unclear | Yes | Yes | 1 | Intermediate | Yes | Unclear |
| Mattila | 0 | 3 | Unclear | Yes | Unclear | Yes | Yes | 7 | Intermediate | No | Yes |
| McKay | 17 | 1 | Unclear | Unclear | Unclear | No | Unclear | 20 | High | Yes | Unclear |
| McKay | 6 | 2 | Unclear | Unclear | Unclear | No | Unclear | 19 | High | Yes | Unclear |
| Melchart | 5 | 2 | No | Yes | Unclear | Yes | Unclear | 8 | Low | Yes | Yes |
| Nicolaides | 6 | 2 | Unclear | Yes | Unclear | No | Unclear | 12 | High | No | Unclear |
| Noel | 0 | 3 | Unclear | Yes | Unclear | Yes | Yes | 11 | Intermediate | No | Unclear |

| Paradise | 14 | 4 | Yes | Unclear | Unclear | Yes | Yes | 30 | High | Yes | Yes |
| Reddihough | 2 | 1 | Yes | Unclear | Yes | No | Unclear | 9 | Intermediate | Yes | Unclear |
| Renjilian | 5 | 4 | Yes | Unclear | Unclear | No | Unclear | 3 | Intermediate | Yes | Unclear |
| Wallace | 4 | 2 | Unclear | Yes | Unclear | Yes | Yes | 9 | Intermediate | Yes | Yes |
| Woodward | 5 | 2 | Unclear | Yes | Unclear | Yes | Yes | 6 | High | Yes | Yes |

IRB = Institutional Review Board.

We considered the available trials of moderate methodological quality (Table 27.6). Measures of variance were available from 26 studies (79%). Concealment of random lists was maintained by 20 investigations (61%). The intent-to-treat principle was met by 16 trials (48%). Altogether, 17 articles provided a CONSORT flowchart. Four studies aimed at blinding outcome assessors.

We examined outcome criteria of high and intermediate reliability in 15 studies each (45%). Studies provided a median of 12 (range 0–65) patient characteristics, enabling comparison of risk profiles among groups. Overall, we found no obvious differences in the dichotomous and continuous baseline measures between randomized subjects and those demanding a certain treatment (Fig. 27.2).

Figure 27.3 illustrates the ratio between the number of patients choosing the control over the experimental intervention in the nonrandomized arms of trials, permitting quantitative data synthesis. In the partially randomized patient preference trial (PRPPT), comprehensive cohort design (CCS), and other trial formats, this ratio ranged from 0.32 to 1.00, 0.51 to 4.13, and 0.28 to 1.11, respectively. In a trial of chemotherapy versus best supportive care for advanced non-small-cell lung cancer (NSCLC), only 5 of 102 patients opting for one or the other treatment preferred best supportive care. The authors later summarized the results of the preference arm (Helsing et al., 1998).

In another trial comparing cognitive with drug therapy for panic disorders, patients who were offered a treatment choice exclusively preferred cognitive therapy. Thus, comparisons were made only between outcomes of randomly allocated and preferred cognitive therapy (Bakker et al., 2000).

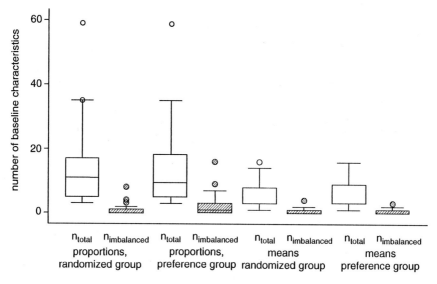

FIGURE 27.2. Number of dichotomous and continuous baseline characteristics and associated numbers of items showing differences between groups at the two-tailed 5% level.

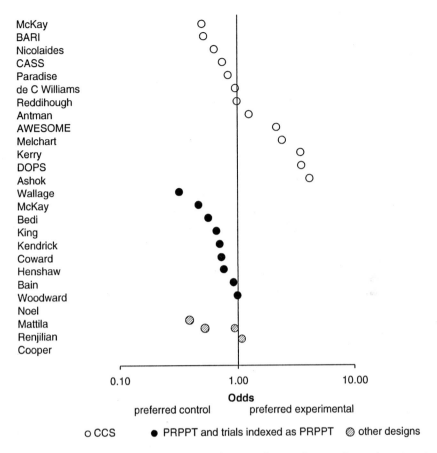

FIGURE 27.3. Ratio of patients preferring the control over the experimental treatment. CCS = comprehensive cohort design; PRPPT = partially randomized patient preference trial.

## Quantitative Analysis

A full comparison of outcomes between randomized and nonrandomized arms could be carried out in 22 studies. Absolute effect sizes were comparable for the two groups (Fig. 27.4).

Of 12 trials investigating binary outcomes (for example, overall survival), 9 showed no differences between experimental and control interventions in either cohort (Fig. 27.5). Cooper observed better acceptability of medical therapy than surgical therapy for heavy menstrual bleeding in both randomized and preference groups (Cooper et al., 1997a,b). Counseling for depression performed better than antidepressants in both cohorts of the hybrid study published by Bedi and coworkers (Bedi et al., 2000; Chilvers et al., 2001; Miller et al., 2003).

Favorable results with vacuum aspiration compared to medical abortion noted in the randomized part of the trial conducted by Henshaw and coworkers (1993)

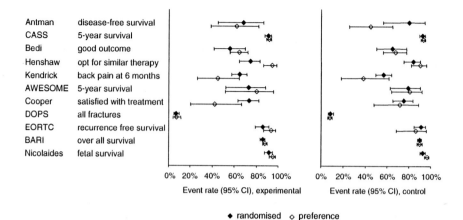

| Antman | disease-free survival |
| CASS | 5-year survival |
| Bedi | good outcome |
| Henshaw | opt for similar therapy |
| Kendrick | back pain at 6 months |
| AWESOME | 5-year survival |
| Cooper | satisfied with treatment |
| DOPS | all fractures |
| EORTC | recurrence free survival |
| BARI | over all survival |
| Nicolaides | fetal survival |

0%  20%  40%  60%  80%  100%
Event rate (95% CI), experimental

0%  20%  40%  60%  80%  100%
Event rate (95% CI), control

♦ randomised   ◊ preference

FIGURE 27.4. Absolute effect sizes (with 95% confidence intervals) among patients receiving the experimental or the control treatment by choice or by chance. CI = confidence interval.

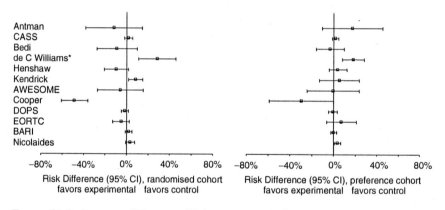

| Antman |
| CASS |
| Bedi |
| de C Williams* |
| Henshaw |
| Kendrick |
| AWESOME |
| Cooper |
| DOPS |
| EORTC |
| BARI |
| Nicolaides |

−80%    −40%    0%    40%    80%
Risk Difference (95% CI), randomised cohort
favors experimental   favors control

−80%    −40%    0%    40%    80%
Risk Difference (95% CI), preference cohort
favors experimental   favors control

FIGURE 27.5. Outcome differences (dichotomous endpoints) between randomized and choice groups. Risk differences were derived from published numbers needed to treat (NNT). CASS = Coronary Artery Surgery Study; AWESOME = Angina With Extremely Serious Operative Mortality Evaluation; DOPS = Danish Osteoporosis Prevention Study; BARI = Bypass Angioplasty Revascularization Investigation.

were not reproduced in patients preferring one or the other treatment. Overall satisfaction was higher in the preference groups. Altogether, 70 of 94 (74.5%) and 83 of 99 (83.8%) women randomized into the medical and surgical arms for abortion would have opted for similar treatment in the future. In the preference arms, these rates were 68 of 72 (94.4%) and 76 of 84 (90.5%), respectively.

Of 10 studies with ordinal or continuous outcomes (mainly quality of life assessments), 8 showed no difference between experimental and control interventions in either group (Fig. 27.6). Bain and coworkers (2001) observed

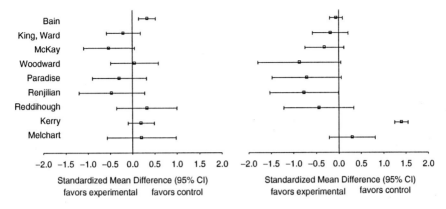

FIGURE 27.6. Outcome differences (continuous measures) between randomized and choice groups. Note that mean differences were standardized to allow global comparison of studies and do not reflect absolute differences in original scales.

favorable results with microwave ablation under local anesthesia compared to general anesthesia for dysfunctional uterine bleeding in the randomized cohort [weighted mean differences (WMD) in a semantic differential scale: 0.42; 95% confidence interval (CI): 0.19–0.64]. Again, this benefit could not be reproduced in the patient-preference cohort (WMD −0.06, 95% CI −0.22 to 0.09) (Coward, 2003).

Only one trial demonstrated a significant difference in standardized mean differences (SMD) of outcome measures in favor of the preference arm that was not observed in the randomized cohort (Kerry et al., 2000). Another six studies were available in which outcomes after treatment allocation could be compared according to random codes or preferences.

Bakker found no differences in the mean number of panic attacks per week after cognitive therapy by allocation or preference (SMD 0.28, 95% CI −0.21 to 0.76) (Bakker et al., 2000). There was also no difference in 1-year survival between subjects receiving etoposide/carboplatin or best supportive care for NSCLC either by chance or choice [risk difference (RD) 8%, 95% CI −14 to 29) (Helsing et al., 1998). The relative risk reduction (RRR) for otitis media episodes per person-year by tympanostomy plus adenectomy versus tympanostomy alone in randomized and nonrandomized groups was estimated at 19% (95% CI −14 to 43) and 25% (95% CI −13 to 50), respectively (Mattila et al., 2003).

Finally, in the German Breast Cancer Study Group trials (GBSG 2 and 3), no differences in survival were noted for six cycles of cyclophosphamide/methotrexate/ fluorouracil (CMF) versus three cycles (randomized: relative risk (RR) 0.9, 95% CI 0.7–1.2; nonrandomized: 0.9, 95% CI 0.6–1.4) or 6 × CMF plus radiotherapy versus 6 × CMF alone (randomized: RR 0.8, 95% CI 0.5–1.3; nonrandomized: 0.8, 95% CI 0.4–1.5). Favorable results with tamoxifen over no tamoxifen were noted only in the nonrandomized group (randomized: RR 0.8, 95% CI 0.5–1.0;

nonrandomized: 0.5, 95% CI 0.3–0.8) (Schmoor et al., 1996, 2000, 2002; Sauerbrei et al., 2000).

## Discussion

The hypothesis of this systematic review was that patients' preferences influence the results of clinical trials. To test this theory, we selected studies in which participants were allocated to treatment groups by choice or chance. We implicitly assumed that respecting preferences generates two independent populations of patients.

The available data do not corroborate this assumption. Random and preference groups were comparable in demographic and risk profiles. We could not reveal a regular pattern of outcome differences between random and preference arms. We were also unable to find evidence for strengthened effects if patients are allowed to choose their treatment option freely. These observations contradict previous theories of additive preference effects in clinical trials.

We could replicate the findings of King and colleagues (2002). Adding some studies not included in the previous review and selecting partly different endpoints did not change the overall results. Indeed, additional information permits a more detailed discussion of the findings.

Only four protocols unambiguously followed the PRPPT rules. As shown in Table 27.3, varying statements about allocation procedures suggest that few investigators comprehended the conceptually subtle, but essential, difference between the PRPPT and the CCS approach; and if they did, the PRPPT schedule was difficult to maintain. Unless the distinct order of informing patients is maintained, the randomized arms of a hybrid trial cannot be free of preference effects (McPherson & Chalmers, 1998). This preference contamination hampers data interpretation.

Patients rarely can or will take over the decision and the responsibility for or against a certain intervention alone, regardless of their doctors' recommendations. Thus, it may be impossible to distinguish between a patient's preference and the doctor's persuasiveness. Poor concordance between the parties, perpetuated by the degree of acceptance of the assigned treatment, makes outcomes unpredictable.

We are aware that a mismatch between the favored, guessed, and actual treatment introduces bias in blinded trials (Halpern, 2003). Because blinding and placebo control are of ancillary importance to the PRPPT design, we do not embark on this discussion.

In the real world, a state of "information vacuum" is the exception rather than the rule. Previous experiences and recommendations by relatives, other patients, and traditional beliefs further contribute to the choice of a certain intervention. We have to admit the power of information, regardless of its validity, as well as its verbal and nonverbal forms of communication. The Internet and the media play a significant role in spreading preliminary knowledge from scientific meetings that may be qualified by further investigations but induces confidence and hope (Schwartz et al., 2002).

We cannot predict how the availability of a new treatment will effect the decisions of patients and whether a hybrid study is still possible in this scenario. On the one hand, patients may preferably desire the new (promising) treatment, prolonging recruitment to randomized arms. On the other hand, the available studies showed a slight trend favoring control over experimental treatments.

Because of the small number of true PRPPTs, current evidence is inadequate to reach meaningful conclusions about the impact of patient preferences on outcomes. Minor deviations in study protocols from the original PRPPT design may have a greater impact than is generally expected.

The current lack in risk and outcome differences between cohorts generated by chance or choice emphasizes our lack of understanding the preference problem. Further conclusions are premature and require scientific approval on a larger scale.

## References

Andrews, G. (1999). Randomized controlled trials in psychiatry: important but poorly accepted. *British Medical Journal*, 319, 562–564.

Antman, K., Suit, H., Amato, D., Corson, J., Wood, W., Proppe, K., et al. (1984). Preliminary results of a randomized trial of adjuvant doxorubicin for sarcomas: lack of apparent difference between treatment groups. *Journal of Clinical Oncology*, 2, 601–608.

Antman, K., Amato, D., Wood, W., Carson, J., Suit, H., Proppe, K., et al. (1985). Selection bias in clinical trials. *Journal of Clinical Oncology*, 3, 1142–1147.

Ashok, P.W., Kidd, A., Flett, G.M., Fitzmaurice, A., Graham, W., Templeton, A. (2002). A randomized comparison of medical abortion and surgical vacuum aspiration at 10-13 weeks gestation. *Human Reproduction*, 17, 92–98.

Bain, C., Cooper, K.G., Parkin, D.E. (2001). A partially randomized patient preference trial of microwave endometrial ablation using local anaesthesia and intravenous sedation or general anaesthesia: a pilot study. *Gynaecological Endoscopy*, 10, 223–228.

Bakker, A., van Dyck, R., Spinhoven, P., van Balkom, A.J.L.M. (1999). Paroxetine, clomipramine, and cognitive therapy in the treatment of panic disorder. *Journal of Clinical Psychiatry*, 60, 831–838.

Bakker, A., Spinhoven, P., van Balkom, A.J., Vleugel, L., van Dyck, R. (2000). Cognitive therapy by allocation versus cognitive therapy by preference in the treatment of panic disorder. *Psychotherapy and Psychosomatics*, 69, 240–243.

BARI Investigators (1996). Comparison of coronary bypass surgery with angioplasty in patients with multivessel disease. *New England Journal of Medicine*, 335, 217–225.

Bedi, N., Chilvers, C., Churchill, R., Dewey, M., Duggan, C., Fielding, K., et al. (2000). Assessing effectiveness of treatment of depression in primary care: partially randomized preference trial. *British Journal of Psychiatry*, 177, 312–318.

Benson, K., Hartz, A.J. (2000). A comparison of observational studies and randomized, controlled trials. *New England Journal of Medicine*, 342, 1878–1886.

Bijker, N., Peterse, J.L., Fentiman, I.S., Julien, J.P., Hart, A.A., Avril, A., et al. (2002). Effects of patient selection on the applicability of results from a randomized clinical trial

(EORTC 10853) investigating breast-conserving therapy for DCIS. *British Journal of Cancer*, 87, 615–620.

Bower, P., Byford, S., Sibbald, B., Ward, E., King, M., Lloyd, M., et al. (2000). Randomized controlled trial of non-directive counselling, cognitive-behaviour therapy, and usual general practitioner care for patients with depression. II. Cost effectiveness. *British Medical Journal*, 321, 1389–1392.

Brewin, C.R., Bradley, C. (1989). Patient preferences and randomized clinical trials. *British Medical Journal*, 299, 313–315.

Brooks, M.M., Jones, R.H., Bach, R.G., Chaitman, B.R., Kern, M.J., Orszulak, T.A., et al. (2000). Predictors of mortality and mortality from cardiac causes in the Bypass Angioplasty Revascularization Investigation (BARI) randomized trial and registry: for the BARI Investigators. *Circulation*, 101, 2682–2689.

CASS Principal Investigators and Their Associates (1984). Coronary artery surgery study (CASS): a randomized trial of coronary artery bypass surgery; comparability of entry characteristics and survival in randomized patients and nonrandomized patients meeting randomization criteria. *Journal of the American College of Cardiology*, 3, 114–128.

Chard, J.A., Lilford, R. J. (1998). The use of equipoise in clinical trials. *Social Science and Medicine*, 47, 891–898.

Chaitman, B.R., Rosen, A.D., Williams, D.O., Bourassa, M.G., Aguirre, F.V., Pitt, B., et al. (1997). Myocardial infarction and cardiac mortality in the Bypass Angioplasty Revascularization Investigation (BARI) randomized trial. *Circulation*, 96, 2162–2170.

Chilvers, C., Dewey, M., Fielding, K., Gretton, V., Miller, P., Palmer, B., et al. (2001). Antidepressant drugs and generic counselling for treatment of major depression in primary care: randomized trial with patient preference arms. *British Medical Journal*, 322, 772–775.

Concato, J., Shah, N., Horwitz, R.I. (2000). Randomized, controlled trials, observational studies, and the hierarchy of research designs. *New England Journal of Medicine*, 342, 1887–1892.

Cooper, K.G., Grant, A.M., Garratt, A.M. (1997a). The impact of using a partially randomized patient preference design when evaluating alternative managements for heavy menstrual bleeding. *British Journal of Obstetrics and Gynaecology*, 104, 1367–1373.

Cooper, K.G., Parkin, D.E., Garratt, A.M., Grant, A.M. (1997b). A randomized comparison of medical and hysteroscopic management in women consulting a gynaecologist for treatment of heavy menstrual loss. *British Journal of Obstetrics and Gynaecology*, 104, 1360–1366.

Coward, D.D. (2002). Partial randomization design in a support group intervention study. *Western Journal of Nursing Research*, 24, 406–421.

Coward, D.D. (2003). Facilitation of self-transcendence in a breast cancer support group. II. *Oncology Nursing Forum*, 30, 291–300.

De C Williams, A.C., Nicholas, M.K., Richardson, P.H., Pither, C.E., Fernandes, J. (1999). Generalizing from a controlled trial: the effects of patient preference versus randomization on the outcome of inpatient versus outpatient chronic pain management. *Pain*, 83, 57–5.

Detre, K.M., Guo, P., Holubkov, R., Califf, R.M., Sopko, G., Bach, R., et al. (1999). Coronary revascularization in diabetic patients: a comparison of the randomized and observational components of the Bypass Angioplasty Revascularization Investigation (BARI). *Circulation*, 99, 633–640.

Feit, F., Brooks, M.M., Sopko, G., Keller, N.M., Rosen, A., Krone, R., et al. (2000). Long-term clinical outcome in the Bypass Angioplasty Revascularization Investigation

Registry: comparison with the randomized trial; BARI Investigators. *Circulation*, 101, 2795–2802.

Gossop, M., Johns, A., Green, L. (1986). Opiate withdrawal: inpatient versus outpatient programmes and preferred versus random assignment to treatment. *British Medical Journal*, 293, 103–104.

Halpern, S.D. (2003). Evaluating preference effects in partially unblinded, randomized clinical trials. *Journal of Clinical Epidemiology*, 56, 109–115.

Helsing, M., Bergman, B., Thaning, L., Hero, U. (1998). Quality of life and survival in patients with advanced non-small cell lung cancer receiving supportive care plus chemotherapy with carboplatin and etoposide or supportive care only: a multicentre randomized phase III trial; Joint Lung Cancer Study Group. *European Journal of Cancer*, 34, 1036–1044.

Henshaw, R.C., Naji, S.A., Russell, I.T., Templeton, A.A. (1993). Comparison of medical abortion with surgical vacuum aspiration: women's preferences and acceptability of treatment. *British Medical Journal*, 307, 714–717.

Howie, F.L., Henshaw, R.C., Naji, S.A., Russell, I.T., Templeton, A.A. (1997). Medical abortion or vacuum aspiration? Two year follow up of a patient preference trial. *British Journal of Obstetrics and Gynaecology*, 104, 829–833.

Jack, W.J.L., Cherry, U., Rodger, A. (1990). Recruitment to a prospective breast conservation trial: why are so few patients randomized? *British Medical Journal*, 301, 83–85.

Jansen, S.J.T., Stiggelbout, A.M., Nooij, M., Kievit, J. (2000). The effect of individually assessed preference weights on the relationship between holistic utilities and nonpreference-based assessment. *Quality of Life Research*, 9, 541–557.

Julien, J.P., Bijker, N., Fentiman, I.S., Peterse, J.L., Delledonne, V., Rouanet, P., et al. (2000). Radiotherapy in breast-conserving treatment for ductal carcinoma in situ: first results of the EORTC randomized phase III trial 10853; EORTC Breast Cancer Cooperative Group and EORTC Radiotherapy Group. *Lancet*, 355, 528–533.

Kaptchuk, T.J. (2001). The double-blind, randomized, placebo-controlled trial: gold standard or golden calf? *Journal of Clinical Epidemiology*, 54, 541–549.

Kassirer, J.P. (1994). Incorporating patients' preferences into medical decisions. *New England Journal of Medicine*, 330, 1895–1896.

Kendrick, D., Fielding, K., Bentley, E., Miller, P., Kerslake, R., Pringle, M. (2001). The role of radiography in primary care patients with low back pain of at least 6 weeks duration: a randomized (unblinded) controlled trial. *Health Technology Assessment*, 5, 1–69.

Kennedy, W.A., Laurier, C., Malo, J.L., Ghezzo, H., L'Archeveque, J., Contandriopoulos, A. P. (2003). Does clinical trial subject selection restrict the ability to generalize use and cost of health services to "real life" subjects? *International Journal of Technology Assessment in Health Care*, 19, 8–16.

Kerry, S., Hilton, S., Patel, S., Dundas, D., Rink, E., Lord, J. (2000). Routine referral for radiography of patients presenting with low back pain: is patients' outcome influenced by GPs' referral for plain radiography? *Health Technology Assessment*, 40(20), 1–121.

King, M., Sibbald, B., Ward, E., Bower, P., Lloyd, M., Gabbay, M., et al. (2000). Randomized controlled trial of non-directive counselling, cognitive-behaviour therapy and usual general practitioner care in the management of depression as well as mixed anxiety and depression in primary care. *Health Technology Assessment*, 4(19), 1–83.

King, M., Nazareth, I., Lampe, F., Bower, P., Chandler, M., Morou, M., et al. (2005). Impact of participant and physician intervention preferences on randomized trials: a systematic review. *Journal of the American Medical Association*, 293, 1089–1099.

Kitchener, H.C., Burns, S., Nelson, L., Myers, A.J., Fletcher, I., Desai, M., et al. (2004). A randomized controlled trial of cytological surveillance versus patient choice between surveillance and colposcopy in managing mildly abnormal cervical smears. *BJOG*, 111, 63–70.

Kotwall, C.A., Mahoney, L.J., Myers, R.E., Decoste, L. (1992). Reasons for non-entry in randomized clinical trials for breast cancer: a single institutional study. *Journal of Surgical Oncology*, 50, 125–129.

Kramer, M.S., Shapiro, S.H. (1984). Scientific challenges in the application of randomized trials. *Journal of the American Medical Association*, 252, 2739–2745.

Lambert, M.F., Wood, J. (2000). Incorporating patient preferences into randomized trials. *Journal of Clinical Epidemiology*, 53, 163–166.

Lilford, R.J. (2003). Ethics of clinical trials from a Bayesian and decision analytic perspective: whose equipoise is it anyway? *British Medical Journal*, 326, 980–981.

MacLehose, R.R., Reeves, B.C., Harvey, I.M., Sheldon, T.A., Russell, I.T., Black, A.M. (2000). A systematic review of comparisons of effect sizes derived from randomized and non-randomized studies. *Health Technology Assessment*, 4(34), 1–154.

Mattila, P.S., Joki-Erkkila, V.P., Kilpi, T., Jokinen, J., Herva, E., Puhakka, H. (2003). Prevention of otitis media by adenoidectomy in children younger than 2 years. *Archives of Otolaryngology Head and Neck Surgery*, 129, 163–168.

McCormack, J., Greenhalgh, T. (2000). Seeing what you want to see in randomized controlled trials: versions and perversions of UKPDS data. *British Medical Journal*, 320, 1720–1723.

McCulloch, P., Taylor, I., Sasako, M., Lovett, B., Griffin, D. (2002). Randomized trials in surgery: problems and possible solutions. *British Medical Journal*, 324, 1448–1451.

McKay, J.R., Alterman, A.I., McLellan, A.T., Snider, E.C., O'Brien, C.P. (1995). Effect of random versus nonrandom assignment in a comparison of inpatient and day hospital rehabilitation for male alcoholics. *Journal of Consulting and Clinical Psychology*, 63, 70–78.

McKay, J.R., Alterman, A.I., McLellan, A.T., Boardman, C.R., Mulvaney, F.D., O'Brien, C. P. (1998). Effect of random versus nonrandom assignment in the evaluation of treatment for cocaine abusers. *Journal of Consulting and Clinical Psychology*, 66, 697–701.

McPherson, K. (1994). The best and the enemy of the good: randomized controlled trials, uncertainty, and assessing the role of patients choice in medical decision making. *Journal of Epidemiology and Community Health*, 48, 6–15.

McPherson, K., Chalmers, I. (1998). Incorporating patient preferences into clinical trials: information about patients' preference must be obtained first. *British Medical Journal*, 317, 78.

McPherson, K., Britton, A.R., Wennberg, J.E. (1997). Are randomized controlled trials controlled? Patient preferences and unblind trials. *Journal of the Royal Society of Medicine*, 90, 652–656.

Melchart, D., Steger, H. G., Linde, K., Makarian, K., Hatahet, Z., Brenke, R., et al. (2002). Integrating patient preferences in clinical trials: a pilot study of acupuncture versus midazolam for gastroscopy. *Journal of Alternative Complementary Medicine*, 8, 265–274.

Miller, P., Chilvers, C., Dewey, M., Fielding, K., Gretton, V., Palmer, B., et al. (2003). Counseling versus antidepressant therapy for the treatment of mild to moderate depression in primary care: economic analysis. *International Journal of Technology Assessment in Health Care*, 19, 80–90.

Moher, D., Schulz, K.F., Altman, D.G., for the CONSORT Group (2001). The CONSORT statement: revised recommendations for improving the quality of reports of parallel-group randomized trials. *Lancet*, 357, 1191–1194.

Morrison, D.A., Sethi, G., Sacks, J., Grover, F., Sedlis, S., Esposito, R., et al. (1999). A multicenter, randomized trial of percutaneous coronary intervention versus bypass surgery in high-risk unstable angina patients: the AWESOME (Veterans Affairs Cooperative Study #385, angina with extremely serious operative mortality evaluation) investigators from the Cooperative Studies Program of the Department of Veterans Affairs. *Controlled Clinical Trials*, 20, 601–619.

Morrison, D.A., Sethi, G., Sacks, J., Henderson, W., Grover, F., Sedlis, S., et al. (2001). Percutaneous coronary intervention versus coronary artery bypass graft surgery for patients with medically refractory myocardial ischemia and risk factors for adverse outcomes with bypass: a multicenter, randomized trial; Investigators of the Department of Veterans Affairs Cooperative Study #385, the Angina With Extremely Serious Operative Mortality Evaluation (AWESOME). *Journal of the American College of Cardiology*, 38, 143–149.

Morrison, D.A., Sethi, G., Sacks, J., Henderson, W., Grover, F., Sedlis, S., et al. (2002a). Percutaneous coronary intervention versus coronary bypass graft surgery for patients with medically refractory myocardial ischemia and risk factors for adverse outcomes with bypass: the VA AWESOME multicenter registry: comparison with the randomized clinical trial. *Journal of the American College of Cardiology*, 39, 266–273.

Morrison, D.A., Sethi, G., Sacks, J., Henderson, W. G., Grover, F., Sedlis, S., et al. (2002b). Percutaneous coronary intervention versus repeat bypass surgery for patients with medically refractory myocardial ischemia: AWESOME randomized trial and registry experience with post-CABG patients. *Journal of the American College of Cardiology*, 40, 1951–1954.

Mosekilde, L., Beck-Nielsen, H., Sørensen, O.H., Nielsen, S.P., Charles, P., Vestergaard, P., et al. (2000). Hormonal replacement therapy reduces forearm fracture incidence in recent postmenopausal women—results of the Danish Osteoporosis Prevention Study. *Maturitas*, 36, 181–193.

Mosekilde, L., Beck-Nielsen, H., Sørensen, O.H., Nielsen, S.P., Charles, P., Vestergaard, P., et al. (2001). Behandling med hormonsubstitutionsterapi nedsætter risikoen for underarmsbrud hos postmenopausale kvinder: Resultater fra Danish Osteoporosis Prevention Study. [Hormone replacement therapy reduces the risk of forearm fracture in postmenopausal women: results of the Danish Osteoporosis Prevention Study]. *Ugeskr Læger*, 163, 7064–7069.

Nicolaides, K., Brizot, M.L., de Patel, F., Snijders, R. (1994). Comparison of chorionic villus sampling and amniocentesis for fetal karyotyping at 10-13 weeks gestation. *Lancet*, 344, 435–439.

Noel, P.H., Larme, A.C., Meyer, J., Marsh, G., Correa, A., Pugh, J.A. (1998). Patient choice in diabetes education curriculum: nutritional versus standard content for type 2 diabetes. *Diabetes Care*, 21, 896–901.

Olschewski, M., Scheurlen, H. (1985). Comprehensive cohort study: an alternative to randomized consent design in a breast preservation trial. *Methods of Information in Medicine*, 24, 131–134.

Paradise, J.L., Bluestone, C.D., Bachman, R.Z., Colborn, D.K., Bernard, B.S., Taylor, F.H., et al. (1984). Efficacy of tonsillectomy for recurrent throat infection in severely affected children: results of parallel randomized and nonrandomized clinical trials. *New England Journal of Medicine*, 310, 674–683.

Paradise, J.L., Bluestone, C.D., Rogers, K.D., Taylor, F.H., Colborn, D.K., Bachman, R.Z., et al. (1990). Efficacy of adenoidectomy for recurrent otitis media in children previously treated with tympanostomy-tube placement: results of parallel randomized and nonrandomized trials. *Journal of the American Medical Association*, 263, 2066–2073.

Peppercorn, J.M., Weeks, J.C., Cook, E.F., Joffe, S. (2004). Comparison of outcomes in cancer patients treated within and outside clinical trials: conceptual framework and structured review. *Lancet*, 363, 263–270.

Plaisier, P.W., Berger, M.Y., van der Hul, R.L., Nijs, H.G.T., den Toom, R., Terpstra, O. T., et al. (1994). Unexpected difficulties in randomizing patients in a surgical trial: a prospective study comparing extracorporeal shock wave lithotripsy with open cholecystectomy. *World Journal of Surgery*, 18, 769–773.

Prescott, R.J., Counsell, C.E., Gillespie, W.J., Grant, A.M., Russell, I.T., Kiauka, S., et al. (1999). Factors that limit the quality, number and progress of randomized controlled trials. *Health Technology Assessment*, 3(20), 1–143.

Rauschecker, H.F., Sauerbrei, W., Gatzemeier, W., Sauer, R., Schauer, A., Schmoor, C., et al. (1998). Eight-year results of a prospective non-randomized study on therapy of small breast cancer: the German Breast Cancer Study Group (GBSG). *European Journal of Cancer*, 34, 315–323.

Reddihough, D.S., King, J., Coleman, G., Catanese, T. (1998). Efficacy of programmes based on conductive education for young children with cerebral palsy. *Developmental and Medicine Child Neurology*, 40, 763–770.

Renjilian, D.A., Perri, M.G., Nezu, A.M., McKelvey, W.F., Shermer, R.L., Anton, S.D. (2001). Individual versus group therapy for obesity: effects of matching participants to their treatment preferences. *Journal of Consulting and Clinical Psychology*, 69, 717–721.

Ross, S., Grant, A., Counsell, C., Gillespie, W., Russell, I., Prescott, R. (1999). Barriers to participation in randomized controlled trials: a systematic review. *Journal of Clinical Epidemiology*, 52, 1143–1156.

Rücker, G. (1989). A two-stage trial design for testing treatment, self-selection and treatment preference effects. *Statistics in Medicine*, 8, 477–485.

Sauerbrei, W., Bastert, G., Bojar, H., Beyerle, C., Neumann, R.L., Schmoor, C., et al. (2000). Randomized 2 × 2 trial evaluating hormonal treatment and the duration of chemotherapy in node-positive breast cancer patients: an update based on 10 years' follow-up; German Breast Cancer Study Group. *Journal of Clinical Oncology*, 18, 94–101.

Schmoor, C., Olschewski, M., Schumacher, M. (1996). Randomized and non-randomized patients in clinical trials: experiences with comprehensive cohort studies. *Statistics in Medicine*, 15, 263–271.

Schmoor, C., Sauerbrei, W., Bastert, G., Schumacher, M. (2000). Role of isolated locoregional recurrence of breast cancer: Results of four prospective studies. *Journal of Clinical Oncology*, 18, 1696–1708.

Schmoor, C., Olschewski, M., Sauerbrei, W., Schumacher, M. (2002). Long-term follow-up of patients in four prospective studies of the German Breast Cancer Study Group (GBSG): a summary of key results. *Onkologie*, 25, 143–150.

Schwartz, L.M., Woloshin, S., Baczek, L. (2002). Media coverage of scientific meetings: too much, too soon? *Journal of the American Medical Association*, 287, 2859–2863.

Sedlis, S.P., Morrison, D.A., Lorin, J.D., Esposito, R., Sethi, G., Sacks, J., et al. (2002). Percutaneous coronary intervention versus coronary bypass graft surgery for diabetic patients with unstable angina and risk factors for adverse outcomes with bypass: outcome of diabetic patients in the AWESOME randomized trial and registry. *Journal of the American College of Cardiology*, 40, 1555–1566.

Sedlis, S.P., Ramanathan, K.B., Morrison, D.A., Sethi, G., Sacks, J., Henderson, W. (2004). Department of Veterans Affairs Cooperative Study #385, Angina With

Extremely Serious Operative Mortality Evaluation (AWESOME) Investigators: outcome of percutaneous coronary intervention versus coronary bypass grafting for patients with low left ventricular ejection fractions, unstable angina pectoris, and risk factors for adverse outcomes with bypass (the AWESOME Randomized Trial and Registry). *American Journal of Cardiology*, 94, 118–120.

Silverman, W.A., Altman, D.G. (1996). Patient's preferences and randomized trials. *Lancet*, 347, 171–174.

Stiggelbout, A.M., de Haes, J.C.J.M. (2001). Patient preference for cancer therapy: an overview of measurement approaches. *Journal of Clinical Oncology*, 19, 220–230.

Wallage, S., Cooper, K.G., Graham, W.J., Parkin, D.E. (2003). A randomized trial comparing local versus general anaesthesia for microwave endometrial ablation. *BJOG*, 110, 799–807.

Ward, E., King, M., Lloyd, M., Bower, P., Sibbald, B., Farrelly, S., et al. (2000). Randomized controlled trial of non-directive counselling, cognitive-behaviour therapy, and usual general practitioner care for patients with depression. I. Clinical effectiveness. *British Medical Journal*, 321, 1383–1388.

Woodward, J., Kelly, S.M. (2004). A pilot study for a randomized controlled trial of water birth versus land birth. *BJOG*, 111, 537–545.

Zelen, M. (1979) A new design for randomized clinical trials. *New England Journal of Medicine*, 300, 1242–1245.

# 28
# Are the Results of Randomized Trials Influenced by Preference Effects? Part II. Why Current Studies Often Fail to Answer this Question

Franz Porzsolt and Dirk Stengel

It is assumed that shared decision making and respecting patients' preferences increases the comfort of both providers and consumers of health services. It is also plausible to expect enhanced effect sizes and improved outcomes with treatment options that match patients' demands.

Two recent systematic reviews challenge this assumption (King et al., 2005). In hybrid studies that incorporated both a randomized and a preference arm, differences were not noted in risk profiles or in outcomes between subjects who were allocated to a treatment group by choice (preference) or chance (randomization).

The correct interpretation of these findings may have significant consequences for research and clinical practice. The matter of debate is whether randomization can generally, sometimes, or never be replaced by allocation according to preference.

## Randomized Trials and Hybrid Designs

By reducing bias, the randomized controlled trial (RCT) takes credit for uncovering causal relations between interventions and outcomes. However, the RCT represents an artificial tool that has little in common with clinical decision making.

We do not want to recapitulate RCT issues that have been extensively discussed in the literature, such as limited external validity (Kaptchuk, 2001; Rothwell, 2005), doctors' efforts to breach random codes (Schulz, 1995), and, with blinding, patients' attempts to find out what treatment they received (Fergusson et al., 2004). It is nevertheless remarkable that so much energy is spent to undermine the architecture of a trial concept that aims at demasking "true" effect sizes. The need for alternative or hybrid formats was recognized early, leading to various design proposals to overcome the reluctance to comply with conventional RCTs (MacLehose et al., 2000).

Three major trial concepts characterized by the following steps have been established in research practice.

## Prerandomization Designs

- Randomize subjects before obtaining informed consent.
- Ask patients of both randomized groups for acceptance of random assignment.
- In case of refusal, treat according to preference.

The prerandomization design (Zelen, 1979, 1990) was developed to enhance recruitment rates in clinical trials with expected imbalanced preferences, that is, most patients were expected to prefer one of the offered treatments. Typical examples are studies that compare an experimental treatment with no treatment (null-arm control) (Riethmüller et al., 1994).

Patients who refuse the treatment assigned by randomization compromise the validity of the study. To circumvent this problem, the original design was modified in that only individuals assigned to the experimental treatment group were informed about randomization. Patients assigned to the control group (receiving standard therapy or no treatment in the absence of an accepted standard) are not informed about their participation in a clinical trial.

Despite unsolved ethical questions, both design variants are inadequate to study preference effects. The original design violates the randomization procedure, whereas in its modification preference effects can occur only in the experimental group (because only these patients provide informed consent) (Porzsolt et al., 2003, 2004).

## Comprehensive Cohort Design and Its Variants (Randomized Trial and Parallel Registries)

The comprehensive cohort design (CCS) (Olschewski & Scheurlen, 1985) and CCS variants (randomized trial and parallel registries) require the following questions.

1. Ask patients if they are willing to participate in an RCT.
2. Randomize subjects who agree.
3. Treat subjects who refuse random allocation according to their preference.

## Partially Randomized Patient Preference Trials

Partially randomized patient preference trials (PRPPTs) have the following criteria (Brewin & Bradley, 1989).

1. Ask for preferred treatment first.
2. If subject is undecided, offer randomization.

The differences between CCS studies and PRPPTs are subtle but essential. Randomization requires both absence of a preference and absence of averseness to allocation by chance. In clinical research, it is almost impossible to determine which condition influences the patient's decision. Patients in a CCS study have a higher chance of being randomized than in a PRPPT, despite a given preference. The primary aim of the CCS is recruitment of patients in a randomized trial. In contrast, the PRPPT design is chosen if the primary goal is to exclude patients with an existing preference from randomization. Consequently, the randomized arms of a CCS study are more frequently contaminated by patients with preferences than the randomized arms of a PRPPT.

Of 33 studies identified in our review, only 4 (12.1%) unambiguously followed the PRPPT schedule, whereas another 7 (21.1%) were called PRPPTs but were more likely to represent CCS studies. At best, only one-third of these studies could reveal preference effects.

## Theoretical Methodological Advantages of Partially Randomized Patient Preference Trials

If conducted properly, the PRPPT segregates patients with preferences from those without preferences. This creates a randomized cohort uncontaminated by latent preference effects and makes it possible to estimate their influence on overall outcomes.

We use a simplification of previous models of additive and interactive preference effects to illustrate this theory (McPherson et al., 1997; McPherson & Chalmers, 1998; Halpern, 2003).

Consider the effect sizes $e_A$ and $e_B$ observed with treatment options A and B in a clinical trial. Not surprisingly, the overall effect size divides up into the active principle (for example, a pharmacological effect) $a_A$ and an additive (or preference) component $p_A(A)$ that only works if the actual treatment meets the patients' expectations and demands. Thus, we observe the following.

$$e_A = a_A + p_A(A) \approx \max_A$$
$$e_B = a_B + p_B(B) \approx \max_B$$

## Effect of Preferences on the Results of "Classic" RCTs

In the unlikely situation of an ideal RCT, where patients have no preferences, the additive components $p_A(A)$ and $p_B(B)$ do not exist. The observed effects are caused by the active principles $a_A$ and $a_B$. The maximum achievable effects, however, are not reached.

In reality most patients who participate in a RCT have a weak preference for treatment A or treatment B. Patients with strong preferences generally refuse to participate in RCTs, regardless of the treatment option they prefer. The special situation of a general preference for a certain treatment option was already discussed in the context of the Zelen design.

Preferences of patients and their doctors limit participation in RCTs (Ross et al., 1999; Sehouli et al., 2005). The stronger the preference, the less likely is the acceptance of randomization. Thus, strong preference cannot be expressed or detected in RCTs.

PRPPTs minimize the contamination of randomized groups and might represent the best available method to study populations with moderate preferences. Again, it is unlikely that strong preferences would be detected in PRPPTs because patients and doctors with strong preferences refuse to participate in the randomized treatment arms.

## Conclusions

Both systematic reviews failed to demonstrate differences in outcomes when randomized and preference-based groups were compared. In addition, no differences in the risk profiles between randomized and preference-based groups were detected. The most likely explanation for these observations is the contamination of randomized groups by preferences, which is supported by evidence presented in Table 27.3 (see Chapter 27).

Preference has been discussed in the academic literature as a potential confounder of clinical trials but has not been mentioned in clinical research practice. The possible reasons are a lack of awareness of the problem and a lack of accepted methods to quantify the influence of results by preferences.

The available evidence suggests that RCTs are contaminated by preferences. This problem cannot be substantiated or solved unless methods to assess the effects of preferences are developed. At this stage of the debate, we can identify the problem and stress the need for action. In answer to our initial question, it may indeed be necessary to replace randomization by preference allocation if a study aims at assessing the effects of preference rather than treatment.

To quantify the impact of preferences on outcomes, preference must remain the single independent variable in a clinical experiment. Treatments can be randomized, whereas preferences cannot. Consequently, three aspects must be considered in an ideal clinical preference trial. First, patients without preferences must be excluded from the study, as they would attenuate effect sizes. Second, all included patients must receive the same treatment regardless of their preference. Otherwise, treatment is introduced as a second variable. Third, patients must not be informed about the treatment they receive to avoid jeopardizing the preference. This implies that the patient cannot distinguish between the treatments under investigation.

Possible design options for such studies are summarized in Figure 28.1. Because these studies abandon informed consent but use information as an experimental variable, they induce ethical conflicts and cannot be realized unless the scientific community and institutional review boards allow exceptions to presently accepted ethical rules. With established trial designs conforming to our current ethical framework, it is difficult if not impossible to reveal preference effects (King et al., 2005).

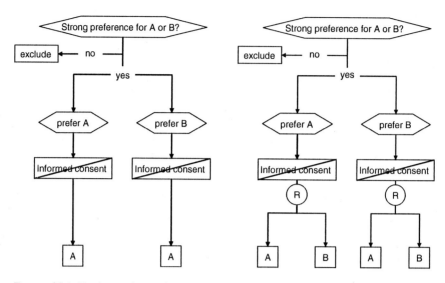

FIGURE 28.1. Design options with preference as the single independent variable. Left. Preference cohort design. Patients without a strong preference for treatment A or B are excluded. All other patients are asked for their preference. Regardless of their preference, they are assigned to treatment A. The treatment decision is not communicated. Right. Preference random design. Patients without a strong preference for treatment A or B are excluded. All other patients are asked for their preference. Without being informed, patients are randomly (R) assigned to treatment A or B. The treatment decision is not communicated. Because patients prefer A or B they must be unable to identify the actually applied study treatment.

Investigating preference effects is not only an academic question. It may change our understanding and the practice of clinical research.

## References

Brewin, C.R., Bradley, C. (1989). Patient preferences and randomized clinical trials. *British Medical Journal*, 299, 313–315.

Fergusson, D., Glass, K.C., Waring, D., Shapiro, S. (2004) Turning a blind eye: the success of blinding reported in a random sample of randomized, placebo controlled trials. *British Medical Journal 2004*, 328–432.

Halpern, S.D. (2003). Evaluating preference effects in partially unblinded, randomized clinical trials. *Journal of Clinical Epidemiology*, 56,109–115.

Kaptchuk, T.J. (2001). The double-blind, randomized, placebo-controlled trial: gold standard or golden calf? *Journal of Clinical Epidemiology*, 54, 541–549.

King, M., Nazareth, I., Lampe, F., Bower, P., Chandler, M., Morou, M., et al. (2005). Impact of participant and physician intervention preferences on randomized trials: a systematic review. *Journal of the American Medical Association*, 293, 1089–1099.

MacLehose, R.R., Reeves, B.C., Harvey, I.M., Sheldon, T.A., Russell, I.T., Black, A.M. (2000). A systematic review of comparisons of effect sizes derived from randomized and non-randomized studies. *Health Technology Assessment*, 4(34), 1–154.

McPherson, K., Chalmers, I. (1998). Incorporating patient preferences into clinical trials: information about patients' preference must be obtained first. *British Medical Journal*, 317, 78.

McPherson, K., Britton, A., Wennberg, J. E. (1997). Are randomized controlled trials controlled? Patient preferences and unblind trials. *Journal of the Royal Society of Medicine*, 90, 652–656.

Olschewski, M., Scheurlen, H. (1985). Comprehensive Cohort Study: an alternative to randomized consent design in a breast preservation trial. *Methods of Information in Medicine*, 24, 131–134.

Porzsolt, F., Kumpf, J., Coppin, C., Pöppel, E. (2003). Stringent application of epidemiologic criteria changes the interpretation of the effects of immunotherapy in advanced renal cell cancer. In: C. William, V. Bramwell, X. Bonfill, J. Cuzick, J.F. Forbes, R. Grant, et al. (Eds). *Evidence-based oncology*. Oxford: British Medical Journal Books.

Porzsolt, F., Schlotz-Gorton, N., Biller-Andorno, N., Thim, A., Meissner, K., Roeckl-Wiedmann, I., et al. (2004). Applying evidence to support ethical decisions: is the placebo really powerless? *Science and Engineering Ethics*, 10, 119–132.

Riethmüller, G., Schneider-Gädicke, E., Schlimok, G., Schmiegel, W., Raab, R., Höffken, K., et al. (1994). Randomized trial of monoclonal antibody for adjuvant therapy of resected Dukes' C colorectal carcinoma: German Cancer Aid 17-1A Study Group. *Lancet*, 343, 1177–1183.

Ross, S., Grant, A., Counsell, C., Gillespie, W., Russell, I., Prescott, R. (1999). Barriers to participation in randomized controlled trials: a systematic review. *Journal of Clinical Epidemiology*, 52, 1143–1156.

Rothwell, P.M. (2005). External validity of randomized controlled trials: "to whom do the results of this trial apply?" *Lancet*, 365, 82–93.

Schulz, K.F. (1995). Subverting randomization in controlled trials. *Journal of the American Medical Association*, 274, 1456–1458.

Sehouli, J., Kostromitskaia, J., Stengel, D., Bois, A. (2005). Why institutions do not participate in ovarian cancer trials: results from a survey in Germany. *Onkologie*, 28, 13–17.

Zelen, M. (1979). A new design for randomized clinical trials. *New England Journal of Medicine*, 300, 1242–1245.

Zelen, M. (1990). Randomized consent designs for clinical trials: an update. *Statistics in Medicine*, 9, 645–656.

# 29
# Suggested Changes in Practice, Research, and Systems: Clinical Economics Point of View

Robert M. Kaplan and Franz Porzsolt

This book is about gaining value for patients in health care. We have covered a lot of territory, ranging from ethical and philosophical issues to the contributions of psychology and clinical medicine. Portions of the book consider problems in clinical practice, such as overdiagnosis, patient preferences, and assessments of quality and safety in health care. We have also considered methods in economic analysis and clinical epidemiology. Considering the collection of chapters, what general lessons have we learned? In this final chapter we summarize some of these issues.

## Mistakes We Have Made

To move forward, we must reexamine where we have been. Health care is the largest sector in the economy in most developed countries (Anderson et al., 2005). We have been unable to control health care costs for a variety of reasons. First, we have had difficulty spending in a responsible way. In the United States, for example, health care costs have grown from 4% of the gross domestic product during the 1960s to nearly 15% today (Smith et al., 2006). Was health care in the 1960s really that bad to justify this dramatic increase in health care costs, or has our system undergone a change in the estimation of the value of health care?

The increase in health care costs is associated with higher prices for products manufactured by companies that provide health benefits for their employees. For example, General Motors (GM), the world's largest automobile producer, is currently on the verge of bankruptcy largely because it has been unable to control expenses. One of the largest controllable components of the GM budget is health insurance for the employees. Many health care services are attractive. However, to control costs in all economic sectors (not only in health care), tough decisions must be made about which services are necessary and which provide best value for patients.

The second problem is overdiagnosis. Improvements in diagnostic technology have led to significant increases in the rate of disease identified within communities. Several chapters in this book discuss the problem of pseudodisease—disease that, although identifiable, does not have any adverse affect on patients if left untreated. In the future, we will be faced with the challenge of selecting not only treatments but diagnostic tests. Patients diagnosed with a disease are likely to demand treatment, even when the value of treatment is expected to be low. Pseudodisease is the diagnostic equivalent of ineffective and potentially harmful treatment; and it therefore deserves attention.

The third problem is the lack of interest in value. Not all treatments afford an equal level of benefit to patients. Some offer only minor benefit, whereas others produce substantial changes in patient outcome. Furthermore, the cost to produce a unit of benefit differs dramatically across treatment options. Until recently, health care decision makers expressed little interest in estimating value for patients. With shrinking budgets and a continually increasing menu of attractive options, it is no longer ethical to advocate for every option. We must concentrate on choices that offer the best value for the communities served. More interest in the emerging value (outcomes research in addition to clinical research) is an essential part of feedback and successful quality management.

Finally, physicians and administrators have often spoken on the behalf of patients. A growing amount of literature suggests that patients may make decisions independently of their health care providers. These patient preferences must find their voice.

## Emerging Problems

Several chapters in this book document abuse of the health care system by both users and providers. There is substantial variability in the use of health care services among countries and even among communities in the same country. Health care providers often order tests and provide treatments that have limited value for patients. Excessive utilization increases the cost of health care without necessarily producing benefits.

Aggressive approaches to diagnosis and treatment result in overestimates of illness in communities. Many people are diagnosed with health problems, and substantial proportions of all populations consume prescription medications. These treatments often result in better patient outcomes. However, the inflation of illness through overdiagnosis also leads to inappropriate use of resources, high costs, and exposure of patients to medical errors and potentially harmful side effects of treatment.

Societies are becoming increasingly concerned about health care costs. Some advocate cost-effectiveness analysis as a means of cutting costs and not necessarily as a method to gain value for money. The purpose of cost-effectiveness analysis is not to save money. In fact, most advocates of these methods would prefer to keep budgets constant or to increase them. The purpose of cost-effectiveness analysis is to save lives, not to save money. Thoughtful analysis can be used to gain the greatest value for the resources available to decision makers.

We believe that more cross-disciplinary discussions are required. Experts often favor the methods they know best. Problems in health care are complex, and they can be solved only by taking a look at the broad prospective offered by multidisciplinary studies. One example is the introduction of economic thinking in health care.

## Economic Thinking

The chapters in this book have explored issues in outcomes research and the challenge of estimating value for patients. We began with the discussion of CLINECS, a concept that brings together thinking from several academic and medical disciplines. A central component of the CLINECS model is the application of economic thinking to problems in medicine and health care. We believe CLINECS thinking may change the way health care is delivered.

### Clinical Economic Thinking

Economics is an established social science. It is well integrated into academia and public policy. However, there has been relatively little penetration of economic thinking into medicine and health care. The one major exception is outcomes research and medical decision making. Economists have a unique way of thinking about problems. There are a variety of ways in which economists might think differently from those trained in other disciplines. We briefly outline some of these ideas and then apply them to health care.

#### Tradeoffs

Advocates in health care often argue that programs require more resources. Cardiologists argue that more tests and procedures should be funded. Oncologists press for greater use of screening, chemotherapy, and new approaches to tumor management. Pediatricians argue that more money must be spent on children. All of the specialists have similar arguments. They need more money.

When budgets are limited, more expenditures in one area may reduce expenditures elsewhere. In other words, funding decisions require tradeoffs. Economists take these tradeoffs very seriously. Much of their science involves a systematic evaluation of the risks and benefits of various alternatives. This can also be applied at the individual level. Selection of treatment options often requires a balance between positive effects and negative consequences. A careful enumeration of risks and benefits and the development of systematic models that assist in making these tradeoffs is an important part of economic science.

Although economists study costs, they define costs more broadly than most people, who think of costs solely in terms of money. Accountants consider how much money must be devoted to each alternative. Economists use the term cost in a broader sense. For economists, a cost is what must be surrendered to obtain a particular alternative. For example, recovery from surgery is a cost of the decision to have an operation. Investment in a cancer-screening program might mean that there are not enough resources to purchase new radiology equipment. Costs describe what is traded off when a decision is made. Some costs are monetary, and some reflect nonmonitary preferences. Monetary costs are relatively easy to quantify. Some of the other costs require new assessment methodologies.

Development of decision models requires a consideration of components of the decision process. Some of these components are subjective, such as the values and quality of life. Some components are economic, including the amount of money required to execute choices. Some aspects of the decisions require the use of epidemiological data to estimate the number of people involved. Furthermore, the decisions require evidence-based data to estimate the potential gains derived from the various treatment alternatives. Throughout this book, we and the other authors have attempted to clarify some of the important components of these decisions. The most important lesson from economic thinking is that health care costs will definitely rise unless tradeoffs are taken seriously.

### Selfishness Is Important

Most people express concern when self-interest in making choices is emphasized. Economists view selfishness differently. They believe that selfishness is required for economies to succeed. For example, individual decision makers optimize their resources by choosing alternatives that give them the most satisfaction at the lowest cost. Markets work best if consumers attend to their own self-interest. For example, if I shop to obtain the lowest price on a product, others will benefit because providers who want my business must offer the best service or product at the lowest cost. This competition forces the price of the product to be lower. Economists do not criticize people for being selfish. Instead, they argue that selfishness, or consumer sovereignty, is not only necessary but desirable. This important feature cannot work in health care services or systems that are publicly financed. Therefore, health care that is completely free may produce more harm than good.

### Importance of Markets

Economists take markets very seriously. For several centuries economists have described the benefits of free market systems. In 1776 Adam Smith, the noted British economist, built on earlier observations to describe the almost magical order created by free market exchange. Smith suggested that transactions were guided by an "invisible hand" (Smith, 1776). Many economists believe that markets are a force of nature. Furthermore, they suggest that attempts to disrupt markets sometimes cause serious problems.

## Health Care and Economic Thinking

One of the difficulties with health care is that many important economic princi-ples are challenged. For example, it is difficult for consumers to maximize their utilities in health care. Instead of making their own decisions, patients often have decisions made for them. They are not able to purchase products that maximize the use of their own resources because many of the important products are controlled by prescription. Although most physicians want to act in the best interests of their patients, it is not clear that they fully understand patient preferences when making these decisions. Tradeoffs, which are so important to economic thinking, are not valued in the same way by health care providers and their patients. Several of the chapters in this book address this issue. Decisions in health care often violate consumer sovereignty and do not involve the systematic use of decision models. Furthermore, the delivery of health care often disrupts natural market forces because they remove the all important consumer (patient) from the decision process. According to economic thinking, there are serious consequences for disrupting market equilibrium. If markets are a force of nature, there is a price to pay for polices that restrict free trade and systematic selfish decision making.

## Outputs Versus Outcomes

To take this thinking into consideration, we must distinguish outputs of health care from outcomes of health care. As noted in Chapter 3, outputs include laboratory results and clinical tests. Outcomes emphasize the effects on quality and quantity of life demonstrated by measures such as the quality-adjusted life-year (QALY). Studies of outputs might consider only the costs of interventions, whereas studies of outcomes attempt to evaluate systematically the tradeoffs using economic modeling. The CLINECS model places greater emphasis on patient preferences and perceptions. It emphasizes the benefits of care from the patients' perspective.

This book lays out various methodologies to begin addressing these problems. It considers the contributions from disciplines including psychology, philosophy and ethics, clinical epidemiology, medicine, and economics. The authors consider problems regarding the safety of health care, the meaning of clinical tests, the value of evidence-based care, and the effectiveness of treatments. Economic perspectives evaluate the relative benefit of various alternatives. Philosophical and ethical contributions probe the value of selecting alternatives from both the individual and the societal perspectives.

## Summary

The delivery of medicine and health care in North America and Europe will continue to evolve. We are hopeful that the perspectives described in this volume can contribute to this debate. The practice of medicine must evolve beyond the simple diagnosis and treatment of disease. Progress in basic and clinical research is essential but no longer sufficient. The new aspect is the added value to patients in day-to-day health care. Resources are limited, and new ways of thinking about problems are required. We hope that this book will contribute to future health care decision making.

# *References*

Anderson, G.F., Hussey, P.S., Frogner, B.K., Waters, H.R. (2005). Health spending in the United States and the rest of the industrialized world. *Health Affairs (Millwood), 24,* 903–914.

Smith, A. (1776). *An inquiry into the nature and causes of the wealth of nations.* London: Printed for W. Strahan, T. Cadell, A.M. Kelley.

Smith, C., Cowan, C., Heffler, S., & Catlin, A. (2006). National health spending in 2004: recent slowdown led by prescription drug spending. *Health Affairs (Millwood), 25,* 186–196.

# Index

Page numbers followed by f and t indicates figure and table respectively